Mineral Composition and Radioactivity of Edible Mushrooms

Mineral Composition and Radioactivity of Edible Mushrooms

Pavel Kalač

Faculty of Agriculture, Department of Applied Chemistry,
University of South Bohemia, CZ-370 05 České Budějovice,
Czech Republic

ELSEVIER

ACADEMIC PRESS
An imprint of Elsevier

Academic Press is an imprint of Elsevier
125 London Wall, London EC2Y 5AS, United Kingdom
525 B Street, Suite 1650, San Diego, CA 92101, United States
50 Hampshire Street, 5th Floor, Cambridge, MA 02139, United States
The Boulevard, Langford Lane, Kidlington, Oxford OX5 1GB, United Kingdom

Notices
Knowledge and best practice in this field are constantly changing. As new research and experience broaden our understanding, changes in research methods, professional practices, or medical treatment may become necessary.

Practitioners and researchers must always rely on their own experience and knowledge in evaluating and using any information, methods, compounds, or experiments described herein. In using such information or methods they should be mindful of their own safety and the safety of others, including parties for whom they have a professional responsibility.

To the fullest extent of the law, neither the Publisher nor the authors, contributors, or editors, assume any liability for any injury and/or damage to persons or property as a matter of products liability, negligence or otherwise, or from any use or operation of any methods, products, instructions, or ideas contained in the material herein.

British Library Cataloguing-in-Publication Data
A catalogue record for this book is available from the British Library

Library of Congress Cataloging-in-Publication Data
A catalog record for this book is available from the Library of Congress

ISBN: 978-0-12-817565-1

Publisher: Charlotte Cockle
Acquisition Editor: Nina Rosa de Araujo Bandeira
Editorial Project Manager: Ana Claudia A. Garcia
Production Project Manager: Vijayaraj Purushothaman
Cover Designer: Matthew Limbert

Typeset by MPS Limited, Chennai, India

Dedication

To my wife Marie for 52 years of steady support and understanding.

Contents

List of figures

List of tables

Biography

Pavel Kalač (1943) is a professor of Agricultural Chemistry at the University of South Bohemia, České Budějovice, Czech Republic, where he has served at the Faculty of Agriculture since 1971. He graduated from the University of Chemistry and Technology in Prague, Czech Republic.

Professor Kalač has published 69 articles registered on the Web of Science, including 36 original articles and reviews in Elsevier journals, particularly in *Food Chemistry* (19) and *Meat Science* (8). He has published three books and numerous articles in Czech that deal with food and feed chemistry. His works frequently cite researchers studying related topics.

With Elsevier books, Kalač published *Edible Mushrooms: Chemical Composition and Nutritional Value* (2016) and *Effects of Forage Feeding on Milk: Bioactive Compounds and Flavor* (2017).

Preface

My attitude remains virtually the same as described in the preface of my previous book *Edible Mushrooms: Chemical Composition and Nutritional Value* published by Elsevier/Academic Press in 2016.

Wild-growing mushrooms have been a part of my life since early childhood. Feelings of being a successful hunter, the esthetic appreciation of mushrooms found in their natural environment, and favorite dishes prepared from them have always given me much joy. Mushroom picking has been my recreational hobby for over 65 years.

Mushrooms became a hobby-research topic during my academic career as a food and feed chemist. My earliest articles published together with colleagues from 1975 during the emerging period of the topic dealt with some trace elements in selected wild-growing species. Over the years, I have collected 100s of articles dealing with the mineral composition and radioactivity of wild-growing and cultivated mushrooms since that time. Only now, in my senior years, I have found the courage to collate the expanding, but highly dispersed information, into a book. My appreciation and thanks are extended to numerous researchers whose efforts and results contributed to the information presented in this book.

Although written primarily for nutritionists, food chemists, and mushroom producers, it is my hope that *Mineral Compostion and Radioactivity of Edible Mushrooms* will also prove to be useful for food and human nutrition science students and mushroom fanciers.

Pavel Kalač

January 22, 2019

In České Budějovice

Acknowledgments

I am particularly indebted to Dr. Javier Guillén Gerada from the University of Extremadura, Cáceres, Spain, for his help with Chapter 5, Radioactivity, dealing with mushroom radioactivity.

Encouragement of Prof. Martin Křížek during the preparation of the manuscript and help from Dr. Martin Šeda during communication with the editors are highly appreciated.

My gratitude is also extended to anonymous reviewers of the book proposal for their positive evaluation and members of the editorial board for their decision to publish the manuscript. Moreover, I highly appreciate the attitude and helpfulness of Elsevier editors Nina Bandeira, Ana Claudia Abad Garcia and Vijayaraj Purushothaman.

Chapter 1

Introduction

The term "mushroom" is commonly used to describe the fruiting body (sporocarp), which is the morphological part of the macrofungus that bears spores. Macrofungi form fruiting bodies that are visible to the naked eye and large enough to be picked up by hand. In the context of this book, the term mushroom relates to the fleshy, edible fruiting bodies (particularly culinary species) either freshly harvested or processed.

The number of mushroom species on Earth is currently estimated to be around 150,000; however, only about 10% are known to science. Over 2000 species are safe for consumption, and about 700 species are known to possess significant pharmacological properties (Wasser, 2010, 2011). Humans have been attracted to mushrooms since ancient times, for instance, the Romans referred to them as "food of the gods." Mushrooms have been consumed worldwide as a delicacy and appreciated for their specific aroma and texture. However, they have become a component of staple sustenance during periods of food shortage, e.g. wars. The consumption of mushrooms has recently increased as a part of a healthy lifestyle due to their low-energy level and convenient fiber content.

The mushroom industry has three main categories: (1) production of cultivated culinary species, (2) wild-growing culinary species, and (3) medicinal mushrooms.

Around 100 species can be cultivated commercially, but only about 20 of them are cultivated on an industrial scale. According to data from the Food and Agriculture Organization (FAOSTAT) given in Table 1.1 the total world production of cultivated mushrooms was nearly 11 million metric tons in 2016, with China being the leading producer by far. The accrual of the production has been very dynamic, 4.2 and 9.9 million metric tons were reported in 2003 and 2013, respectively. *Agaricus bisporus* (white or button mushrooms, brown mushrooms, crimini, cremini, portobello) is the most cultivated species, followed by *Lentinula edodes* (usually called shiitake by its Japanese common name), several species of genus *Pleurotus* (particularly *P. ostreatus*, oyster mushroom, hiratake), *Flammulina velutipes* (golden needle mushroom, enokitake), *Grifola frondosa* (ram's head, maitake), *Volvariella volvacea* (straw mushroom), *Hericium erinaceus* (lion's mane mushroom, yamabushitake), and others. Some 45% of the produced mushrooms are

Mineral Composition and Radioactivity of Edible Mushrooms.
DOI: https://doi.org/10.1016/B978-0-12-817565-1.00001-7

TABLE 1.1 Production statistics of cultivated edible mushrooms including truffles in 2016 (FAOSAT) of countries with production above 50,000 metric tons.

Country	Production (metric tons)	Percentage of global production
China	7,797,929	72.26
Italy	683,620	6.34
United States	419,630	3.89
The Netherlands	300,000	2.78
Poland	260,140	2.41
Spain	197,010	1.83
Iran	150,063	1.39
Canada	133,935	1.24
France	101,949	0.95
United Kingdom	99,813	0.92
Germany	72,141	0.67
Ireland	70,000	0.65
Japan	65,579	0.61
Australia	50,387	0.47
World	10,790,859	100.0

culinary processed in the fresh state. The rest are preserved, mostly by canning and drying, with a ratio of about 10:1.

Information on mushroom consumption has been very scarce.

Consumption of wild-growing species is preferred to cultivated mushrooms in many countries in Central and Eastern Europe due to their more savorous properties and species diversity. Furthermore, mushroom picking in forests and grasslands has been a lasting cultural heritage, while more recently it has become a highly valued recreational activity. Mushrooms in their natural habitat are appreciated for their esthetic value. Some fanciers devote great effort to seeking and harvesting mushrooms without consuming them. Such an attitude is quite different from that in countries where wild mushrooms have been ignored as "toadstools." For instance, picking mushrooms is a "national hobby" in the Czech Republic. It is interesting to note that Czech composer Václav Hájek (1937–2014), a great fancier of mushrooms, composed hundreds of opuses on individual mushroom species. In the Czech Republic about 70% of the population collect mushrooms, with a statistical mean of 5–8 kg of fresh mushrooms per household or 2–3 kg per capita yearly, although some individuals consume more than 10 kg yearly. The actual consumption is lower due to the removal of inedible parts and those damaged by animals or insect larvae. Information on the harvest and consumption of wild-growing species worldwide has been based on guessing.

Most pickers collect wild-growing mushrooms as a delicacy for their own consumption. However, collecting mushrooms has also been an economic activity for some rural populations.

Medicinal mushrooms have an established history in traditional ancient therapies. Medicinal traditions from Japan, China, and Korea have particularly stressed the importance of *Ganoderma lucidum* (ling zhi or reishi) and *L. edodes*. *Inonotus obliquus*, *Fomitopsis officinalis*, and *Piptoporus betulinus* have been used for the treatment of several ailments in rural populations of Russia. Recently, extensive research of many effective components of mushrooms, in particular polysaccharides, revealed many medicinal benefits, including antitumor, antioxidant, immunomodulating, cardiovascular, hepatoprotective, antidiabetic, and other effects of medicinal and culinary-medicinal mushroom species (Chang & Wasser, 2012; Chatterjee et al., 2017; Wasser, 2010, 2011). Medicinal mushrooms produce beneficial effects as drugs and as nutraceuticals (or functional foods) consumed as part of a healthy diet. Moreover, a novel class of medicinal mushroom products is available in the form of dietary supplements (Jayachandran, Xiao, & Xu, 2017; Rathore, Prasad, & Sharma, 2017; Roncero-Ramos & Delgado-Andrade, 2017).

Many mushroom species are inedible, deleterious, or toxic. The macrofungi alike plants are fixed to their positions what makes impossible to escape from an attack by fungivores, ranging from insects to mammals. It has led to the evolution of several defense strategies to deter the pests. Mushroom fruiting bodies often produce pungent or bitter compounds and even toxins to deter fungivores. However, this book does not discuss these groups or medicinal mushrooms.

Generally, the nutritional benefits of edible mushrooms have been overrated. Critical reviews with numerous references have been published (Bernaś, Jaworska, & Lisiewska, 2006; Kalač, 2009, 2013; Wang et al., 2014) and data available until 2015 were collated in a book (Kalač, 2016).

Overall, according to Kalač, the dry matter (DM) of mushrooms is low, usually 8–14 g 100 g^{-1} of the fresh matter (FM). DM of 10 g 100 g^{-1} FM (10%) has been commonly used for the conversion between DM and FM if the actual DM is unknown. Usual proximal compositions are 20–25, 2–3, and 5–12 g 100 g^{-1} DM for crude protein, crude fat, and ash (minerals), respectively. Various carbohydrates form the rest of DM. Due to their very low DM and fat content, mushrooms are a low-energy food item. The calculated energy value mostly ranges between 300 and 400 kcal (approx. 1250–1670 kJ) kg^{-1} FM. Nevertheless, such data are overestimated because a considerable proportion of polysaccharides is indigestible.

Previous data on protein content were overestimated by about one-third; however, this misinformation has been steadily passed on. Nevertheless, the nutritional value of mushroom protein seems to be higher compared to most plant proteins. They also contain a limited amount of methionine, an essential amino acid in humans. Mushrooms rank among food items with marginal nutritional roles of their lipids (fats). Within polysaccharides, glycogen forms energy reserves, and nitrogen-containing chitin is the predominant component of the cell walls and dietary fiber. The level of fiber ranges around 25–30 g 100 g^{-1} DM with about half being in an insoluble form. The widely disseminated information concerning the high vitamin levels of mushrooms, particularly B vitamins, has to be corrected. Mushrooms appear to be a good dietary source of ergosterol, the precursor of vitamin D_2 (ergocalciferol), and vitamin B_{12}. The contents of other vitamins are comparable or lower than those of many vegetables.

1.1 Mineral composition and radioactivity

The crude ash of mushrooms consist of seven major mineral elements (calcium, chlorine, magnesium, phosphorus, potassium, sodium and sulfur), quantitatively highly prevailing, and tens of trace elements generally occurring at the level up to 5 mg 100 g^{-1} FM (i.e., about up to 50 mg 100 g^{-1} DM) for each of them. Cultivated mushrooms usually contain 5–12 g of ash per 100 g DM (i.e., approximately 0.5–1.2 g 100 g^{-1} FM). This extent is typical for cultivated species, whereas contents above 20 g 100 g^{-1} DM occur in some wild-growing species. Generally, the ash content of mushrooms is higher than or comparable to that of most vegetables. However, the ash composition can differ markedly among edible mushrooms and vegetables.

Mushroom ash is formed mainly by potassium and phosphorus, with usual levels of 2–4 and 0.5–1 g 100 g^{-1} DM, respectively, whereas sodium and calcium contents are very low. Some edible mushroom species are able to accumulate great levels of trace elements—including detrimental ones such as arsenic, cadmium, lead, or mercury—from the underlying substrates. The content of detrimental trace elements may exceed acceptable limits.

Available information, particularly on detrimental and essential trace elements, has expanded greatly during the past few decades. The data from numerous literature were collated and evaluated in several reviews (Falandysz & Borovička, 2013; Kalač, 2010; Kalač & Svoboda, 2000). The current state of knowledge on major and trace elements in edible mushroom species will be provided in Chapter 3, Major essential elements, and Chapter 4, Trace elements, respectively.

The information on edible mushroom radioactivity has been widely diffused within European countries during the years following the disaster at the Chernobyl Nuclear Power Plant, Ukraine, in 1986. Opinion of the public has often overrated the health risk of mushroom intake. Nevertheless, some wild-growing mushroom species really showed higher level of radioactivity than whatever food items. The elevated level of nuclear fission products has continued in the stricken regions and will still affect mushrooms from these areas over the next decades. Earlier data on mushroom radioactivity were evaluated in reviews with numerous references (Duff & Ramsey, 2008; Kalač, 2001).

Most data on both minerals and radioactivity deal with fresh fruiting bodies. However, fresh mushrooms rank among the most perishable food items, with a very short shelf life of only 1–3 days at ambient temperature. Deterioration after harvesting is caused by high water content, high respiration rate, and lack of physical protection to avoid water loss and microbial attack, which is extensive mainly in wild-growing species often microbially contaminated by fungivores (e.g., snails, insects, or rodents). Such quick deterioration has been an obstacle for manufacturers, sellers, and consumers. Short-term cold storage of fresh fruiting bodies packed under a modified atmosphere, drying, canning, or deep-freezing have been commonly used for mushroom preservation. Generally, information on changes in mineral content and composition and in radioactivity during preservation, storage, and various culinary treatments has been limited. This book aims to provide this information.

1.2 Basic mycological terms

Scientific (Latin) names are used in the text of this book because common names (e.g., boletes, cepes, chantarelles, or truffles) are widely known for only the most consumed species, whereas less frequently consumed mushroom species have local common names.

However, mycological taxonomy and terminology goes through changes caused by the application of molecular approaches. New genera have been established and traditional classifications have changed considerably. For instance, widely harvested *Xerocomus badius* Fr. (synonyms *Boletus badius* (Fr.) Gilb., *Ixocomus badius* (Fr.) Quél., *Suillus badius* (Fr.) Kuntze, and others) was recently classified as *Imleria badia* (Fr.). Current novel classifications would be lucid for mushroom taxonomists, but would not make much sense to most readers. Widely used traditional scientific names will therefore be used in the text. Some synonyms have been included in the Index of Mushroom Species; however, there is some uncertainty; does the traditional classification of some analyzed species correlate with the current categorization?

The fruiting body is the sexual part of a macrofungus bearing spores. The bodies are mostly above ground, but can also be formed under the ground (e.g., truffles) or growing on living trees or dead wood. They vary in size, shape, and coloration among species. Fruiting bodies growing from spacious mycelia (hyphae) are formed by the process of fructification. Mycelium is the vegetative part of a fungus and consist of a mass of branched hyphae. The basic terminology of a fruiting body is given in Fig. 1.1. The lifetime of the bulk of fruiting bodies in nature is only about 10–14 days. In some species (e.g., genus *Coprinus*) the life span is very short, even ephemeral. On the contrary, some fruiting bodies growing on trees (e.g., polypores) remain for months and even years.

Mushrooms are heterotrophic eukaryotic organisms. They can be divided into three classes according to their prevailing nutritional (trophic) strategy or ecological preferences. *Mycorrhizal* (symbiotic) species live in a close, mutually profitable relationship with their host vascular plant, usually the roots of a tree. *Saprobic* (saprotrophic, saprophytic) species, commonly called saprophytes, derive their nutrients from various dead organic matters. Some species of this group are exploited for cultivation, while mycorrhizal species have not yet been successfully cultivated on a large scale. The third group, *parasitic* species, lives on other species in a nonsymbiotic relationship such as ligniperdous mushrooms on living trees.

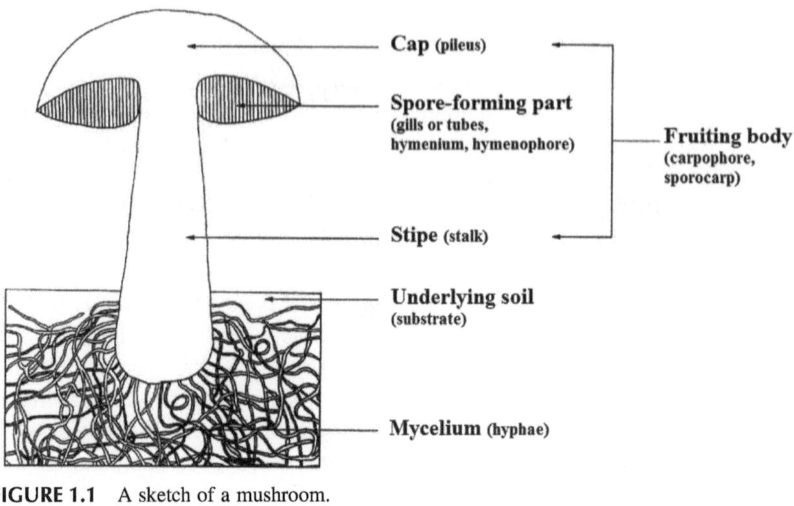

FIGURE 1.1 A sketch of a mushroom.

References

Bernaś, E., Jaworska, G., & Lisiewska, Z. (2006). Edible mushrooms as a source of valuable nutritive constituents. *Acta Scientiarum Polonorum, Technologia Alimentaria, 5*, 5–20.

Chang, S. T., & Wasser, S. P. (2012). The role of culinary-medicinal mushrooms on human welfare with a pyramid model for human health. *International Journal of Medicinal Mushrooms, 14*, 95–134.

Chatterjee, S., Sarma, M. K., Deb, U., Steinhauser, G., Walther, C., & Gupta, D. K. (2017). Mushrooms: From nutrition to mycoremediation. *Environmental Science and Pollution Research, 24*, 19480–19493.

Duff, M. C., & Ramsey, M. L. (2008). Accumulation of radiocesium by mushrooms in the environment: A literature review. *Journal of Environmental Radioactivity, 99*, 912–932.

Falandysz, J., & Borovička, J. (2013). Macro and trace mineral constituents and radionuclides in mushrooms: Health benefits and risks. *Applied Microbiology and Biotechnology, 97*, 477–501.

Jayachandran, M., Xiao, J., & Xu, B. (2017). A critical review on health promoting benefits of edible mushrooms through gut microbiota. *International Journal of Molecular Sciences, 18*, Art. Nr. 1934.

Kalač, P. (2001). A review of edible mushroom radioactivity. *Food Chemistry, 75*, 29–35.

Kalač, P. (2009). Chemical composition and nutritional value of European species of wild growing mushrooms: A review. *Food Chemistry, 113*, 9–16.

Kalač, P. (2010). Trace element contents in European species of wild growing edible mushrooms: A review for the period 2000-2009. *Food Chemistry, 122*, 2–15.

Kalač, P. (2013). A review of chemical composition and nutritional value of wild-growing and cultivated mushrooms. *Journal of the Sciences of Food and Agriculture, 93*, 209–218.

Kalač, P. (2016). *Edible Mushrooms. Chemical Composition and Nutritional Value.* Amsterdam: Elsevier/Academic Press, ISBN 978-0-12-804455-1.

Kalač, P., & Svoboda, L. (2000). A review of trace element concentrations in edible mushrooms. *Food Chemistry, 69*, 273–281.

Rathore, H., Prasad, S., & Sharma, S. (2017). Mushroom nutraceuticals for improved nutrition and better human health: A review. *PharmaNutrition, 5*, 35–46.

Roncero-Ramos, I., & Delgado-Andrade, C. (2017). The beneficial role of edible mushrooms in human health. *Current Opinion in Food Science, 14*, 122–128.

Wang, X. M., Zhang, J., Wu, L. H., Zhao, Y. L., Li, T., Li, J. Q., ... Liu, H. G. (2014). A mini-review of chemical composition and nutritional value of edible wild-grown mushroom from China. *Food Chemistry, 151*, 279–285.

Wasser, S. P. (2010). Medicinal mushroom science: History, current status, future trends, and unsolved problems. *International Journal of Medicinal Mushrooms, 12*, 1–16.

Wasser, S. P. (2011). Current findings, future trends, and unsolved problems in studies of medicinal mushrooms. *Applied Microbiology and Biotechnology, 89*, 1323–1332.

Chapter 2

Overall outline of mineral composition

2.1 Factors affecting mineral element levels in fruiting bodies

2.1.1 Overall information

Wide variability in the content of individual minerals within a species has been reported in mushrooms since the beginning of their analyses in the 1970s. Such variability is notably higher than that in vegetables and other agricultural crops. Generally, element contents in fruiting bodies are species-dependent, whereas genus-dependence is sometimes stated, but with limited conclusiveness. Substrate composition is an important factor, but great differences exist in the uptake of individual metals as reported in pioneering works in the 1980s (Gast, Jansen, Bierling, & Haanstra, 1988; Tyler, 1982).

The age of the fruiting body and its size are of less importance than the substrate composition. Some authors reported higher trace element contents in younger fruiting bodies. This is explained by the transport of an element from the mycelium to the fruiting body during the initial stage of fructification. During the consequent accrual of the fruiting body mass, the element level dilutes. For instance, Nasr, Malloch, and Arp (2012) classified 27 tested mycorrhizal species into four groups with regards to changes in their mercury content from emergence to senescence.

The proportion of an element originating from atmospheric depositions seems likewise to be limited due to the short lifetime of the fruiting bodies of most mushroom species, ususally being only 10–14 days; however, in some species, for example, *Coprinus* spp., this is considerably shorter. Therefore the effects of depositions can be taken into consideration in long-living fruiting bodies, that is, mostly those growing on wood.

So far sporadic reports provide information on changes in mineral composition of fruiting bodies growing in the same stand, that is, under the same geochemical conditions, but over consecutive years. However, these reports are based on probability and not certainty that the analyzed fruiting bodies originate from the same mycelium. For example, the biological factors possibly related to mycelium and year-to-year fluctuating weather conditions have

Mineral Composition and Radioactivity of Edible Mushrooms.
DOI: https://doi.org/10.1016/B978-0-12-817565-1.00002-9

affected variability or similarity in the level of various elements in *Boletus edulis* (Zhang et al., 2010), in caps of *Macrolepiota procera* (Gucia, Jarzyńska, Kojta, & Falandysz, 2012), and in conditionally edible (after detoxification of hallucinogens by parboiling) caps and stipes of *Amanita muscaria* (Lipka, Saba, & Falandysz, 2018).

In the author's opinion, element levels in wild-growing mushrooms considerably elevate with the increasing age of mycelium and protracted interval between the fructifications. This hypothesis has not yet been proven experimentally in the natural environment, nevertheless, repeated reports dealing with cultivated species support it. The highest element contents are observed in the first harvest flush of cultivated *Agaricus bisporus* (e.g., Koyyalamudi, Jeong, Manavalan, Vysetti, & Pang, 2013). The levels reported in wild-growing *A. bisporus* have been considerably higher than those in the cultivated counterparts. This may be explained not only by the differences in substrate composition and contamination, but also by age of the mycelium, which may be years up to a number of decades in nature compared to only several months in a cultivation plant.

Furthermore, many elements are distributed unevenly within the fruiting bodies. The highest levels are often observed in the spore-forming part (hymenophore), less in the flesh of the cap, and the lowest in stipe. However, the level of some elements is higher in stipes than in caps. The available data on the distribution will be discussed for the individual elements in Chapter 3, Major essential elements, and Chapter 4, Trace elements.

2.1.2 Bioaccumulation of mineral elements

A note on terminology: the term bioconcentration should be used for aquatic environments, while bioaccumulation applies for terrestrial lifeforms including mushrooms. Nevertheless, the former term is common in the literature dealing with mushrooms and will, thus, be frequently used in this book.

Geomycology, an interdisciplinary field, has emerged recently and is defined as "the scientific study of the roles of fungi in processes of fundamental importance to geology" (Gadd, Rhee, Stephenson, & Wei, 2012). The discipline deals with nutrient and element cycling, rock and mineral transformations, bioweathering, mycogenic biomineral formation, and interactions of fungi with clay minerals and metals. Synoptic information on the topic is available in reviews by Gadd (2007) and Gadd et al. (2012).

Like plants and microbes, fungi are involved in soil mineral weathering and element cycling. Their mycelia colonize organic and mineral soils and produce various chemical compounds, for example, organic acids. The acids leach nutrients such as major minerals from mineral surfaces. The released elements can then be translocated to the host plants. In addition to hyphae, rhizomorphs with root-like structures spread over a huge area of a forest also participate in the uptake of mineral elements.

Many papers have reported that the content of various elements increases in fruiting bodies from polluted areas compared with those from unpolluted rural sites, which have been taken as background values. Moreover, geologically specific substrates, for example, mercuriferous or seleniferous soils, can affect the mineral composition of mushrooms.

Great differences in the level of many major and trace elements exist among fruiting bodies within a species, but collected from distant sites (e.g., Falandysz et al., 2011). An interesting view is the recent report by Bosiacki, Siwulski, Sobieralski, and Krzebietke (2018). Wild-growing *A. bisporus* was sampled from 55 sites of various types across Poland during the period of 2010–15. Each sample consisted of 10–20 fruiting bodies. Surprisingly high ranges of eight metals were observed (Table 2.1). Cluster analysis of cadmium, lead, nickel, and chromium contents showed the highest similarity of the element levels from urban forests and meadows. The highest levels of these contaminants were determined in an industrial region.

Different proportions of various forms (e.g., exchangeable, absorbable, organic-matter–bound, etc.) of the elements present in underlying soils seem to be an important factor affecting the level of bioaccumulation in fruiting bodies (Nogaj et al., 2012).

TABLE 2.1 Ranges in the content of eight trace metals (mg kg^{-1} dry matter) in samples of wild-growing *Agaricus bisporus* collected from 55 sites across Poland.

Element	Range
Cadmium	0.68–6.14
Chromium	0.38–6.93
Copper	1.90–102
Iron	33.0–432
Manganese	2.86–387
Nickel	0.20–3.09
Lead	0.98–42.8
Zinc	31.9–125

Source: Adapted from Bosiacki, M., Siwulski, M., Sobieralski, K., & Krzebietke, S. (2018). The content of selected heavy metals in fruiting bodies of *Agaricus bisporus* (Lange) Imbach. wild growing in Poland. *Journal of Elementology, 23*, 875–886.

Numerous papers reported considerably elevated levels of contaminating elements in fruiting bodies collected in polluted areas. In *Boletus appendiculatus* (syn. *Boletus aereus*) Kuthan (1979) found 14–36, 2–10, 1–3, and 0.2–0.5 mg kg^{-1} DM (dry matter) of lead in distances <10, 30–80, 80–120, and 250–500 m from the shoulder of a main road in Bulgaria. The increased contents of cadmium, lead, and zinc were reported in several mushroom species picked along a French motorway (Cuny, van Haluwyn, & Pesch, 2001). Considerably increased levels of these main deleterious metals (i.e., cadmium, mercury, and lead) occur in mushrooms growing within towns and notably in the vicinity of both former and operating metal smelters or mining areas, metal-ore–rich areas, and landfills of sewage sludge. For references until 2009 see Kalač and Svoboda (2000) and Kalač (2010). Further references will be given for individual elements in Chapter 4, Trace elements.

In Finland, great amounts of wood ash are produced, which are partly recycled as forest fertilizer. However, the high level of cadmium in the ash (usually 1–30 mg kg^{-1}) is a serious disadvantage. Surprisingly, no increase in cadmium content (Lodenius, Soltanpour-Gargari, & Tulisalo, 2002) or a further 12 elements (Moilanen et al., 2006) was observed in mushrooms after several years following the ash application.

Interesting results were published in Sweden (Movitz, 1980). No significant differences in cadmium levels were found between herbarium mushroom samples during the period of 1890–1926 and samples collected from the same sites at the end of the 1970s.

The ability to accumulate an element from substrate to fruiting body is expressed by the bioconcentration factor (BCF; also called the bioaccumulation factor or transfer factor), the ratio of an element content in the fruiting body to the content in the underlying substrate, both values in DM. If the BCF value is >1, an element is bioaccumulated, at value <1 it is bioexcluded. Some mushroom species, called hyperaccumulators, are able to bioaccumulate in their fruiting bodies an element with BCF value of order many hundreds or even several thousands, for example, silver in *Amanita strobiliformis* (Borovička, Řanda, Jelínek, & Dunn, 2007). High ability to bioaccumulate cadmium or mercury is characteristic for numerous mushroom species, while lead is bioexcluded.

In this context, more information on which substrate horizons individual species take their nutrients is needed. The ability to absorb and accumulate trace elements directly from rock fragments in the *shiro* (Japanese name for a complex soil community of mycorrhizae, soil microbes, and host-tree roots) was observed in *Tricholoma matsutake* (Vaario et al., 2015). The uppermost layer up to 10 cm depth has usually been sampled and analyzed for mineral elements. This layer of forest substrate contains mainly organic debris. Mycelium of saprobic species, nutrients which originate from organic matter, is generally located in the litter layers rich in humus, usually at or very close to the substrate surface. On the contrary, mycelium of mycorrhizal species is dispersed in the mineral layer where roots of the host plant are growing, that is, at lower horizons. For instance, mycelium of mycorrhizal *Suillus luteus* is associated with the mineral horizons of podzol soils (Rosling et al., 2003). Nasr and Arp (2011) distributed the tested mushrooms in reference to species-specific substrate preferences into five groups in relation to mercury bioaccumulation.

High-accumulating ability of several mushroom species promoted their screening as bioindicators of heavy metals, mainly during the 1980s. Numerous works were reviewed (Wondratschek & Röder, 1993) coming to the conclusion that no mushroom species can be considered as an exact indicator of environmental pollution with deleterious elements. Such attitude remains valid until now in spite of from time to time emerging suggestion of a species.

2.2 Chemistry and biochemistry of mineral elements in fruiting bodies

Mechanisms sustaining metal tolerance in mycorrhizal fungi were reviewed by Bellion, Courbot, Jacob, Blaudez, and Chalot (2006). The mushrooms participate in crucial symbiotic relationships with plants that grow on contaminated sites and alleviate the metal toxicity for their host plants. A large proportion of some metals, particularly zinc, copper, and cadmium, was found to be fixed in mycorrhizas, thus, forming a biological barrier that reduces the movement of the metals to the tissues of host plants. The participating mechanisms can be described as extracellular and intracellular. The former mechanisms are mainly implied for the avoidance of metal entry, whereas the latter systems aim to reduce the metal burden in the cytosol.

Within extracellular chelation and cell-wall binding, di- and tricarboxylic acids, particularly oxalic and citric acids, are excreted by mushroom cells to chelate metal ions. However, mushrooms also excrete other compounds, for example, specific proteins able to sequester metal ions. Binding of metals to the fungal cell walls is enabled by numerous binding sites, such as free carboxyl, amino, hydroxyl, phosphate, and sulfhydryl (mercapto) groups. Choma et al. (2018) isolated an alkali-soluble polysaccharide from cell walls of *B. edulis* containing primarily α-(1$\rightarrow$3)-D-glucan chains substituted with α-(1$\rightarrow$3)-D-mannans. Tests of biosorption properties of the polysaccharide showed high ability to accumulate lead and cadmium, with only medium efficacy for nickel and zinc.

Despite the described mechanisms, large amounts of metals may enter into the mushroom cells. Metallothioneins, low-molecular weight, and cysteine and metal-rich proteins containing sulfur-rich metal clusters play crucial role in intracellular complexation of metals. Tripeptide glutathione is another compound participating in intracellular chelation.

Collin-Hansen, Pedersen, Andersen, and Steinnes (2007) were the first authors to report on the occurrence of phytochelatins, a family of cysteine-rich oligopeptides, in mushrooms, namely in *B. edulis*. Some mushrooms have an ability to initiate an efficient antioxidant defense system against some metals, such as was observed in *M. procera* toward nickel (Ni^{2+}) (Baptista, Ferreira, Soares, Coelho, & Bastos, 2009). However, knowledge concerning the mechanisms of metal transfer in intracellular compartments of mushroom cells is lacking.

Recognition of the factors affecting the bioaccumulation of elements, particularly potentially toxic ones, in the mycelium and fruiting bodies of mushrooms is also important for the mycoremediation of soils. For overall information on soil mycoremediation see a review of Ali et al. (2017). This topic is, however, beyond the scope of this book.

Information on speciation, that is, various chemical forms of essential and toxic elements occurring in edible mushrooms, has been very limited. Results of general traits will be given in this section, whereas specific data for the individual elements are discussed in Chapter 4, Trace elements.

Wuilloud, Kannamkumarath, and Caruso (2004a) extracted dried *A. bisporus*, *B. edulis*, and *Lentinula edodes* in three ways—as hot-water, alkaline, and acidic extractions—followed by size-exclusion chromatography separation enabling to determine molecular-weight distribution patterns. There were observed differences in the fractionation patterns of arsenic, cadmium, lead, mercury, silver, and tin depending on mushroom species and the extraction medium. Most of the elements were associated with high-molecular weight fractions. Similar conclusions were reported for the speciation of bismuth, cobalt, copper, iodine, iron, molybdenum, nickel, selenium, and zinc in *B. edulis* (Wuilloud, Kannamkumarath, & Caruso, 2004b).

Collin-Hansen, Andersen, and Steinnes (2003, 2005a, 2005b), Collin-Hansen et al. (2007), Collin-Hansen, Yttri, Andersen, Berthelsen, and Steinnes (2002) studied the chemical forms of several metals in selected mushroom species growing in the heavily polluted vicinity of two metal smelters in Norway. Levels of metallothionein-like (MT-like) proteins were analyzed in five edible and two inedible species. Cd, Zn-MT-like proteins were detected in all the samples, while only 72% of the samples contained detectable levels of Cu-MT-like proteins. Concentration of the MT-like proteins did not reflect variations in the metal contents (2002). Sequencing of a novel cadmium-binding protein isolated from *B. edulis* showed that the protein does not belong to the metallothionein family (2003). Molecular defense systems, determined by the activity of antioxidant enzymes superoxide dismutase, and catalase and by the level of glutathione and heat shock protein 70 kDa, were induced in *B. edulis* growing in the areas polluted with cadmium, zinc, copper, and mercury. However, the defense mechanisms were insufficient for protection against the harmful effects of severe metal stress (2005a). Moreover, low levels of mercury and probably of the other three metals damaged the DNA and lipids in *B. edulis* (2005b). Peptides of the phytochelatin family, binding a large fraction of cadmium, were detected in caps of *B. edulis* growing on substrates with an excess of cadmium, zinc, copper and mercury (2007).

2.3 Losses of minerals during mushroom preservation and cooking

Information on changes in the mineral composition of mushrooms during various preservation methods and cooking treatments has been very limited. Only data with a common attitude will be given in this section, while information dealing with individual elements will be discussed in Chapter 3, Major essential elements, and Chapter 4, Trace elements.

Washing and peeling of *A. bisporus* decreased the contents of cadmium, lead, copper, and zinc by 30%–40% of the initial level (Źródłowski, 1995). Such reductions seem to be very high; however, no further information on the effects these factors is available.

Chen et al. (2017) investigated effects of hot-air drying at 60°C for 12 h (HD) and freeze drying (FD) on speciation of cadmium, chromium, and lead in *L. edodes*. They separated six fractions (water-soluble, exchangeable, bound to carbonates, bound to iron and manganese oxides, bound to organic matter, and residual) using Tessier's sequential extraction procedure. Cadmium was present mainly in water-soluble form in fresh and HD samples, and as exchangeable after FD. Chromium prevailed in organic and residual fractions in fresh and FD mushrooms, while a more balanced distribution was observed after HD. Lead occurred mainly in the organic fraction in fresh mushrooms; HD resulted in exchangeable fraction and FD in residual one. Soaking of dried *L. edodes* at 65°C for 2 h significantly decreased the contents of all three elements in four of six fractions.

During blanching of *A. bisporus* in a bath containing table salt, citric acid, and sodium bisulfite ($NaHSO_3$) at 95°C–100°C for 15 min, decreases of 45%, 36%, 23%, and 4% from the initial content was observed for manganese, iron, zinc, and copper, respectively (Coşkuner & Özdemir, 1997). Blanching of the same species in solutions of table salt and various concentrations of citric acid or ethylene diamine tetraacetic acid (EDTA) at 95°C–100°C for 15 min did not significantly affect contents of these four elements. However, a considerable decrease of copper and iron was observed during the blanching in solutions of EDTA at a concentration of 0.5–8.0 g L^{-1} (Coşkuner & Özdemir, 2000).

Common culinary treatments, such as soaking the mushrooms in a 0.3% table-salt solution for up to 15 min at ambient temperature and boiling in the same solution for up to 60 min, were investigated in fresh, air-dried, freeze-dried, and frozen slices of *Xerocomus badius*. Short-time boiling (blanching) was found to be a more efficient operation than soaking to decrease the content of cadmium, lead, and mercury. The metals were leached to a great extent from the most destroyed tissues of frozen mushroom slices, but less so from fresh or freeze-dried tissues. The most extensive leaching was observed for cadmium, with the lowest being for mercury (Svoboda, Kalač, Špička, & Janoušková, 2002).

Changes in the content of 17 trace elements in fresh caps of *Amanita fulva* caused by blanching in boiling water for 15 min and following pickling in a vinegar solution at room temperature for 30 days was reported by Drewnowska et al. (2017). Blanching highly decreased (57%–86%) the level of As, Cd, Co, Cu, Mn, Ni, Pb, Rb, and Tl, and less (24%–40%) of Ba, Cr, U, and Zn, while it did not affect the contents of Ag and Sr. Pickled caps as compared with the fresh counterparts showed very high reduction (>80%–99%) of As, Cd, Mn, Pb, Rb, Tl, and Zn, a high decrease (56%–72%) of Co, Cu, and Ni, whereas Ba and Cr decreased at a smaller rate (7.5%–14%).

It may then be deduced that both blanching and pickling of mushrooms can effectively decrease the levels of most of detrimental metals, but, at the same time, deprive the meal from a proportion of the essential elements. However, the available data are insufficient for any generalized conclusions.

Within the emerging preservation technologies, Fernandes et al. (2016) tested the effects of gamma rays or electron-beam irradiation on the mineral profiles of *B. edulis*, *Hydnum repandum*, and *M. procera*. The applied irradiation doses did not show a systematic effect on the macro- and microelement profiles, except for the dose of 10 kGy.

There is specific information concerning the contents of 14 elements in 5 species of canned mushrooms produced in Spain (Rubio et al., 2018). Unfortunately, changes in the element content caused by canning were not tested in the survey. The results are given in Table 2.2 (note that the values are expressed in wet weight).

2.4 Consumer health implications

There exist some differences among national lists of marketable mushroom species with regards to their edibility. For instance, *Gyromitra esculenta*, *Paxillus involutus*, and *Tricholoma equestre* are banned in some countries and are allowable in others.

While hundreds of papers report data on the mineral element contents in various species of both wild-growing and cultivated edible mushrooms, only minimal information has been available until now on the bioaccessibility and bioavailability of the elements. Bioaccessibility can be defined as the quantity of a nutrient, toxin, or other substances which is released from a food matrix in the gastrointestinal tract and becomes available for absorption. The bioavailability is defined as the degree to which a nutrient, toxin, or other substance become available for body use or deposition after exposure. Under oral exposure, bioavailability generally includes absorption, body utilization, and/or deposition.

TABLE 2.2 Mean content and standard deviation (mg kg^{-1} wet weight) of 14 trace elements in canned mushrooms ($n = 20$ per species) prepared in Spain (Rubio et al., 2018).

Element	*Agaricus bisporus*	*Lactarius deliciosus*	*Lentinula edodes*	*Pholiota nameko*	*Pleurotus ostreatus*
Aluminum	16.8 ± 6.76	18.2 ± 6.37	16.8 ± 5.99	19.3 ± 6.92	18.1 ± 4.13
Boron	0.34[a] ± 0.18	0.49 ± 0.15	0.41 ± 0.13	0.46 ± 0.17	0.43 ± 0.16
Barium	0.51[a] ± 0.20	0.77 ± 0.37	0.77 ± 0.31	0.80 ± 0.49	0.62 ± 0.21
Cadmium	0.002	0.006	0.009[a]	0.002	0.004
Chromium	0.07[a] ± 0.03	0.16 ± 0.21	0.15 ± 0.13	0.10 ± 0.05	0.17 ± 0.13
Copper	1.54 ± 0.71	1.64 ± 1.07	1.53 ± 0.77	1.73 ± 0.94	1.99 ± 1.12
Iron	5.14[a] ± 1.91	10.9 ± 4.36	10.5 ± 3.08	10.9 ± 3.2	11.0 ± 3.27
Lead	0.07 ± 0.06	0.08 ± 0.04	0.09 ± 0.04	0.08 ± 0.03	0.1 ± 0.1
Lithium	0.66 ± 1.19	1.26 ± 1.08	0.80 ± 1.10	0.67 ± 1.22	0.84 ± 1.15
Molybdenum	0.02	0.02	0.02	0.03	0.02
Nickel	0.12 ± 0.09	0.13 ± 0.08	0.16 ± 0.12	0.13 ± 0.08	0.18 ± 0.11
Strontium	0.90[a] ± 0.80	2.08 ± 0.75	2.15 ± 1.79	2.20 ± 1.14	2.63 ± 1.68
Vanadium	0.09 ± 0.07	0.08 ± 0.03	0.07 ± 0.04	0.08 ± 0.04	0.08 ± 0.04
Zinc	2.55 ± 0.94	2.32 ± 0.71	2.23 ± 0.83	1.93 ± 0.59	2.91 ± 1.08

[a]*Means with statistical differences ($P < .05$) between mushrooms canned in glass jars and metallic containers.*
Source: Reprinted by permission from *Springer Nature.*

Several compounds binding various elements to poorly digestible complexes are well-known in foods of plant origin. Among them, phytic acid plays a large role due to its being a polyvalent compound binding particularly bi- and trivalent metal cations to poorly soluble salts, phytates. At neutral pH value its ability to bind metals decreases in the order of: Cu > Zn > Ni > Co > Mn > Fe > Ca. In reports dealing with the phytic acid content in edible mushrooms, 160–360 mg 100 g^{-1} were observed in eight tropical species in Nigeria (Aletor, 1995), 338, 1815, and 385 mg 100 g^{-1}, in caps, stipes and tubers, respectively, of *Pleurotus tuber-regium* (Akindahunsi & Oyetayo, 2006) and 11–19 mg 100 g^{-1} in five wild-growing species from India (Gaur, Rao, & Kushwaha, 2016). Unfortunately, it is not clear from any of the three articles whether the contents are given in fresh or DM. Oxalic acid binds calcium to insoluble calcium oxalate. The contents of oxalic acid in mushrooms range in hundreds and thousands mg 100 g^{-1} DM. The highest levels were observed in *A. bisporus*, *A. bitorquis*, and *A. campestris* (for overall data, see Kalač, 2016). The formation of poorly bioavailable complexes is naturally desirable in toxic elements, while it is unwanted in essential ones.

Bioavailability of an element can be estimated via in vivo and in vitro methods. The former involves the use of animals or human beings, while the latter methods usually simulate gastrointestinal digestion followed by the determination of dialyzable mineral fraction passing across a semipermeable membrane.

Kinetics of four major (K, Mg, Ca, Na) and three trace elements (Cu, Fe, Zn) extraction in artificial digestive juices from 12 wild-growing and cultivated species were reported by Kała et al. (2017). Artificial saliva (pH 7.0) and artificial intestinal juice (pH 8.0) were used. The cleaned fruiting bodies were freeze-dried. The mushroom samples were incubated at normal human body temperature for 1 min in the artificial saliva and for 15, 60, or 120 min in the gastric juice. Overall, the simulation showed that the tested metals were released into the artificial gastric juice in relatively high proportions, and from *Leccinum scabrum* and *Auricularia polytricha* in a limited extent. Nevertheless, the rate of absorption of the released elements into the tissues and organs of the human body has to be elucidated by further research.

As results from the previous sections and will be described in more detail in Chapter 3, Major essential elements, and Chapter 4, Trace elements, an element content and its chemical species in the consumed mushrooms are affected by numerous factors. Due to insufficient data on element species and bioavailability, legislation limits for deleterious elements and recommended intake for essential ones are given for total element content, with the exceptions for mercury (total and organic) and chromium (potentially essential Cr^{III}, while deleterious Cr^{VI}).

Average daily requirements and tolerable daily intakes of major and trace elements for adults are given in Tables 3.1 and 4.1, respectively, and in the text accompanying the tables. According to the WHO materials, values of provisional tolerable weekly intake are 0.015, 0.0058, 0.004, and 0.025 mg kg^{-1} bodyweight for deleterious arsenic, cadmium, total mercury, and lead, respectively. However, the limits are provisional and are updated/withdrawn in accordance with growing knowledge.

The limits of 0.2 and 0.3 mg kg^{-1} fresh matter for cadmium and lead, respectively, are now valid for mushrooms in the European Union (EEC Directive 2001/22/EC). Due to high consumption of wild-growing species, the Czech Republic has set more elaborated legislation until it joined the EU in 2004. Statutory limits of 3.0, 5.0, 2.0, and 10.0 mg kg^{-1} DM were valid for arsenic, total mercury, cadmium, and lead, respectively, in wild-growing species. Moreover, the limits of 4.0, 80, 80, and 80 mg kg^{-1} DM were formerly appointed for chromium, copper, iron, and zinc, respectively. However, the limits for cultivated mushrooms were considerably lower, at only 1.0 mg kg^{-1} DM for total mercury and cadmium.

A single main meal of 300 g of fresh mushrooms (i.e., about 30 g of DM) is commonly considered in the literature for evaluation of potential risk of deleterious elements consumed in mushrooms. Such a serving seems to be rather high as 200–250 g appears to be more realistic.

Many reports present data on element contents separately for caps and stipes, and possibly for more parts of the fruiting bodies. Such data are of limited value for nutritional/health evaluation in species, complete fruiting bodies of which are consumed, because information on weight proportions of separated anatomical parts in fresh matter are mostly lacking.

2.5 Analytical determination of mineral elements

As results from the previous sections, mineral element levels in fruiting bodies are affected by numerous factors and usually vary widely within a species. Representative sampling is, therefore, necessary. The low number of fruiting bodies analyzed either separately or as a pool sample cannot give believable data on mineral composition. As many as 15 fruiting bodies should be used. Unfortunately, information on the number of analyzed fruiting bodies is lacking in some papers. It seems that the only one fruiting body was analyzed in some reports because a very low level of standard deviation reflects only variability of instrumental measurements of the same sample and, therefore, lacking in differences among more fruiting bodies. Only reports with at least five analyzed fruiting bodies per species are collated in Chapter 3, Major essential elements, and Chapter 4, Trace elements.

Samples are sometimes separated into groups of young, fully developed, and aging fruiting bodies. Fruiting bodies are often split into caps and stipes, at times into the spore-forming part (hymenophore), rest of cap flesh, and stipe. Nevertheless, information on some nonconsumable parts, for example, the peel of caps in some species (*M. procera*, some *Agaricus* spp., *Suillus* spp.) are removed, is commonly lacking.

A specific problem can arise due to an incorrect determination of mushroom species. Such confusion may occur in very similar species, for instance in *T. equestre*, which is interchangeable with several related species (Rzymski & Klimaszyk, 2018).

After picking, the bottom part of the stipe with rest of the substrate is eliminated from the sampled fruiting body. The body is cleaned of the remaining soil with a plastic knife, brush, or distilled water and then sliced. The cleaning operation is particularly necessary in underground species and species growing in sandy substrates. The slices are dried either at ambient temperature or in an oven at various temperatures in the range of 40°C–105°C until dry. Freeze-drying is an alternative. The dried material is then powdered. Usage of fresh mushrooms without drying is reported only exceptionally.

Dry mineralization, eliminating organic matter by ashing at temperature up to about 450°C, is not virtually used now. The mushroom powder is usually digested (mineralized) in concentrated nitric acid or in a mixture of nitric acid/dihydrogen peroxide or nitric acid/perchloric acid in closed Teflon containers, assisted with microwave treatment. The digest is then diluted to an appropriate volume. Deep eutectic solvent using choline chloride and oxalic acid was recently proposed for the dissolution of mushroom samples for the determination of selenium and arsenic ions (Zounr, Tuzen, & Khuhawar, 2018). Some quantification methods [e.g., X-rays, fluorescence spectrometry, or instrumental neutron activation analysis (NAA)] use the powdered form without mineralization.

Various measurement techniques have been used for the determination of mineral elements in mushrooms, these being chiefly:

- electrothermal atomization atomic absorption spectrometry for many elements,
- cold vapor atomic absorption spectrometry (CV-AAS) for total mercury,
- hydride generation atomic absorption spectrometry (HG-AAS) for arsenic, antimony, selenium, tellurium, and possibly germanium,
- inductively coupled plasma–atomic emission spectrometry (ICP-AES) for multielemental analyses,
- inductively coupled plasma–mass spectrometry (ICP-MS) for trace elements and isotopic analyses,
- anodic stripping voltammetry (ASV),
- neutron activation analysis (NAA),
- spectrophotometry for determination of phosphorus forming yellow complex with molybdenate-vanadate reagent,
- X-ray fluorescence spectrometry.

Selection of the analytical processes including the final measuring method is crucial for the credibility of the results. Choice of an inappropriate process can result in highly biased data. For instance, determination of total mercury using ICP-AES at wavelength 194.163 nm gives incorrect results compared with CV-AAS (Jarzyńska & Falandysz, 2011). Similarly, ICP-AES determination of selenium gives inaccurate results unlike measurements using HG-AAS (Jarzyńska, Kojta, Drewnowska, & Falandysz, 2012).

Various certified reference materials (CRMs) of plant origins have been used. Nevertheless, mushroom matrices differ in their composition from plant ones, for example, in chitin instead of cellulose. Development of mushroom CRMs is, therefore, welcomed. Chew, Sim, Ng, Shin, and Lee (2016) prepared such a mushroom powder with certified values for arsenic, cadmium, calcium, and lead determination.

Within the European Union, the Institute for Reference Materials and Measurements organized two proficiency tests, designated as IMEP-116 and IMEP-39, for the determination of inorganic arsenic and total arsenic, cadmium, lead, and mercury in mushrooms. Some 62 laboratories from 36 countries participated within the latter test. Laboratory results were rated with a z-score in accordance with ISO 13528. The z-score compares the participant's deviation from the reference value of a determined element with the standard deviation for proficiency assessment used as a common quality criterion. The proportion of satisfactory z-scores ranged from 64% (for inorganic arsenic) to 84% (total mercury) (Cordeiro et al., 2015).

High sensitivity of recent analytical instruments, particularly those using inductively coupled plasma, enables to determine tens of elements including those present at very low concentrations. Some papers published during the past few years have provided comprehensive data for several mushroom species or various variants within a species. Evaluation of such datasets requires advanced statistical methods such as principal component analysis and heatmaps. The existing results contribute to the explanation of relations among variables; however, they do not allow generalizing conclusions.

References

Akindahunsi, A. A., & Oyetayo, F. L. (2006). Nutrient and antinutrient distribution of edible mushroom, *Pleurotus tuber-regium* (Fries) Singer. *LWT*, *39*, 548–553.

Aletor, V. A. (1995). Compositional studies on edible tropical species of mushrooms. *Food Chemistry*, *54*, 265–268.

Ali, A., Guo, D., Mahar, A., Wang, P., Shen, F., Li, R. H., & Zhang, Z. Q. (2017). Mycoremediation of potentially toxic trace elements – A biological tool for soil cleanup: A review. *Pedosphere*, *27*, 205–222.

Baptista, P., Ferreira, S., Soares, E., Coelho, V., & Bastos, M. (2009). Tolerance and stress response of *Macrolepiota procera* to nickel. *Journal of Agricultural and Food Chemistry*, *57*, 7145–7152.

Bellion, M., Courbot, M., Jacob, C., Blaudez, D., & Chalot, M. (2006). Extracellular and cellular mechanisms sustaining metal tolerance in ectomycorrhizal fungi. *FEMS Microbiology Letters*, *254*, 173–181.

Borovička, J., Řanda, Z., Jelínek, E., & Dunn, C. E. (2007). Hyperaccumulation of silver by *Amanita strobiliformis* and related species of the section *Lepidella*. *Mycological Research, 111*, 1339–1344.

Bosiacki, M., Siwulski, M., Sobieralski, K., & Krzebietke, S. (2018). The content of selected heavy metals in fruiting bodies of *Agaricus bisporus* (Lange) Imbach. wild growing in Poland. *Journal of Elementology, 23*, 875–886.

Chen, C., Chen, G., Wang, S., Pei, F., Hu, Q., & Zhao, L. (2017). Speciation changes of three toxic elements in *Lentinus edodes* after drying and soaking. *Journal of Food Processing and Preservation, 41*, e12772.

Chew, G., Sim, L. P., Ng, S. Y., Shin, R. Y. C., & Lee, T. K. (2016). Development of a mushroom powder Certified Reference Material for calcium, arsenic, cadmium and lead measurements. *Food Chemistry, 190*, 293–299.

Choma, A., Nowak, K., Komaniecka, I., Waśko, A., Pleszczyńska, M., Siwulski, M., & Wiater, A. (2018). Chemical characterization of alkali-soluble polysaccharides isolated from a *Boletus edulis* (Bull.) fruiting body and their potential for heavy metal biosorption. *Food Chemistry, 266*, 329–334.

Collin-Hansen, C., Andersen, R. A., & Steinnes, E. (2003). Isolation of N-terminal sequencing of a novel cadmium-binding protein from *Boletus edulis*. *Journal de Physique IV France, 107*, 311–314.

Collin-Hansen, C., Andersen, R. A., & Steinnes, E. (2005a). Molecular defense systems are expressed in the king bolete (*Boletus edulis*) growing near metal smelters. *Mycologia, 97*, 973–983.

Collin-Hansen, C., Andersen, R. A., & Steinnes, E. (2005b). Damage to DNA and lipids in *Boletus edulis* exposed to heavy metals. *Mycological Research, 109*, 1386–1396.

Collin-Hansen, C., Pedersen, S. A., Andersen, R. A., & Steinnes, E. (2007). First report on phytochelatin in a mushroom: Induction of phytochelatins by metal exposure in *Boletus edulis*. *Mycologia, 99*, 161–174.

Collin-Hansen, C., Yttri, K. E., Andersen, R. A., Berthelsen, B. O., & Steinnes, E. (2002). Mushrooms from two metal-contaminated areas in Norway: Occurrence of metals and metallothionein-like proteins. *Geochemistry: Exploration, Environment, Analysis, 2*, 121–130.

Cordeiro, F., Llorente-Mirandes, T., López-Sánchez, J. F., Rubio, R., Sánchez-Agullo, A., Raber, G., et al. (2015). Determination of total cadmium, lead, arsenic, mercury and inorganic arsenic in mushrooms: Outcome of IMEP-116 and IMEP-39. *Food Additives and Contaminants A, 32*, 54–67.

Coşkuner, Y., & Özdemir, Y. (1997). Effect of canning processes on the element content of cultivated mushrooms (*Agaricus bisporus*). *Food Chemistry, 60*, 559–562.

Coşkuner, Y., & Özdemir, Y. (2000). Acid and EDTA blanching effects on the essential element content of mushrooms (*Agaricus bisporus*). *Journal of the Science of Food and Agriculture, 80*, 2074–2076.

Cuny, D., van Haluwyn, C., & Pesch, R. (2001). Biomonitoring of trace elements in air and soil compartments along the major motorway in France. *Water, Air, and Soil Pollution, 125*, 273–289.

Drewnowska, M., Falandysz, J., Chudzińska, M., Hanć, A., Saba, M., & Barałkiewicz, D. (2017). Leaching of arsenic and sixteen metallic elements from *Amanita fulva* mushrooms after food processing. *LWT – Food Science and Technology, 84*, 861–866.

Falandysz, J., Frankowska, A., Jarzyńska, G., Dryżałowska, A., Kojta, A. K., & Zhang, D. (2011). Survey on composition and bioconcentration potential of 12 metallic elements in King Bolete (*Boletus edulis*) mushroom that emerged at 11 spatially distant sites. *Journal of Environmental Science and Health B, 46*, 231–246.

Fernandes, Â., Barreira, J. C. M., Antonio, A. L., Rafalski, A., Morales, P., Férnandez-Ruiz, V., ... Ferreira, I. C. F. R. (2016). Gamma and electron-beam irradiation for wild mushrooms conservation: Effects on macro- and micro-elements. *European Food Research and Technology*, *242*, 1169–1175.

Gadd, G. M. (2007). Geomycology: Biogeochemical transformation of rocks, minerals, metals and radionuclides by fungi, bioweathering and biotransformation. *Mycological Research*, *111*, 3–49.

Gadd, G. M., Rhee, Y. J., Stephenson, K., & Wei, Z. (2012). Geomycology: Metals, actinides and biominerals. *Environmental Microbiology Reports*, *4*, 270–296.

Gast, C. H., Jansen, E., Bierling, J., & Haanstra, L. (1988). Heavy metals in mushrooms and their relationship with soil characteristics. *Chemosphere*, *17*, 789–799.

Gaur, T., Rao, P. B., & Kushwaha, K. P. S. (2016). Nutritional and anti-nutritional components of some selected edible mushroom species. *Indian Journal of Natural Products and Resources*, *7*, 155–161.

Gucia, M., Jarzyńska, G., Kojta, A. K., & Falandysz, J. (2012). Temporal variability in 20 chemical elements content of Parasol Mushroom (*Macrolepiota procera*) collected from two sites over a few years. *Journal of Environmental Science and Health B*, *47*, 81–88.

Jarzyńska, G., & Falandysz, J. (2011). The determination of mercury in mushroomss by CV-AAS and ICP-AES techniques. *Journal of Environmental Science and Health A*, *46*, 569–573.

Jarzyńska, G., Kojta, A. K., Drewnowska, M., & Falandysz, J. (2012). Notes on selenium in mushrooms data determined by inductively coupled plasma atomic emission spectroscopy (ICP-AES) and hydride generation atomic absorption spectroscopy (HG-AAS) techniques. *African Journal of Agricultural Research*, *7*, 5233–5237.

Kała, K., Krakowska, A., Sułkowska-Ziaja, K., Szewczyk, A., Reczyński, W., Opoka, W., & Muszyńska, B. (2017). Kinetics of extracted bioactive components from mushrooms in artificial digestive juices. *International Journal of Food Properties*, *20*, 1796–1817.

Kalač, P. (2010). Trace element contents in European species of wild growing edible mushrooms: A review for the period 2000-2009. *Food Chemistry*, *122*, 2–15.

Kalač, P. (2016). *Edible mushrooms. Chemical composition and nutritional value*. Amsterdam: Elsevier/Academic Press.

Kalač, P., & Svoboda, L. (2000). A review of trace element concentrations in edible mushrooms. *Food Chemistry*, *69*, 273–281.

Koyyalamudi, S. R., Jeong, S. C., Manavalan, S., Vysetti, B., & Pang, G. (2013). Micronutrient mineral content of the fruiting bodies of Australian cultivated *Agaricus bisporus* white button mushrooms. *Journal of Food Composition and Analysis*, *31*, 109–114.

Kuthan, J. (1979). [Assessment of lead content in *Boletus aereus* along a main road in Bulgaria]. *Česká Mykologie*, *33*, 58–59. (in German).

Lipka, K., Saba, M., & Falandysz, J. (2018). Preferential accumulation of inorganic elements in *Amanita muscaria* from North-eastern Poland. *Journal of Environmental Science and Health A*, *53*, 968–974.

Lodenius, M., Soltanpour-Gargari, A., & Tulisalo, E. (2002). Cadmium in forest mushrooms after application of wood ash. *Bulletin of Environmental Contamination and Toxicology*, *68*, 211–216.

Moilanen, M., Fritze, H., Nieminen, M., Sirpa, P., Issakainen, J., & Piispanen, J. (2006). Does wood ash application increase heavy metal accumulation in forest berries and mushrooms? *Forest Ecology and Management*, *226*, 153–160.

Movitz, J. (1980). [High levels of cadmium in Swedish wild mushrooms]. *VarFöda*, *32*, 270–278. (in Swedish).

Nasr, M., & Arp, P. A. (2011). Hg concentrations and accumulations in fungal fruiting bodies, as influenced by forest soil substrates and moss carpets. *Applied Geochemistry*, *26*, 1905–1917.

Nasr, M., Malloch, D. W., & Arp, P. A. (2012). Quantifying Hg within ectomycorrhizal fruiting bodies, from emergence to senescence. *Fungal Biology*, *116*, 1163–1177.

Nogaj, E., Kowol, J., Kwapuliński, J., Brodziak-Dopierała, B., Paukszto, A., Rochel, R., ... Mirosławski, J. (2012). Contribution of bioavailable forms of chosen metals in soil to heavy-metal contamination of wild mushrooms. *Polish Journal of Environmental Studies*, *21*, 165–169.

Rosling, A., Landeweert, R., Lindahl, B. D., Larsson, K.-H., Kuyper, T. W., Taylor, A. ,F. S., & Finlay, R. D. (2003). Vertical distribution of ectomycorrhizal fungal taxa in a podzol soil profile. *New Phytologist*, *159*, 775–783.

Rubio, C., Martínez, C., Paz, S., Gutiérrez, A. J., González-Weller, D., Revert, C., ... Hardisson, A. (2018). Trace elements and toxic metal intake from the consumption of canned mushrooms in Spain. *Environmental Monitoring and Assessment*, *190*. Available from https://doi.org/10.1007/s10661-018-6614-6, Art. Nr. 237.

Rzymski, P., & Klimaszyk, P. (2018). Edible or not? Systematic review and critical viewpoint on *Tricholoma equestre* toxicity. *Comprehensive Reviews in Food Science and Food Safety*, *17*, 1309–1324.

Svoboda, L., Kalač, P., Špička, J., & Janoušková, D. (2002). Leaching of cadmium, lead and mercury from fresh and differently preserved edible mushroom, *Xerocomus badius*, during soaking and boiling. *Food Chemistry*, *79*, 41–45.

Tyler, G. (1982). Accumulation and exclusion of metals in *Collybia peronata* and *Amanita rubescens*. *Transactions of the British Mycological Society*, *79*, 239–245.

Vaario, L. M., Pennanen, T., Lu, J., Palmén, J., Stenman, J., Leveinen, J., ... Kitunen, V. (2015). *Tricholoma matsutake* can absorb and accumulate trace elements directly from rock fragments in the shiro. *Mycorrhiza*, *25*, 325–334.

Wondratschek, I., & Röder, U. (1993). Monitoring of heavy metals in soils by higher fungi. In B. Markert (Ed.), *Plants as biomonitors. Indicators for heavy metals in the terrestrial environment* (pp. 345–363). Weinheim: VCH.

Wuilloud, R. G., Kannamkumarath, S. S., & Caruso, J. A. (2004a). Speciation of essential and toxic elements in edible mushrooms: Size-exclusion chromatography separation with on-line UV-inductively coupled plasma mass spectrometry detection. *Applied Organometallic Chemistry*, *18*, 156–165.

Wuilloud, R. G., Kannamkumarath, S. S., & Caruso, J. A. (2004b). Multielemental speciation analysis of fungi porcini (*Boletus edulis*) mushroom by size exclusion liquid chromatography with sequential on-line UV-ICP-MS detection. *Journal of Agricultural and Food Chemistry*, *52*, 1315–1322.

Zhang, D., Frankowska, A., Jarzyńska, G., Kojta, A. K., Drewnowska, M., Wydmańska, D., ... Falandysz, J. (2010). Metals of King Bolete (*Boletus edulis* Bull.:Fr.) collected at the same site over two years. *African Journal of Agricultural Research*, *5*, 3050–3055.

Zounr, R. A., Tuzen, M., & Khuhawar, M. Y. (2018). Determination of selenium and arsenic ions in edible mushroom samples by novel chloride-oxalic deep eutectic solvent extraction using graphite furnace-atomic absorption spectrometry. *Journal of AOAC International*, *101*, 593–600.

Źródłowski, Z. (1995). The influence of washing and peeling of mushrooms *Agaricus bisporus* on the level of heavy metals contamination. *Polish Journal of Food and Nutrition Science*, *45*, 26–33.

Chapter 3

Major essential elements

The crude ash of mushrooms consists of seven major mineral elements, quantitatively highly prevailing, and of tens of trace elements generally occurring at a level up to 50 mg kg^{-1} FM (i.e., about up to 500 mg kg^{-1} DM) for each. Data on trace elements are given in Chapter 4, Trace elements, and information on radioactive isotopes is covered in Chapter 5, Radioactivity.

Mushrooms usually contain 50–120 g of ash per kg DM (i.e., approximately 5–12 g kg^{-1} FM). Such an extent is typical for cultivated species, whereas contents above 200 g kg^{-1} DM occur in some wild-growing species. These differences probably result from the great variability of substrates in nature. The variability in ash contents seems to be lower than in the other main components of mushrooms, for example, in crude protein or carbohydrates (Kalač, 2016).

The major mineral elements (in alphabetical order) are calcium, chlorine, magnesium, phosphorus, potassium, sodium, and sulfur. The last element is included in food chemistry among minerals even though in mushrooms it occurs mostly in organic forms. All these elements are essential for the normal functioning of various physiological processes in humans. Recent average daily requirements of four major elements (i.e., calcium, magnesium, phosphorous, potassium) recommended by the European Food Safety Authority (EFSA, 2017) are given in Table 3.1. The assessments of sodium and chlorine (as chloride) are ongoing and are meant for publication by the EFSA in 2019.

The literature data since 2010 on the element contents collated in Tables 3.2–3.6 are mean values expressed in g kg^{-1} DM. However, relative standard deviations are commonly high. Only data on at least five fruiting bodies per species, analyzed either separately or as a pooled sample, are inserted into the tables. Superscripts C and S are used for the contents in caps and stipes, respectively. The superscripts are given in order of the increasing contents (e.g., $X^{C,S}$ if the level of an element is higher in stipes than in caps).

The first report on mineral composition of mushrooms appeared in 1907 in a book by J. Zellner (Zellner, 1907). Data of Friese (1929) pose a singular journal article from the very incipiency of this research topic. More reliable

Mineral Composition and Radioactivity of Edible Mushrooms.
DOI: https://doi.org/10.1016/B978-0-12-817565-1.00003-0

TABLE 3.1 Average requirements (mg day^{-1}) of major elements for adults (≥18 years) according to EFSA (2017).

Element	Males	Females
Calcium	1000 (18–24 years) 950 (≥25 years)	1000 (18–24 years) 950 (≥25 years)
Magnesium	350	300
Phosphorus	550	550
Potassium	3500	3500

data started to become available from the mid-1970s with the development of advanced instruments and analytical methods. Pioneering data on the major elements in more than 400 mushroom species, not exceeded as a whole until now, published laboratory of Professor Ruth Seeger in the University of Würzburg, Germany in the late 1970s and the 1980s. The vast proportion of the available data on both major and trace elements from the last two decades originates from Polish and Turkish laboratories.

3.1 Calcium (Ca)

Seeger and Hüttner (1981), in their comprehensive study, analyzed 1018 samples of 406 wild-growing edible, inedible, and toxic mushroom species. Contents of calcium between 0.1 and 0.5 g kg^{-1} DM were determined in 57% of the samples and the mean value was 0.49 ± 0.06 g kg^{-1} DM. The highest level was observed in the *Polyporaceae* family, while the *Russulaceae* and *Lycoperdaceae* families had particularly low levels.

Data on calcium mean contents published since 2010 are collated in Table 3.2. The contents range between about 0.05 and more than 1.0 g kg^{-1} DM. The most frequent levels are 0.05–0.75 g kg^{-1} DM for both cultivated and wild-growing fruiting bodies. Nevertheless, wide ranges are apparent within species with numerous data such as in cultivated *Lentinula edodes* and wild-growing *Boletus edulis*, *Cantharellus cibarius*, or *Xerocomus badius*. As results from Table 3.2, the reported distribution of calcium between caps and stipes varies both among mushroom species and within species.

The highest reported contents during the observed period were 3.62, 2.71, 2.48, and 2.33 g kg^{-1} DM in *Helvella leucopus* (Sarikurkcu, Tepe, Solak, & Cetinkaya, 2012), *X. badius* growing in an alkaline flotation tailing site (Mleczek et al., 2016), *Boletus pseudoscaber* (Dimitrijevic et al., 2016), and in cultivated *Grifola frondosa* (Niedzielski et al., 2017), respectively.

TABLE 3.2 Data on the mean content (g kg^{-1} dry matter) of calcium in fruit bodies of wild-growing mushrooms collected from unpolluted (X), geologically specific (●), and anthropogenically contaminated (▲) sites and in cultivated species, published since 2010.

Species	<0.05	0.05–0.1	0.1–0.2	0.2–0.3	0.3–0.5	0.5–0.75	0.5–1.0	>1.0	References
Wild growing									
Agaricus arvensis						X			Ayaz et al. (2011)
Agaricus bisporus		X							Gąsecka et al. (2018)
Agaricus campestris					$X^{C,S}$		$▲^{C}$	X, $▲^{S}$	Sarikurkcu et al. (2012), Zsigmond et al. (2018)
Agaricus lanipes				X					Gezer et al. (2016)
Agrocybe cylindracea								X	Sarikurkcu et al. (2012)
Albatrellus ovinus				$X^{C,S}$					Mędyk et al. (2017)
Amanita fulva	X^{C}		X^{S}						Falandysz, Drewnowska, Chudzińska, and Barałkiewicz (2017)
Amanita ponderosa						X			Salvador, Martins, Vicente, and Caldeira (2018)
Armillariella mellea		X	X						Gąsecka et al. (2018), Zavastin et al. (2018)
Auricularia auricula-judae						X			Gąsecka et al. (2018)

(*Continued*)

TABLE 3.2 Data on the mean content (g kg^{-1} dry matter) of calcium in fruit bodies of wild-growing mushrooms collected from unpolluted (X), geologically specific (●), and anthropogenically contaminated (▲) sites and in cultivated species, published since 2010. (Continued)

Species	<0.05	0.05–0.1	0.1–0.2	0.2–0.3	0.3–0.5	0.5–0.75	0.5–1.0	>1.0	References
Boletus appendiculatus			X				X^{Sm}	X^{Cm}	Alaimo et al. (2018), Dimitrijevic et al. (2016), Wang, Zhang, Li, Wang, and Liu (2015)
Boletus bruneissimus			X^{S}				X^{C}		Wang et al. (2015)
Boletus edulis	X	X, X^{C}	X, X^{S}	X	X, $X^{S,C}$		X	X	Ayaz et al. (2011), Brzezicha-Cirocka, Mędyk, Falandysz, and Szefer (2016), Cvetkovic, Mitic, Stankov-Jovanovic, Dimitrijevic, and Nikolic-Mandic (2015), Dimitrijevic et al. (2016), Falandysz et al. (2011), Frankowska, Ziółkowska, Bielawski, and Falandysz (2010), Mędyk et al. (2017), Mleczek et al. (2013, 2015), Turfan et al. (2018), Wang et al. (2015, 2015b), Zavastin et al. (2018), Zhang et al. (2010)
Boletus griseus					X	$X^{S,C}$			Liu, Zhang, Li, Shi, and Wang (2012), Wang et al. (2015)
Boletus impolitus			X						Dimitrijevic et al. (2016)

Boletus luridus					$X^{S,C}$				Wang et al. (2015)
Boletus pallidus					$X^{C,S}$				Wang et al. (2015)
Boletus pseudoscaber								X	Dimitrijevic et al. (2016)
Boletus rubellus				X^{C}			X^{S}		Wang et al. (2015)
Boletus speciosus	X		$X^{S,C}$						Liu et al. (2012), Wang et al. (2015)
Boletus tomentipes		X^{S}	X^{C}		X^{C}	X^{S}			Wang et al. (2015, 2015a)
Boletus umbriniporus		X^{S}	X^{C}						Wang et al. (2015)
Calvatia gigantea					X				Gąsecka et al. (2018)
Cantharellus cibarius		X		X	X		X	X	Ayaz et al. (2011), Cvetkovic et al. (2015), Drewnowska and Falandysz (2015), Falandysz and Drewnowska (2015), Gąsecka et al. (2018), Mleczek et al. (2013), Zavastin et al. (2018)
Cantharellus tubaeformis								X	Ayaz et al. (2011), Brzezicha-Cirocka et al. (2016)
Clitopilus prunulus								X^{m}	Alaimo et al. (2018),
Craterellus cornucopioides			X						Turfan et al. (2018)
Fistulina hepatica					X				Gąsecka et al. (2018)
Flammulina velutipes					X^{C}				Zeng, Suwandi, Fuller, Doronila, and Ng (2012)

(*Continued*)

TABLE 3.2 Data on the mean content (g kg^{-1} dry matter) of calcium in fruit bodies of wild-growing mushrooms collected from unpolluted (X), geologically specific (●), and anthropogenically contaminated (▲) sites and in cultivated species, published since 2010. (Continued)

Species	<0.05	0.05–0.1	0.1–0.2	0.2–0.3	0.3–0.5	0.5–0.75	0.5–1.0	>1.0	References
Gomphidius glutinosus				X^S					Mędyk et al. (2017)
Grifola frondosa			X						Gąsecka et al. (2018)
Helvella leucopus								X	Sarikurkcu et al. (2012)
Hericium erinaceus									
Hydnum repandum		X			X				Ayaz et al. (2011), Jedidi et al. (2017)
Laccaria laccata								X	Ayaz et al. (2011)
Lactarius deliciosus			X	X					Jedidi et al. (2017), Mleczek et al. (2013), Turfan et al. (2018)
Lactarius hygrophoroides	X								Liu et al. (2012),
Lactarius piperatus						X			Cvetkovic et al. (2015)
Laetiporus sulphureus	X				X				Gąsecka et al. (2018), Turfan et al. (2018)
Leccinum aurantiacum		X				X			Brzezicha-Cirocka et al. (2016), Mleczek et al. (2013)
Leccinum duriusculum		X^C	X^S						Jarzyńska and Falandysz (2012a)
Leccinum griseum			$X^{S,C}$						Jarzyńska and Falandysz (2012b)

Leccinum scabrum		X	X, $X^{S,C}$	X					Falandysz (2018), Gąsecka et al. (2018), Mędyk et al. (2017), Mleczek et al. (2015)
Leccinum versipelle				X					Mędyk et al. (2017), Mleczek et al. (2015)
Lentinus cladopus								X	Mallikarjuna et al. (2013)
Lepista nuda						X			Ayaz et al. (2011)
Lepista gilva				X					Gąsecka et al. (2018)
Leucopaxillus giganteus				X					Liu et al. (2012)
Lycoperdon perlatum		X	X						Brzezicha-Cirocka et al. (2016), Mędyk et al. (2017)
Lyophyllum fumosum					X				Gąsecka et al. (2018)
Macrocybe gigantea					X				Liu et al. (2012)
Macrolepiota procera			X, X^C	$X^{C,S}$	X^S	X^S			Gąsecka et al. (2018), Gucia et al. (2012), Jarzyńska, Gucia, Kojta, Rezulak, and Falandysz (2011), Kojta et al. (2011), Kułdo et al. (2014), Stefanović et al. (2016)
Marasmius oreades				X				X	Cvetkovic et al. (2015), Turfan et al. (2018)
Melanoleuca arcuata				X					Liu et al. (2012)
Morchella conica			X						Turfan et al. (2018)

(Continued)

TABLE 3.2 Data on the mean content (g kg^{-1} dry matter) of calcium in fruit bodies of wild-growing mushrooms collected from unpolluted (X), geologically specific (●), and anthropogenically contaminated (▲) sites and in cultivated species, published since 2010. (Continued)

Species	<0.05	0.05–0.1	0.1–0.2	0.2–0.3	0.3–0.5	0.5–0.75	0.5–1.0	>1.0	References
Morchella deliciosa				X					Liu et al. (2012)
Morchella elata								X^{C}	Zeng et al. (2012)
Morchella esculenta							X	X	Gąsecka et al. (2018), Rossbach et al. (2017), Sarikurkcu et al. (2012)
Mycena haematopus			X						Liu et al. (2012)
Pleurotus djamor					X				Mallikarjuna et al. (2013)
Pleurotus eryngii		X^{C}							Zeng et al. (2012)
Pleurotus ostreatus			X						Tel-Çayan, Öztürk, Duru, Yabanli, and Türkoğlu (2017)
Ramaria botrytis		X							Turfan et al. (2018)
Sparassis crispa			X						Gąsecka et al. (2018)
Suillus bovinus			X	X^{C}	X^{S}				Gąsecka et al. (2018), Mędyk et al. (2017)
Suillus luteus		X^{C}	X		$X^{C,S}$				Zeng et al. (2012), Mędyk et al. (2017), Mleczek et al. (2013)
Suillus variegatus		X^{C}	X^{S}						Szubstarska, Jarzyńska, and Falandysz (2012)
Terfezia claveryi					X		X		Kivrak (2015), Vahdani et al. (2017)

Terfezia olbiensis					X				Kivrak (2015)
Tirmania nivea						X			Vahdani et al. (2017)
Tricholoma equestre		X	X						Gąsecka et al. (2018), Jedidi et al. (2017)
Tricholoma fracticum	X								Tel-Çayan et al. (2017)
Tricholoma matsutake				X	X				Li et al. (2013), Liu et al. (2012)
Tricholoma terreum					X				Turfan et al. (2018)
Xerocomus badius	X, ▲^{S}	X^{C},X, ▲^{S}	X, X$^{C\ S}$	X^{S}	X			▲	Dimitrijevic et al. (2016), Kojta, Jarzyńska, and Falandysz (2012), Kojta and Falandysz (2016), Mleczek et al. (2013, 2015, 2016), Proskura et al. (2017)
Xerocomus chrysenteron					X				Dimitrijevic et al. (2016)
Xerocomus subtomentosus			X^{S,C}	X^{C}	X^{S}				Jarzyńska, Chojnacka, Dryżalowska, Nnorom, and Falandysz (2012), Mędyk et al. (2017)
Cultivated									
A. arvensis						X			Rzymski et al. (2017)
A. bisporus (unspecified)					X				Gaur, Rao, and Kushwaha (2016)
									(*Continued*)

TABLE 3.2 Data on the mean content (g kg^{-1} dry matter) of calcium in fruit bodies of wild-growing mushrooms collected from unpolluted (X), geologically specific (●), and anthropogenically contaminated (▲) sites and in cultivated species, published since 2010. (Continued)

Species	<0.05	0.05–0.1	0.1–0.2	0.2–0.3	0.3–0.5	0.5–0.75	0.5–1.0	>1.0	References
A. bisporus (brown)			X			X			Bach, Helm, Bellettini, Maciel, and Haminiuk (2017), Rzymski et al. (2017)
A. bisporus (white)			X	X	X			X	Bach et al. (2017), Jedidi et al. (2017), Mleczek et al. (2018), Rzymski et al. (2017)
Agaricus subrufescens				X			X		Bach et al. (2017), Rzymski et al. (2017)
A. cylindracea			X						Niedzielski et al. (2017)
A. auricula-judae								X	Mleczek et al. (2018)
Auricularia polytricha			X						Niedzielski et al. (2017)
Auricularia thailandica							X		Bandara et al. (2017)
Calocybe indica				X					Gaur et al. (2016)
Clitocybe maxima				X					Niedzielski et al. (2017)
F. velutipes	X				X				Bach et al. (2017), Niedzielski et al. (2017)
G. frondosa								X	Niedzielski et al. (2017)
H. erinaceus			X						Niedzielski et al. (2017), Turfan et al. (2018)

L. sulphureus					X				Niedzielski et al. (2017)
Lentinula edodes	X		X		X	X	X	X	Bach et al. (2017), Gaur et al. (2016), Gonçalves et al. (2014), Mallikarjuna et al. (2013), Mleczek et al. (2017, 2018), Turfan et al. (2018)
M. gigantea									Gaur et al. (2016)
Pholiota nameko					X				Niedzielski et al. (2017)
P. djamor			X						Bach et al. (2017)
P. eryngii		X							Bach et al. (2017), Gonçalves et al. (2014)
Pleurotus florida							X		Mallikarjuna et al. (2013)
P. ostreatus		X				X			Bach et al. (2017), Gonçalves et al. (2014), Mleczek et al. (2018), Turfan et al. (2018)
Pleurotus sajor-caju				X					Gaur et al. (2016)
Trametes versicolor							X		Niedzielski et al. (2017)
Tremella fuciformis					X				Mleczek et al. (2018), Niedzielski et al. (2017)
Volvariella volvacea								X	Mleczek et al. (2018)

C, Caps; *S*, stipes; *Xm*, median value.

TABLE 3.3 Data on the mean content (g kg^{-1} dry matter) of magnesium in fruit bodies of wild-growing mushrooms collected from unpolluted (X), geologically specific (●), and anthropogenically contaminated (▲) sites and in cultivated species, published since 2010.

Species	<0.5	0.5–1.0	1.0–1.25	1.25–1.5	1.5–1.75	1.75–2.0	2.0–2.5	References
Wild growing								
Agaricus arvensis			X					Ayaz et al. (2011)
Agaricus bisporus		X						Gąsecka et al. (2018)
Agaricus campestris		▲^{S}	X^{S}	▲^{C}		X^{C}	X	Sarikurkcu et al. (2012), Zsigmond et al. (2018)
Agaricus lanipes		X						Gezer et al. (2016)
Agrocybe cylindracea							X	Sarikurkcu et al. (2012)
Albatrellus ovinus		$X^{S,C}$						Mędyk et al. (2017)
Amanita fulva		X^{S}	X^{C}					Falandysz et al. (2017)
Amanita ponderosa		X						Salvador et al. (2018)
Armillariella mellea		X						Gąsecka et al. (2018), Zavastin et al. (2018)
Auricularia auricula-judae		X						Gąsecka et al. (2018)
Boletus appendiculatuss	X^{Sm}	$X^{S,C}$, X, X^{Cm}						Alaimo et al. (2018), Sun, Chang, Bao, and Zhuang (2017), Wang et al. (2015)
Boletus bicolor		X						Sun et al. (2017)

Boletus bruneissimus		$X^{S,C}$						Wang et al. (2015)
Boletus edulis	X, $X^{S,C}$	X, X^{C}, X^{S}	X^{C}					Ayaz et al. (2011), Brzezicha-Cirocka et al. (2016), Cvetkovic et al. (2015), Falandysz et al. (2011), Frankowska et al. (2010), Mędyk et al. (2017), Mleczek et al. (2013, 2015), Sun et al. (2017), Wang et al. (2015, 2015b), Zavastin et al. (2018), Zhang et al. (2010)
Boletus flammans		X						Sun et al. (2017)
Boletus griseus	X,X^{S}	X^{C}, X						Liu et al. (2012), Sun et al. (2017), Wang et al. (2015)
Boletus luridus	X^{S}	X^{C}						Wang et al. (2015)
Boletus pallidus		X^{S}	X^{C}					Wang et al. (2015)
Boletus rubellus		$X^{S,C}$						Wang et al. (2015)
Boletus sinicus		X						Sun et al. (2017)
Boletus speciosus	X	$X^{S,C}$, X						Liu et al. (2012), Sun et al. (2017), Wang et al. (2015),
Boletus tomentipes	$X^{S,C}$	X^{S}	X^{C}					Wang et al. (2015, 2015a)
Boletus umbriniporus	$X^{S,C}$							Wang et al. (2015)
Calvatia gigantea		X						Gąsecka et al. (2018)

(*Continued*)

TABLE 3.3 Data on the mean content (g kg^{-1} dry matter) of magnesium in fruit bodies of wild-growing mushrooms collected from unpolluted (X), geologically specific (●), and anthropogenically contaminated (▲) sites and in cultivated species, published since 2010. (Continued)

Species	<0.5	0.5–1.0	1.0–1.25	1.25–1.5	1.5–1.75	1.75–2.0	2.0–2.5	References
Cantharellus cibarius	X	X	X					Ayaz et al. (2011), Brzezicha-Cirocka et al. (2016), Cvetkovic et al. (2015), Drewnowska and Falandysz (2015), Falandysz and Drewnowska (2015), Gąsecka et al. (2018), Mleczek et al. (2013), Zavastin et al. (2018)
Cantharellus tubaeformis		X						Ayaz et al. (2011)
Clitopilus prunulus				X^m				Alaimo et al. (2018)
Fistulina hepatica		X						Gąsecka et al. (2018)
Flammulina velutipes		X^C						Zeng et al. (2012)
Gomphidium glutinosus			X^S			X^C		Mędyk et al. (2017)
Grifola frondosa	X							Gąsecka et al. (2018)
Helvella leucopus							X	Sarikurkcu et al. (2012)
Hydnum repandum		X						Ayaz et al. (2011)
Laccaria laccata		X						Ayaz et al. (2011)
Lactarius deliciosus	X				X			Jedidi et al. (2017), Mleczek et al. (2013)
Lactarius hygrophoroides	X							Liu et al. (2012)

Lactarius piperatus	X							Cvetkovic et al. (2015)
Laetiporus sulphureus		X						Gąsecka et al. (2018)
Leccinum aurantiacum		X	X					Brzezicha-Cirocka et al. (2016), Mleczek et al. (2013)
Leccinum crocipodium		X						Sun et al. (2017)
Leccinum duriusculum		X^S	X^C					Jarzyńska and Falandysz (2012a)
Leccinum griseum		X^S	X^C					Jarzyńska and Falandysz (2012b)
Leccinum scabrum	X	X, $X^{S,C}$						Falandysz (2018), Gąsecka et al. (2018), Mędyk et al. (2017), Mleczek et al. (2015)
Leccinum versipelle		X						Mędyk et al. (2017)
Lentinus cladopus	X							Mallikarjuna et al. (2013)
Lepista gilva	X							Gąsecka et al. (2018)
Lepista nuda			X					Ayaz et al. (2011)
Leucopaxillus giganteus	X							Liu et al. (2012)
Lycoperdon perlatum						X		Brzezicha-Cirocka et al. (2016), Mędyk et al. (2017)
Lyophyllum fumosum		X						Gąsecka et al. (2018)
Macrocybe gigantea		X						Liu et al. (2012)

(Continued)

TABLE 3.3 Data on the mean content (g kg^{-1} dry matter) of magnesium in fruit bodies of wild-growing mushrooms collected from unpolluted (X), geologically specific (●), and anthropogenically contaminated (▲) sites and in cultivated species, published since 2010. (Continued)

Species	<0.5	0.5–1.0	1.0–1.25	1.25–1.5	1.5–1.75	1.75–2.0	2.0–2.5	References
Macrolepiota procera		X, X^S	$X^{S,C}$	X^C	X^C			Gąsecka et al. (2018), Gucia et al. (2012), Jarzyńska et al. (2011), Kojta et al. (2011), Kułdo et al. (2014), Stefanović et al. (2016)
Marasmius oreades			X					Cvetkovic et al. (2015)
Melanoleuca arcuata	X							Liu et al. (2012)
Morchella elata		X^C						Zeng et al. (2012)
Morchella deliciosa	X							Liu et al. (2012)
Morchella esculenta		X	X	X				Gąsecka et al. (2018), Rossbach et al. (2017), Sarikurkcu et al. (2012)
Mycena haematopus	X							Liu et al. (2012)
Pleurotus djamor	X							Mallikarjuna et al. (2013)
Pleurotus eryngii		X^C						Zeng et al. (2012)
Pleurotus ostreatus		X						Tel-Çayan et al. (2017)
Sparassis crispa	X							Gąsecka et al. (2018)
Suillus bovinus	X	X^S	X^C					Gąsecka et al. (2018), Mędyk et al. (2017)

Suillus luteus	X	X^{C}	X^{S}					Zeng et al. (2012), Mędyk et al. (2017), Mleczek et al. (2013)
Suillus variegatus	X^{S}	X^{C}						Szubstarska et al. (2012)
Terfezia claveryi		X		X				Kivrak (2015), Vahdani et al. (2017)
Terfezia olbiensis			X					Kivrak (2015)
Tricholoma equestre	X						X	Gąsecka et al. (2018), Jedidi et al. (2017)
Tricholoma fracticum	X							Tel-Çayan et al. (2017)
Tricholoma matsutake	X							Li et al. (2013), Liu et al. (2012)
Xerocomus badius	X, X^{S}, $▲^{S}$	$X^{C,S}$, ▲, $▲^{C}$	$X^{C,S}$					Kojta et al. (2012), Kojta and Falandysz (2016), Mleczek et al. (2013, 2015, 2016), Proskura et al. (2017)
Xerocomus subtomentosus		X^{S}	X^{C}	X^{C}				Jarzyńska et al. (2012), Mędyk et al. (2017)
Cultivated								
A. arvensis				X				Rzymski et al. (2017)
A. bisporus (unspecified)	X							Gaur et al. (2016)

(*Continued*)

TABLE 3.3 Data on the mean content (g kg^{-1} dry matter) of magnesium in fruit bodies of wild-growing mushrooms collected from unpolluted (X), geologically specific (●), and anthropogenically contaminated (▲) sites and in cultivated species, published since 2010. (Continued)

Species	<0.5	0.5–1.0	1.0–1.25	1.25–1.5	1.5–1.75	1.75–2.0	2.0–2.5	References
A. bisporus (brown)			X	X				Bach et al. (2017), Jedidi et al. (2017), Rzymski et al. (2017)
A. bisporus (white)			X	X				Bach et al. (2017), Mleczek et al. (2018), Rzymski et al. (2017)
Agaricus subrufescens			X			X		Bach et al. (2017), Rzymski et al. (2017)
A. cylindracea		X						Niedzielski et al. (2017)
A. auricula-judae			X					Mleczek et al. (2018)
Auricularia polytricha		X						Niedzielski et al. (2017)
Auricularia thailandica		X						Bandara et al. (2017)
Calocybe indica	X							Gaur et al. (2016)
Clitocybe maxima		X						Niedzielski et al. (2017)
F. velutipes		X			X			Bach et al. (2017), Niedzielski et al. (2017)
G. frondosa				X				Niedzielski et al. (2017)
Hericium erinaceus		X						Niedzielski et al. (2017)

L. sulphureus	X							Niedzielski et al. (2017)
Lentinula edodes	X		X		X		X	Bach et al. (2017), Gaur et al. (2016), Mallikarjuna et al. (2013), Mleczek et al. (2017, 2018)
M. gigantea	X							Gaur et al. (2016)
Pholiota nameko		X						Niedzielski et al. (2017)
P. djamor					X			Bach et al. (2017)
P. eryngii			X					Bach et al. (2017)
Pleurotus florida	X							Mallikarjuna et al. (2013)
P. ostreatus				X		X	X	Bach et al. (2017), Gonçalves et al. (2014), Mleczek et al. (2018)
Pleurotus sajor-caju	X							Gaur et al. (2016)
Trametes versicolor		X						Niedzielski et al. (2017)
Tremella fuciformis	X		X					Mleczek et al. (2018), Niedzielski et al. (2017)
Volvariella volvacea		X						Mleczek et al. (2018)

C, Caps; *S*, stipes; *Xm*, median value.

TABLE 3.4 Data on the mean content (g kg^{-1} dry matter) of phosphorus in fruit bodies of wild-growing mushrooms collected from unpolluted (X), geologically specific (●), and anthropogenically contaminated (▲) sites and in cultivated species, published since 2010.

Species	<2.5	2.5–5.0	5.0–6.0	6.0–7.0	7.0–8.0	8.0–9.0	9.0–10.0	>10	References
Wild growing									
Agaricus arvensis								X	Ayaz et al. (2011)
Agaricus campestris						$▲^{S}$		$X^{S,C}$, $▲^{C}$	Zsigmond et al. (2018)
Agaricus lanipes				X					Gezer et al. (2016)
Amanita fulva	X^{S}					X^{C}			Falandysz et al. (2017)
Amanita ponderosa	X								Salvador et al. (2018)
Boletus appendiculatus	X^{S}		X^{C}		X				Dimitrijevic et al. (2016), Wang et al. (2015)
Boletus bruneissimus		$X^{S,C}$							Wang et al. (2015)
Boletus edulis	X,X^{S}	X, X^{S}	X^{C}	X, X^{C}					Ayaz et al. (2011), Cvetkovic et al. (2015), Turfan et al. (2018), Wang et al. (2015, 2015b)
Boletus griseus		X^{S}			X^{C}				Wang et al. (2015)
Boletus impolitus								X	Dimitrijevic et al. (2016)
Boletus luridus		X^{S}		X^{C}					Wang et al. (2015)
Boletus pallidus			X^{S}					X^{C}	Wang et al. (2015)
Boletus pseudoscaber								X	Dimitrijevic et al. (2016)

Boletus regius							X		Dimitrijevic et al. (2016)
Boletus rubellus		X^{S}	X^{C}						Wang et al. (2015)
Boletus speciosus	X^{S}		X^{C}						Wang et al. (2015)
Boletus tomentipes		X^{S}	$X^{S,C}$	X^{C}					Wang et al. (2015, 2015a)
Boletus umbriniporus	X^{S}		X^{C}						Wang et al. (2015)
Cantharellus cibarius		X							Ayaz et al. (2011), Cvetkovic et al. (2015), Drewnowska and Falandysz (2015), Falandysz and Drewnowska (2015)
Cantharellus tubaeformis		X							Ayaz et al. (2011)
Craterellus cornucopioides	X								Turfan et al. (2018)
Flammulina velutipes						X^{C}			Zeng et al. (2012)
Hydnum repandum			X						Ayaz et al. (2011)
Laccaria laccata				X					Ayaz et al. (2011)
Lactarius deliciosus	X								Turfan et al. (2018)
Lactarius piperatus									Cvetkovic et al. (2015)
Laetiporus sulphureus	X								Turfan et al. (2018)
Leccinum crocipodium				X					Dimitrijevic et al. (2016)
Leccinum duriusculum	X^{S}		X^{C}						Jarzyńska and Falandysz (2012a)

(*Continued*)

TABLE 3.4 Data on the mean content (g kg^{-1} dry matter) of phosphorus in fruit bodies of wild-growing mushrooms collected from unpolluted (X), geologically specific (●), and anthropogenically contaminated (▲) sites and in cultivated species, published since 2010. (Continued)

Species	<2.5	2.5–5.0	5.0–6.0	6.0–7.0	7.0–8.0	8.0–9.0	9.0–10.0	>10	References
Leccinum scabrum	X^S				X^C				Falandysz (2018)
Lentinus cladopus	X								Mallikarjuna et al. (2013)
Lepista nuda								X	Ayaz et al. (2011)
Macrolepiota procera		X^S		X^S				X^C	Gucia et al. (2012), Kojta et al. (2011), Kułdo et al. (2014)
Marasmius oreades		X						X	Cvetkovic et al. (2015), Turfan et al. (2018)
Morchella conica				X					Turfan et al. (2018)
Morchella elata								X^C	Zeng et al. (2012)
Morchella esculenta								X	Rossbach et al. (2017)
Pleurotus djamor					X				Mallikarjuna et al. (2013)
Pleurotus eryngii						X^C			Zeng et al. (2012)
Ramaria botrytis	X								Turfan et al. (2018)
Suillus luteus			X^C						Zeng et al. (2012)
Terfezia claveryi	X				X				Kivrak (2015), Vahdani et al. (2017)
Terfezia olbiensis	X								Kivrak (2015)
Tirmania nivea					X				Vahdani et al. (2017)
Tricholoma terreum		X							Turfan et al. (2018)

Xerocomus badius		●, X	▲^{S}		▲^{C}			X^{S,C}	Dimitrijevic et al. (2016), Kojta et al. (2012), Mleczek et al. (2016), Proskura et al. (2017)
Xerocomus chrysenteron		X							Dimitrijevic et al. (2016)
Xerocomus subtomentosus		X^{S}				X^{C}			Jarzyńska et al. (2012)
Cultivated									
A. arvensis								X	Rzymski et al. (2017)
Agaricus bisporus (unspecified)		X							Gaur et al. (2016)
A. bisporus (brown)								X	Bach et al. (2017), Rzymski et al. (2017)
A. bisporus (white)								X	Bach et al. (2017), Mleczek et al. (2018), Rzymski et al. (2017)
Agaricus subrufescens								X	Bach et al. (2017), Rzymski et al. (2017)
Agrocybe cylindracea								X	Niedzielski et al. (2017)
Auricularia auricula-judae	X								Mleczek et al. (2018)
Auricularia polytricha								X	Niedzielski et al. (2017)
Auricularia thailandica		X							Bandara et al. (2017)
Calocybe indica			X						Gaur et al. (2016)
Clitocybe maxima								X	Niedzielski et al. (2017)
F. velutipes							X	X	Bach et al. (2017), Niedzielski et al. (2017)
Grifola frondosa								X	Niedzielski et al. (2017)

(*Continued*)

TABLE 3.4 Data on the mean content (g kg^{-1} dry matter) of phosphorus in fruit bodies of wild-growing mushrooms collected from unpolluted (X), geologically specific (●), and anthropogenically contaminated (▲) sites and in cultivated species, published since 2010. (Continued)

Species	<2.5	2.5–5.0	5.0–6.0	6.0–7.0	7.0–8.0	8.0–9.0	9.0–10.0	>10	References
Hericium erinaceus	X							X	Niedzielski et al. (2017), Turfan et al. (2018)
L. sulphureus								X	Niedzielski et al. (2017)
Lentinula edodes	X	X			X			X	Bach et al. (2017), Gaur et al. (2016), Mallikarjuna et al. (2013), Mleczek et al. (2017, 2018), Turfan et al. (2018)
Macrocybe gigantea					X				Gaur et al. (2016)
Pholiota nameko								X	Niedzielski et al. (2017)
P. djamor				X					Bach et al. (2017)
Pleurotus eryngyi					X				Bach et al. (2017)
Pleurotus florida				X					Mallikarjuna et al. (2013)
Pleurotus ostreatus		X		X	X				Bach et al. (2017), Mleczek et al. (2018), Turfan et al. (2018)
Pleurotus sajor-caju		X							Gaur et al. (2016)
Trametes versicolor								X	Niedzielski et al. (2017)
Tremella fuciformis	X							X	Mleczek et al. (2018), Niedzielski et al. (2017)
Volvariella volvacea		X							Mleczek et al. (2018)

C, Caps; *S*, stipes.

TABLE 3.5 Data on the mean content (g kg^{-1} dry matter) of potassium in fruit bodies of wild-growing mushrooms collected from unpolluted (X), geologically specific (●), and anthropogenically contaminated (▲) sites and in cultivated species, published since 2010.

Species	<10	10–20	20–25	25–30	30–35	35–40	40–50	>50	References
Wild growing									
Agaricus arvensis					X				Ayaz et al. (2011)
Agaricus bisporus		X							Gąsecka et al. (2018)
Agaricus campestris						X^S, $▲^{S,C}$	X^C	X	Sarikurkcu et al. (2012), Zsigmond et al. (2018)
Agaricus lanipes			X						Gezer et al. (2016)
Agrocybe cylindracea						X			Sarikurkcu et al. (2012)
Albatrellus ovinus						$X^{C,S}$			Mędyk et al. (2017)
Amanita fulva								$X^{S,C}$	Falandysz et al. (2017)
Amanita ponderosa				X					Salvador et al. (2018)
Armillariella mellea		X							Gąsecka et al. (2018)
Auricularia auricula-judae	X								Gąsecka et al. (2018)
Boletus appendiculatus	X^S	X^C, X	X^{Sm}		X^{Cm}				Alaimo et al. (2018), Dimitrijevic et al. (2016), Wang et al. (2015)
Boletus bruneissimus		$X^{S,C}$							Wang et al. (2015)

(*Continued*)

TABLE 3.5 Data on the mean content (g kg^{-1} dry matter) of potassium in fruit bodies of wild-growing mushrooms collected from unpolluted (X), geologically specific (●), and anthropogenically contaminated (▲) sites and in cultivated species, published since 2010. (Continued)

Species	<10	10–20	20–25	25–30	30–35	35–40	40–50	>50	References
Boletus edulis	X, $X^{S,C}$	X,X^{S}	X, X^{C}	X, X^{C}					Ayaz et al. (2011), Brzezicha-Cirocka et al. (2016), Cvetkovic et al. (2015), Dimitrijevic et al. (2016), Falandysz et al. (2011), Frankowska et al. (2010), Mędyk et al. (2017), Mleczek et al. (2013), Turfan et al. (2018), Wang et al. (2015), Zhang et al. (2010)
Boletus griseus	X	$X^{S,C}$							Liu et al. (2012), Wang et al. (2015)
Boletus impolitus		X							Dimitrijevic et al. (2016)
Boletus luridus	X^{S}	X^{C}							Wang et al. (2015)
Boletus pallidus		$X^{S,C}$							Wang et al. (2015)
Boletus pseudoscaber			X						Dimitrijevic et al. (2016)
Boletus regius		X							Dimitrijevic et al. (2016)
Boletus rubellus		$X^{S,C}$							Wang et al. (2015)
Boletus speciosus	X, $X^{S,C}$								Liu et al. (2012), Wang et al. (2015)
Boletus tomentipes		$X^{S,C}$							Wang et al. (2015)
Boletus umbriniporus	X^{S}	X^{C}							Wang et al. (2015)

Calvatia gigantea	X								Gąsecka et al. (2018)
Cantharellus cibarius			X		X		X		Ayaz et al. (2011), Brzezicha-Cirocka et al. (2016), Cvetkovic et al. (2015), Drewnowska and Falandysz (2015), Falandysz and Drewnowska (2015), Gąsecka et al. (2018), Mleczek et al. (2013)
Cantharellus tubaeformis					X				Ayaz et al. (2011)
Clitopilus prunulus								X^{m}	Alaimo et al. (2018),
Craterellus cornucopioides	X								Turfan et al. (2018)
Fistulina hepatica			X						Gąsecka et al. (2018)
Flammulina velutipes			X^{C}						Zeng et al. (2012)
Gomphidius glutinosus							X^{S}	X^{C}	Mędyk et al. (2017)
Grifola frondosa	X								Gąsecka et al. (2018)
Helvella leucopus								X	Sarikurkcu et al. (2012)
Hydnum repandum				X		X			Ayaz et al. (2011), Jedidi et al. (2017)
Laccaria laccata					X				Ayaz et al. (2011)
Lactarius deliciosus	X		X						Jedidi et al. (2017), Mleczek et al. (2013), Turfan et al. (2018)

(Continued)

TABLE 3.5 Data on the mean content (g kg^{-1} dry matter) of potassium in fruit bodies of wild-growing mushrooms collected from unpolluted (X), geologically specific (●), and anthropogenically contaminated (▲) sites and in cultivated species, published since 2010. (Continued)

Species	<10	10–20	20–25	25–30	30–35	35–40	40–50	>50	References
Lactarius hygrophoroides	X								Liu et al. (2012)
Lactarius piperatus					X				Cvetkovic et al. (2015)
Laetiporus sulphureus	X	X							Gąsecka et al. (2018), Turfan et al. (2018)
Leccinum aurantiacum			X		X				Brzezicha-Cirocka et al. (2016), Mleczek et al. (2013)
Leccinum crocipodium		X							Dimitrijevic et al. (2016)
Leccinum duriusculum		X^S				X^C			Jarzyńska and Falandysz (2012a)
Leccinum griseum			X^S		X^C				Jarzyńska and Falandysz (2012b)
Leccinum scabrum		X, X^S			X	X^C			Falandysz (2018), Gąsecka et al. (2018), Mędyk et al. (2017)
Leccinum versipelle				X					Mędyk et al. (2017)
Lentinus cladopus	X								Mallikarjuna et al. (2013)
Lepista gilva		X							Gąsecka et al. (2018)
Lepista nuda				X					Ayaz et al. (2011)
Leucopaxillus giganteus	X								Liu et al. (2012)

Lycoperdon perlatum				X					Brzezicha-Cirocka et al. (2016), Mędyk et al. (2017)
Macrocybe gigantea	X								Liu et al. (2012)
Macrolepiota procera		X, X^S		X^S	X^C	$X^{C,S}$	X^C		Gąsecka et al. (2018), Gucia et al. (2012), Jarzyńska et al. (2011), Kojta et al. (2011), Kułdo et al. (2014), Stefanović et al. (2016)
Marasmius oreades	X				X				Cvetkovic et al. (2015), Turfan et al. (2018)
Melanoleuca arcuata	X								Liu et al. (2012)
Morchella conica	X								Turfan et al. (2018)
Morchella elata			X^C						Zeng et al. (2012)
Morchella esculenta		X			X	X			Gąsecka et al. (2018), Rossbach et al. (2017), Sarikurkcu et al. (2012)
Morchella deliciosa	X								Liu et al. (2012),
Mycena haematopus	X								Liu et al. (2012),
Pleurotus djamor						X			Mallikarjuna et al. (2013)
Pleurotus eryngii		X^C							Zeng et al. (2012)
Ramaria botrytis	X								Turfan et al. (2018)
Sparassis crispa		X							Gąsecka et al. (2018)
Suillus bovinus	X		X^S	X^C					Gąsecka et al. (2018), Mędyk et al. (2017)

(Continued)

TABLE 3.5 Data on the mean content (g kg^{-1} dry matter) of potassium in fruit bodies of wild-growing mushrooms collected from unpolluted (X), geologically specific (●), and anthropogenically contaminated (▲) sites and in cultivated species, published since 2010. (Continued)

Species	<10	10–20	20–25	25–30	30–35	35–40	40–50	>50	References
Suillus luteus		X	X^C			X^S			Zeng et al. (2012), Mędyk et al. (2017), Mleczek et al. (2013)
Suillus variegatus		X^S		X^C					Szubstarska et al. (2012)
Terfezia claveryi		X	X						Kivrak (2015), Vahdani et al. (2017)
Terfezia olbiensis			X						Kivrak (2015)
Tirmania nivea			X						Vahdani et al. (2017)
Tricholoma equestre		X							Gąsecka et al. (2018), Jedidi et al. (2017)
Tricholoma matsutake	X								Li et al. (2013), Liu et al. (2012)
Tricholoma terreum	X								Turfan et al. (2018)
Xerocomus badius	▲	X	X	$▲^{S,C}$	X^S	X^C		$X^{S,C}$	Dimitrijevic et al. (2016), Kojta et al. (2012), Kojta and Falandysz (2016), Mleczek et al. (2013, 2016), Proskura et al. (2017)
Xerocomus chrysenteron		X							Dimitrijevic et al. (2016)
Xerocomus subtomentosus					$X^{S,C}$		$X^{S,C}$		Jarzyńska et al. (2012), Mędyk et al. (2017)

Cultivated									
A. arvensis					X				Rzymski et al. (2017)
A. bisporus (brown)					X	X			Bach et al. (2017), Rzymski et al. (2017)
A. bisporus (white)					X	X	X		Bach et al. (2017), Jedidi et al. (2017), Mleczek et al. (2018), Rzymski et al. (2017)
Agaricus subrufescens		X				X			Bach et al. (2017), Rzymski et al. (2017)
A. cylindracea				X					Niedzielski et al. (2017)
A. auricula-judae	X								Mleczek et al. (2018)
Auricularia polytricha						X			Niedzielski et al. (2017)
Auricularia thailandica		X							Bandara et al. (2017)
Clitocybe maxima		X							Niedzielski et al. (2017)
F. velutipes				X		X			Bach et al. (2017), Niedzielski et al. (2017)
G. frondosa					X				Niedzielski et al. (2017)
Hericium erinaceus	X			X					Niedzielski et al. (2017), Turfan et al. (2018)
L. sulphureus		X							Niedzielski et al. (2017)

(*Continued*)

TABLE 3.5 Data on the mean content (g kg^{-1} dry matter) of potassium in fruit bodies of wild-growing mushrooms collected from unpolluted (X), geologically specific (●), and anthropogenically contaminated (▲) sites and in cultivated species, published since 2010. (Continued)

Species	<10	10–20	20–25	25–30	30–35	35–40	40–50	>50	References
Lentinula edodes	X	X	X	X					Bach et al. (2017), Gonçalves et al. (2014), Mallikarjuna et al. (2013), Mleczek et al. (2017, 2018), Turfan et al. (2018)
Pholiota nameko		X							Niedzielski et al. (2017)
P. djamor				X					Bach et al. (2017)
P. eryngii		X							Bach et al. (2017), Gonçalves et al. (2014)
Pleurotus florida			X						Mallikarjuna et al. (2013)
Pleurotus ostreatus	X		X	X					Bach et al. (2017), Gonçalves et al. (2014), Mleczek et al. (2018), Turfan et al. (2018)
Trametes versicolor		X							Niedzielski et al. (2017)
Tremella fuciformis		X				X			Mleczek et al. (2018), Niedzielski et al. (2017)
Volvariella volvacea	X								Mleczek et al. (2018)

C, Caps; *S*, stipes; *Xm*, median value.

TABLE 3.6 Data on the mean content (g kg^{-1} dry matter) of sodium in fruit bodies of wild-growing mushrooms collected from unpolluted (X), geologically specific (●), and anthropogenically contaminated (▲) sites and in cultivated species, published since 2010.

Species	<0.05	0.05–0.1	0.1–0.2	0.2–0.3	0.3–0.4	0.4–0.5	0.5–0.75	>0.75	References
Wild growing									
Agaricus arvensis							X		Ayaz et al. (2011)
Agaricus bisporus	X								Gąsecka et al. (2018)
Agaricus campestris				$X^{S,C}$				$▲^{C,S}$	Zsigmond et al. (2018)
Agaricus lanipes				X					Gezer et al. (2016)
Albatrellus ovinus		$X^{C,S}$							Mędyk et al. (2017)
Amanita fulva			X^{C}	X^{S}					Falandysz et al. (2017)
Amanita ponderosa								X	Salvador et al. (2018)
Armillariella mellea						X			Gąsecka et al. (2018)
Auricularia auricula-judae		X							Gąsecka et al. (2018)
Boletus appendiculatus		X		X^{S}, X^{Sm}			X^{C}, X^{Cm}		Alaimo et al. (2018), Dimitrijevic et al. (2016), Wang et al. (2015)
Boletus bruneissimus				X^{S}		X^{C}			Wang et al. (2015)

(*Continued*)

TABLE 3.6 Data on the mean content (g kg^{-1} dry matter) of sodium in fruit bodies of wild-growing mushrooms collected from unpolluted (X), geologically specific (●), and anthropogenically contaminated (▲) sites and in cultivated species, published since 2010. (Continued)

Species	<0.05	0.05–0.1	0.1–0.2	0.2–0.3	0.3–0.4	0.4–0.5	0.5–0.75	>0.75	References
Boletus edulis	X^{C}	X, X^{S}	$X^{S,C}$	X, X^{C}	X,X^{S}	X	X		Ayaz et al. (2011), Brzezicha-Cirocka et al. (2016), Cvetkovic et al. (2015), Dimitrijevic et al. (2016), Falandysz et al. (2011), Frankowska et al. (2010), Mleczek et al. (2013), Wang et al. (2015, 2015b), Zhang et al. (2010)
Boletus griseus				X^{S}	X^{C}		X		Liu et al. (2012), Wang et al. (2015)
Boletus impolitus		X							Dimitrijevic et al. (2016)
Boletus luridus		X^{S}	X^{C}						Wang et al. (2015)
Boletus pallidus							$X^{S,C}$		Wang et al. (2015)
Boletus pseudoscaber						X			Dimitrijevic et al. (2016)
Boletus rubellus				X^{C}	X^{S}				Wang et al. (2015)
Boletus speciosus		X	$X^{S,C}$						Liu et al. (2012), Wang et al. (2015)
Boletus tomentipes			$X^{S,C}$						Wang et al. (2015, 2015a)
Boletus umbriniporus						$X^{C,S}$			Wang et al. (2015)
Calvatia giganteum		X							Gąsecka et al. (2018)

Cantharellus cibarius	X	X		X			X		Ayaz et al. (2011), Brzezicha-Cirocka et al. (2016), Cvetkovic et al. (2015), Drewnowska and Falandysz (2015), Falandysz and Drewnowska (2015), Gąsecka et al. (2018), Mleczek et al. (2013)
Cantharellus tubaeformis							X		Ayaz et al. (2011)
Clitopilus prunulus								X^{m}	Alaimo et al. (2018)
Fistulina hepatica		X							Gąsecka et al. (2018)
Flammulina velutipes							X^{C}		Zeng et al. (2012)
Gomphidius glutinosus		X^{S}	X^{C}						Mędyk et al. (2017)
Grifola frondosa			X						Gąsecka et al. (2018)
Hydnum repandum							X	X	Ayaz et al. (2011), Jedidi et al. (2017)
Laccaria laccata							X		Ayaz et al. (2011)
Lactarius deliciosus			X					X	Jedidi et al. (2017), Mleczek et al. (2013)
Lactarius hygrophoroides			X						Liu et al. (2012)
Lactarius piperatus						X			Cvetkovic et al. (2015)
Laetiporus sulphureus	X								Gąsecka et al. (2018)

(Continued)

TABLE 3.6 Data on the mean content (g kg^{-1} dry matter) of sodium in fruit bodies of wild-growing mushrooms collected from unpolluted (X), geologically specific (●), and anthropogenically contaminated (▲) sites and in cultivated species, published since 2010. (Continued)

Species	<0.05	0.05–0.1	0.1–0.2	0.2–0.3	0.3–0.4	0.4–0.5	0.5–0.75	>0.75	References
Leccinum aurantiacum		X		X					Brzezicha-Cirocka et al. (2016), Mleczek et al. (2013)
Leccinum duriusculum					X^{C}			X^{S}	Jarzyńska and Falandysz (2012a)
Leccinum griseum							$X^{C,S}$		Jarzyńska and Falandysz (2012b)
Leccinum scabrum	X			X^{C}				X, X^{S}	Falandysz (2018), Gąsecka et al. (2018), Mędyk et al. (2017)
Leccinum versipelle		X							Mędyk et al. (2017)
Lentinus cladopus				X					Mallikarjuna et al. (2013)
Lepista gilva	X								Gąsecka et al. (2018)
Lepista nuda						X			Ayaz et al. (2011)
Leucopaxillus giganteus					X				Liu et al. (2012)
Lycoperdon perlatum	X	X							Brzezicha-Cirocka et al. (2016), Mędyk et al. (2017)
Lyophyllum fumosum			X						Gąsecka et al. (2018)
Macrocybe gigantea							X		Liu et al. (2012)

Macrolepiota procera		X, X^C	X^C	X^C	X^S	X^S	X^S		Gąsecka et al. (2018), Gucia et al. (2012), Jarzyńska et al. (2011), Kojta et al. (2011), Kułdo et al. (2014), Stefanović et al. (2016)
Marasmius oreades								X	Cvetkovic et al. (2015)
Melanoleuca arcuata						X			Liu et al. (2012)
Morchella deliciosa						X			Liu et al. (2012)
Morchella elata							X^C		Zeng et al. (2012)
Morchella esculenta			X	X					Gąsecka et al. (2018), Rossbach et al. (2017)
Mycena haematopus			X						Liu et al. (2012)
Pleurotus djamor							X		Mallikarjuna et al. (2013)
Pleurotus eryngii							X^C		Zeng et al. (2012)
Pleurotus ostreatus				X					Tel-Çayan et al. (2017)
Sparassis crispa	X								Gąsecka et al. (2018)
Suillus bovinus	X					$X^{S,C}$			Gąsecka et al. (2018), Mędyk et al. (2017)

(*Continued*)

TABLE 3.6 Data on the mean content (g kg^{-1} dry matter) of sodium in fruit bodies of wild-growing mushrooms collected from unpolluted (X), geologically specific (●), and anthropogenically contaminated (▲) sites and in cultivated species, published since 2010. (Continued)

Species	<0.05	0.05–0.1	0.1–0.2	0.2–0.3	0.3–0.4	0.4–0.5	0.5–0.75	>0.75	References
Suillus luteus	X		X^{C}	$X^{C,S}$					Zeng et al. (2012), Mędyk et al. (2017), Mleczek et al. (2013)
Suillus variegatus	X^{C}	X^{S}							Szubstarska et al. (2012)
Terfezia claveryi	X								Kivrak (2015)
Terfezia olbiensis	X								Kivrak (2015)
Tricholoma equestre							X	X	Gąsecka et al. (2018), Jedidi et al. (2017)
Tricholoma fracticum				X					Tel-Çayan et al. (2017)
Tricholoma matsutake				X	X				Li et al. (2013), Liu et al. (2012)
Xerocomus badius		X	X^{C}, ▲	X, $▲^{C}$	X^{S}	X^{C}	X^{S}	$▲^{S}$	Dimitrijevic et al. (2016), Kojta et al. (2012), Kojta and Falandysz (2016), Mleczek et al. (2013, 2016), Proskura et al. (2017)
Xerocomus chrysenteron			X						Dimitrijevic et al. (2016)
Xerocomus subtomentosus							$X^{C,S}$	$X^{S,C}$	Jarzyńska et al. (2012), Mędyk et al. (2017)

Cultivated									
A. arvensis			X						Rzymski et al. (2017)
A. bisporus (brown)					X		X		Bach et al. (2017), Jedidi et al. (2017), Rzymski et al. (2017)
A. bisporus (white)					X		X		Bach et al. (2017), Mleczek et al. (2018), Rzymski et al. (2017)
Agaricus subrufescens		X					X		Bach et al. (2017), Rzymski et al. (2017)
Agrocybe cylindracea	X								Niedzielski et al. (2017)
A. auricula-judae			X						Mleczek et al. (2018)
Auricularia polytricha						X			Niedzielski et al. (2017)
Auricularia thailandica			X						Bandara et al. (2017)
Clitocybe maxima		X							Niedzielski et al. (2017)
F. velutipes				X				X	Bach et al. (2017), Niedzielski et al. (2017)
G. frondosa			X						Niedzielski et al. (2017)
Hericium erinaceus		X							Niedzielski et al. (2017)

(Continued)

TABLE 3.6 Data on the mean content (g kg^{-1} dry matter) of sodium in fruit bodies of wild-growing mushrooms collected from unpolluted (X), geologically specific (●), and anthropogenically contaminated (▲) sites and in cultivated species, published since 2010. (Continued)

Species	<0.05	0.05–0.1	0.1–0.2	0.2–0.3	0.3–0.4	0.4–0.5	0.5–0.75	>0.75	References
L. sulphureus			X						Niedzielski et al. (2017)
Lentinula edodes		X	X					X	Bach et al. (2017), Gonçalves et al. (2014), Mallikarjuna et al. (2013), Mleczek et al. (2017, 2018)
Pholiota nameko				X					Niedzielski et al. (2017)
P. eryngii		X							Bach et al. (2017), Gonçalves et al. (2014)
Pleurotus florida					X				Mallikarjuna et al. (2013)
P. ostreatus	X		X						Bach et al. (2017), Gonçalves et al. (2014), Mleczek et al. (2018)
Trametes versicolor			X						Niedzielski et al. (2017)
Tremella fuciformis	X		X						Mleczek et al. (2018), Niedzielski et al. (2017)
Volvariella volvacea								X	Mleczek et al. (2018)

C, Caps; *S*, stipes; *Xm*, median value.

Several papers reported bioconcentration factors (BCFs) for calcium. Values in the range of 0.91–4.9 were observed for *C. cibarius* collected from four sites (Falandysz & Drewnowska, 2015), 0.68 for both caps and stipes of *Macrolepiota procera* (Kułdo, Jarzyńska, Gucia, & Falandysz, 2014) and 0.76 and 1.28 for caps and stipes, respectively, of *X. badius* (Proskura, Podlasińska, & Skopicz-Radkiewicz, 2017). Differences probably exist among mushroom species; however, calcium is not an accumulated element.

Calcium does not generally rank among elements deficient in human nutrition. Information on biofortification of cultivated mushroom species has, therefore, been virtually lacking. Tabata and Ogura (2003) reported an increase of calcium content in *Auricularia nigricans* by 1.1–1.5 times if cultivated on a sawdust medium supplemented with 1%–5% calcium phosphate or calcium carbonate compared to nonsupplemented variants.

Overall, the calcium content in mushrooms is considerably lower than that found in most of vegetables.

3.2 Chlorine (Cl)

Data on the chlorine content in mushrooms have been virtually lacking. In an initial survey, Stijve, Diserens, Oberson, and de Meijer (1998) determined wide range from 0.1 to 14.4 g kg^{-1} DM in 23 wild-growing species. The highest content of 14.4 g kg^{-1} DM was observed in *Lepista inversa*, followed by 5.1–7.1 g kg^{-1} DM in *Laccaria amethystina*. Similar values were determined in *Amanita caesarea*, *Agaricus arvensis*, and in cultivated *Agaricus bisporus*; however, these results were from only two analyzed fruiting body samples. Levels of 1.34 ± 0.42 g kg^{-1} DM were reported for *X. badius* and mean values in the range of 0.17–7.02 g kg^{-1} DM were determined in four inedible or toxic species (Cejpková et al., 2016). Turfan, Pekşen, Kibar, and Ünal (2018) observed a range of 0.18–4.00 g kg^{-1} DM in eight wild-growing and three cultivated species with the minimum reported in cultivated *Hericium erinaceus* and the maximum in wild *Craterellus cornucopioides*.

These sporadic values of clorine are lower, or comparable, with vegetables.

3.3 Magnesium (Mg)

The initial data on magnesium in mushrooms were published by Seeger and Beckert (1979), who analyzed 1047 samples of 402 wild-growing species. The most frequent range was 0.8–1.8 g kg^{-1} DM. The highest level was observed in the *Coprinaceae* family, and the lowest was in *Boletaceae*. Magnesium was distributed in 10 species as follows: spore-forming part (gills or tubes) > stipes = flesh of caps = spores.

Data on magnesium contents published since 2010 are provided in Table 3.3. The contents range between <0.5 and 2.5 g kg^{-1} DM; the usual range is, however, <0.5–1.5 g kg^{-1} DM. Higher levels were reported only sporadically, namely 4.56, 3.89, 3.48, and 3.24 g kg^{-1} DM in cultivated *L. edodes* (Gonçalves, de Souza, Rocha, Medeiros, & do Couto Jacob, 2014), *Tirmania nivea* (Vahdani, Rastegar, Rahimzadeh, Ahmadi, & Karmostaji, 2017), cultivated *Pleurotus eryngii* (Gonçalves et al., 2014), and *Hydnum repandum* (Jedidi, Ayoub, Philippe, & Bouzouita, 2017), respectively. Similarly as for calcium, wide ranges were determined in species with numerous reports such as *M. procera* or cultivated *L. edodes* and *Pleurotus ostreatus*.

Values of BCF from four sites varied widely between 10 and 40 for *C. cibarius* (Falandysz & Drewnowska, 2015), whereas lower mean levels were observed in *M. procera* and *X. badius*. In the former species, these were 9.2 and 4.9 (Kułdo et al., 2014), while in the latter they were 3.45 and 1.76 (Proskura et al., 2017) for caps and stipes, respectively. Various species most probably have different abilities to bioaccumulate magnesium. Magnesium seems to be either evenly distributed in caps and stipes, or somewhat higher levels are observed in caps than in stipes.

Magnesium has not been rated in human nutrition among the deficient elements. Similarly as for calcium, information on biofortification of cultivated species with magnesium has been virtually lacking. The magnesium content in *Auricularia nigricans* increased 1.7–2.2-times compared with the control variant in fruiting bodies produced on sawdust supplemented with 0.5% of magnesium salts (carbonate, sulfate, or chloride) or with magnesium hydroxide (Tabata & Ogura, 2003). There occur wide ranges of magnesium contents in several species with more data (Table 3.3). It can be supposed that such variability can be caused by different levels of available magnesium in substrates.

Overall, the magnesium content in mushrooms is lower than in most vegetables.

3.4 Phosphorus (P)

Phosphorus in mushrooms has been formerly determined only rarely due to the laborious methods of quantification. A comprehensive study using a spectrofotometric method of determination was carried out by Quinche (1997) with 825 samples. Mean levels of total phosphorus content were 6.1 and 13.7 g kg^{-1} DM in 51 mycorrhizal and 42 saprobic species, respectively. These values significantly differed. Usual contents were 5–7 g kg^{-1} DM in the popular mushrooms of the *Boletaceae* family, and 13–23 g kg^{-1} DM in the genus *Lepista*. Maximum levels ranging between 17.5 and 35.9 g kg^{-1} DM were observed in *Lepista sordida*. Mean contents varied between 10 and 20 g kg^{-1} DM in the popular *Agaricus* spp.

Reports on phosphorus content in mushrooms increased as soon as inductively coupled plasma–optical emission spectroscopy (ICP-OES) and ICP–atomic emission spectroscopy (ICP-AES) instruments became available. Data on phosphorus contents published since 2010 are collated in Table 3.4. The contents range widely between <2.5 and >10 g kg^{-1} DM. Levels above 10 g kg^{-1} DM often occur in cultivated species. An extremely high content of 26.9 g kg^{-1} DM was observed in cultivated *Grifola frondosa* (Niedzielski et al., 2017). As results from Table 3.4, show the reported contents in caps are mostly higher than in stipes. For instance, the ratio of phosphorus content in caps to stipes in *B. edulis* from six sites varied between 1.62 and 2.57 (Wang et al., 2015b).

Similarly as for calcium and magnesium, wide ranges of phosphorus content occur in species with more available data such as *B. edulis* and *M. procera* (Table 3.4). Moreover, considerable variations in phosphorus levels within a species were observed. For example, contents between 4.36 ± 1.15 and 9.01 ± 2.33 g kg^{-1} DM in caps and between 2.15 ± 0.41 and 3.89 ± 0.97 g kg^{-1} DM in stipes were determined in *B. edulis* collected from six sites (Wang et al., 2015b).

Mushrooms are able to bioaccumulate phosphorus extensively in their fruiting bodies from the underlying substrates. Quinche (1997) reported BCF between 5 and 50 for various species. Wide ranges were observed even within individual species, for example, 20.2–50.6 for *Lepista nuda* and 7.2–32.4 for *Lycoperdon perlatum.* High BCF values of 57 and 31 were found for caps and stipes, respectively, of *M. procera* (Kułdo et al., 2014), and values in the range of 31–54 for *C. cibarius* from four sites were reported (Falandysz & Drewnowska, 2015).

Maciejczyk et al. (2015) reported the phosphorus profile of methanolic extracts of 14 dried edible mushroom species using ^{31}P nuclear magnetic resonance spectroscopy. Phosphodiesters (most likely DNA) prevailed, followed by phospholipids. Polyphosphates and, surprisingly, accompanied phosphonates were detected as minor constituents in several species.

Mushrooms can be evaluated as a relatively rich source of phosphorus, more potent than numerous vegetables. However, information on the element's bioavailability from mushroom meals remains lacking.

3.5 Potassium (K)

Potassium comprises the majority part of ash in mushrooms. Seeger (1978), in a pioneering investigation, reported potassium content in the range of 1.5–117 g kg^{-1} DM in 410 wild-growing species. The distribution of potassium within fruiting bodies were uneven with the decreasing order of cap > stipe > spore-forming part (gills or tubes) > spores.

Recent literature data are provided in Table 3.5. The most frequent contents are between <10 to 35 g kg^{-1} DM in both wild-growing and cultivated species, although higher levels often occur. Similarly to in the above discussed major elements, wide ranges were reported in species with numerous data, for example, in *C. cibarius*, *M. procera*, and *X. badius* (see Table 3.5). Distribution of potassium between caps and stipes seems to be balanced in some species, while in others the contents are higher in caps than in stipes. Extremely high levels of 402 and 125 g kg^{-1} DM were determined by Sarikurkcu et al. (2012) in culinary low-valued *Russula brevipes* (syn. *Russula delica*) and in *H. leucopus*, respectively, and Gąsecka, Siwulski, and Mleczek (2018) reported 222 g kg^{-1} DM in *Lyophyllum fumosum*.

Potassium is highly bioaccumulated in fruiting bodies from the underlying substrate, for example, Seeger (1978) reported BCF 20–40. Recent papers report considerably higher values. Mean values of 104 and 119 were observed for *X. badius* caps and stipes, respectively (Proskura et al., 2017), values of 300 (caps) and 140 (stipes) were found for *M. procera* (Kułdo et al., 2014), and in the range of 300–3400 for complete fruiting bodies of *C. cibarius* (Falandysz & Drewnowska, 2015).

The potassium content in mushrooms, both wild and cultivated, is comparable with certain kinds of vegetables that are rich in this element e.g. spinach, cauliflower, cabbage, lettuce or tomato. Mushrooms can, thus, supplement the diets of patients with chronic potassium deficiency. On the contrary, potential detrimental effects of potassium must be taken into consideration for some individuals, particularly in cases of renal insufficiency.

Further information on natural radioactive isotope ^{40}K is given in Section 5.3.1.

3.6 Sodium (Na)

A comprehensive study analyzing 465 edible, inedible, and toxic species reported the most frequent sodium contents being between 0.1 and 0.4 g kg^{-1} DM (Seeger, Trumpfheller, & Schweinshaut, 1983). Sodium levels amounted only approximately to 1% of potassium contents. The highest contents were observed in the *Coprinaceae* family, while above-average levels were also reported in the *Agaricaceae* family. *Agaricus bitorquis* was the species with the highest mean sodium content of 3.47 g kg^{-1} DM.

In a further study focused on sodium, Vetter (2003) similarly determined usual mean contents of 0.1–0.4 g kg^{-1} DM. The contents were virtually independent on taxonomic position and type of nutrition [mycorrhizal, saprobic or growing on wood (xylophagous)].

Recent data on sodium contents are collated in Table 3.6. The most frequent levels are 0.05–0.75 g kg^{-1} DM, that is, the same as for calcium. Similarly as in other major elements, wide ranges occur within species with numerous data such as in *B. edulis*, *M. procera*, and *X. badius.* The highest mean contents reported during the observed period were 3.27 and 2.04 g kg^{-1} DM in cultivated *L. edodes* (Mallikarjuna et al., 2013) and in *Xerocomus subtomentosus* (Mędyk, Grembecka, Brzezicha-Cirocka, & Falandysz, 2017), respectively. Sodium distribution in caps and stipes varies among species. There are species with balanced content and those with differences.

Sodium is bioaccumulated in fruiting bodies from the underlying substrate. There were reported BCF values 12.1 and 28.6 in *X. badius* (Proskura et al., 2017), 50 and 110 in *M. procera* (Kułdo et al., 2014), for caps and stipes, respectively. Considerably lower BCF values of 4.1–9.5 were observed in *C. cibarius* collected from four sites (Falandysz & Drewnowska, 2015).

Overall, the sodium content of mushrooms is lower or comparable with vegetables. Sodium intake should be kept down in human nutrition, therefore mushrooms are advantageous due to their low levels of the element.

3.7 Sulfur (S)

Mean total sulfur content 2.2 ± 1.1 g kg^{-1} DM was found in eight wild species ranging between 0.9 and 4.4 g kg^{-1} DM in *Amanita rubescens* and *Xerocomus chrysenteron*, respectively. While the differences in sulfur content were highly significant among the tested species, insignificant differences were observed between caps and stipes (Rudawska & Leski, 2005). In a more recent article from Canada (Nasr, Malloch, & Arp, 2012) on 304 samples of 27 wild, edible, inedible, and toxic species, the mean total sulfur content 2.63 ± 0.91 g kg^{-1} DM was reported. The minimum and maximum levels of 0.73 and 13.87 g kg^{-1} DM were observed in *H. repandum* and *B. edulis*, respectively. A similar range of 0.95–12.5 g kg^{-1} DM reported Turfan et al. (2018) in eight wild-growing and three cultivated species with the minimum being in wild *Laetiporus sulphureus* and the maximum in *B. edulis*. The high level of 10.2 g kg^{-1} DM was observed in *Marasmius oreades*. Zsigmond et al. (2018) determined mean values between 2.8 and 5.6 g kg^{-1} DM in *Agaricus campestris* growing in urban and peri-urban areas. The levels in caps were somewhat higher than in stipes.

The reported values of sulfur content in mushroms are comparable with vegetables, but lower than those in pulses. Sulfur occurs in mushrooms chiefly in sulfur-containing amino acids including ergothioneine. Various organic sulfur compounds, for example, lentinic acid or lenthionine, are characteristic for *L. edodes*.

3.8 Conclusion

Information on the usual contents of the five major mineral elements in mushrooms, both cultivated and wild-growing, is given in Table 3.7. Potassium and phosphorus are the highly prevailing elements, whereas calcium and sodium comprise a very low proportion of ash. The contents expressed per fresh matter would be approximately 10 times lower. Data for chlorine and sulfur are insufficient to make a reasonable generalization.

TABLE 3.7 Usual contents (g kg^{-1} dry matter) of major mineral elements in mushrooms.

Element	Content
Calcium	0.05–0.75
Magnesium	<0.5–1.5
Phosphorus	<2.5–>10
Potassium	<10–35
Sodium	0.05–0.75

Data for chlorine and sulfur have been very sporadic.

When compared to most vegetables, mushrooms are richer in potassium and phosphorus and lower in magnesium, sodium, and calcium. However, the ability to bioaccumulate a certain element is obviously affected by the particular species and the level of the bioavailable element in the underlying substrate. These factors lead to wide variability in the content of particular elements in the fruiting bodies within a species. The existing data suggest a very extensive rate of bioaccumulation for potassium, a high rate for phosphorus, and virtually no rate for calcium.

Unfortunately, information on the bioavailability of the major elements from mushroom meals is lacking.

References

Alaimo, M. G., Dongarrà, G., La Rosa, A., Tamburo, E., Vasquez, G., & Varrica, D. (2018). Major and trace elements in *Boletus aereus* and *Clitopilus prunulus* growing on volcanic and sedimentary soils of Sicily (Italy). *Ecotoxicology and Environmental Safety*, *157*, 182–190.

Ayaz, F. A., Torun, H., Colak, A., Sesli, E., Millson, M., & Glew, R. H. (2011). Macro- and microlement contents of fruiting bodies of wild-edible mushrooms growing in the East Black Sea region of Turkey. *Food and Nutrition Sciences*, *2*, 53–59.

Bach, F., Helm, C. V., Bellettini, M. B., Maciel, G. M., & Haminiuk, C. W. I. (2017). Edible mushrooms: A potential source of essential amino acids, glucans and minerals. *International Journal of Food Science and Technology*, *52*, 2382–2392.

Bandara, A. R., Karunarathna, S. C., Mortimer, P. E., Hyde, K. D., Khan, S., Kakumyan, P., & Xu, J. (2017). First successful domestication and determination of nutritional and antioxidant properties of the red ear mushroom *Auricularia thailandica* (*Auriculariales, Basidiomycota*). *Mycological Progress*, *16*, 1029–1039.

Brzezicha-Cirocka, J., Mędyk, M., Falandysz, J., & Szefer, P. (2016). Bio- and toxic elements in edible wild mushrooms from two regions of potentially different environmental conditions in eastern Poland. *Environmental Science and Pollution Research*, *23*, 21517–21522.

Cejpková, J., Gryndler, M., Hršelová, H., Kotrba, P., Řanda, Z., Synková, I., & Borovička, J. (2016). Bioaccumulation of heavy metals, metalloids, and chlorine in ectomycorrhizae from smelter-polluted area. *Environmental Pollution*, *218*, 176–185.

Cvetkovic, J. S., Mitic, V. D., Stankov-Jovanovic, V. P., Dimitrijevic, M. V., & Nikolic-Mandic, S. D. (2015). Elemental composition of wild edible mushrooms from Serbia. *Analytical Letters*, *48*, 2017–2121.

Dimitrijevic, M. V., Mitic, V. D., Cvetkovic, J. S., Stankov Jovanovic, V. P., Mutic, J. J., & Nikolic Mandic, S. D. (2016). Update on element content profiles in eleven wild edible mushrooms from family *Boletaceae*. *European Food Research and Technology*, *242*, 1–10.

Drewnowska, M., & Falandysz, J. (2015). Investigation on mineral composition and accumulation by popular edible mushroom common chantarelle (*Cantharellus cibarius*). *Ecotoxicology and Environmental Safety*, *113*, 9–17.

EFSA (European Food Safety Authority). (2017). *Dietary reference values for nutrients. Summary report*. 92 pp. doi: 10.2903/sp.efsa.2017.e15121.

Falandysz, J. (2018). Mineral constituents in *Leccinum scabrum from* lowland locations in the central Europe and their relation to concentration in forest topsoil. *Journal of Environmental Science and Health B*, *53*, 546–560.

Falandysz, J., & Drewnowska, M. (2015). Macro and trace elements in Common Chanterelle (*Cantharellus cibarius*) mushroom from the European background areas in Poland: Composition, accumulation, dietary exposure and data review for species. *Journal of Environmental Science and Health B*, *50*, 374–387.

Falandysz, J., Drewnowska, M., Chudzińska, M., & Barałkiewicz, D. (2017). Accumulation and distribution of metallic elements and metalloids in edible *Amanita fulva* mushrooms. *Ecotoxicology and Environmental Safety*, *137*, 265–271.

Falandysz, J., Frankowska, A., Jarzyńska, G., Dryżalowska, A., Kojta, A. K., & Zhang, D. (2011). Survey on composition and bioconcentration potential of 12 metallic elements in King Bolete (*Boletus edulis*) mushroom that emerged at 11 spatially distant sites. *Journal of Environmental Science and Health B*, *46*, 231–246.

Frankowska, A., Ziółkowska, J., Bielawski, L., & Falandysz, J. (2010). Profile and bioconcentration of minerals in King Bolete (*Boletus edulis*) from the Płocka Dale in Poland. *Food Additives and Contaminants B*, *3*, 1–6.

Friese, W. (1929). [Mineral composition of mushrooms]. *Zeitschrift für Untersuchung der Lebensmittel*, *57*, 604–613. (in German).

Gąsecka, M., Siwulski, M., & Mleczek, M. (2018). Evaluation of bioactive compounds content and antioxidant properties of soil-growing and wood-growing edible mushrooms. *Journal of Food Processing and Preservation*, *42*, e13386. Available from https://doi.org/10.1111/jfpp.13386, 10 pp.

Gaur, T., Rao, P. B., & Kushwaha, K. P. S. (2016). Nutritional and anti-nutritional components of some selected edible mushroom species. *Indian Journal of Natural Products and Resources*, *7*, 155–161.

Gezer, K., Kaygusuz, O., Herken, E. N., Dodurga, Y., Koizhaiganova, M., & Seçme, M. (2016). Evaluation of the nutritional composition of wild edible mushroom *Agaricus lanipes* (F.H. Møller & Jul. Schäff.) Hlaváček. *Bangladesh Journal of Botany*, *45*, 161–166.

Gonçalves, J. M., de Souza, M. D. C., Rocha, R. C. C., Medeiros, R. J., & do Couto Jacob, S. (2014). Macro and trace elements in edible mushrooms, Shiitake, Shimeji and Cardoncello from Petrópolis, Rio de Janeiro, Brazil. *Ciência Rural*, *44*, 943–949.

Gucia, M., Jarzyńska, G., Rafal, E., Roszak, M., Kojta, A. K., Osiej, I., & Falandysz, J. (2012). Multivariete analysis of mineral constituents of edible Parasol Mushroom (*Macrolepiota procera*) and soils beneath fruiting bodies collected from Northern Poland. *Environmental Science and Pollution Research*, *19*, 416–431.

Jarzyńska, G., & Falandysz, J. (2012a). Trace elements profile of Slate Bolete (*Leccinum durius-culum*) mushroom and associated upper soil horizon. *Journal of Geochemical Exploration, 121*, 69–75.

Jarzyńska, G., & Falandysz, J. (2012b). Metallic elements profile of Hazel (Hard) Bolete (*Leccinum griseum*) mushroom and associated upper soil horizon. *African Journal of Biotechnology, 11*, 4588–4594.

Jarzyńska, G., Chojnacka, A., Dryżalowska, A., Nnorom, I. C., & Falandysz, J. (2012). Concentrations and bioconcentration factors of minerals in Yellow-cracking Bolete (*Xerocomus subtomentosus*) mushroom collected in Noteć Forest, Poland. *Journal of Food Science, 77*, H202–H206.

Jarzyńska, G., Gucia, M., Kojta, A. K., Rezulak, K., & Falandysz, J. (2011). Profile of trace elements in Parasol Mushroom (*Macrolepiota procera*) from Tucholskie Forest. *Journal of Environmental Science and Health B, 46*, 741–751.

Jedidi, I. K., Ayoub, I. K., Philippe, T., & Bouzouita, N. (2017). Chemical composition and nutritional value of three Tunisian wild edible mushrooms. *Journal of Food Measurement and Characterization, 11*, 2069–2075.

Kalač, P. (2016). *Edible mushrooms. Chemical composition and nutritional value*. Amsterdam: Elsevier/Academic Press, ISBN 978-0-12-804455-1.

Kivrak, I. (2015). Analytical methods applied to assess chemical composition, nutritional value and in vitro bioactivities of *Terfezia olbiensis* and *Terfezia claveryi* from Turkey. *Food Analytical Methods, 8*, 1279–1293.

Kojta, A. K., & Falandysz, J. (2016). Metallic elements (Ca, Hg, Fe, K, Mn, Na, Zn) in the fruiting bodies of *Boletus badius*. *Food Chemistry, 200*, 206–214.

Kojta, A. K., Gucia, M., Jarzyńska, G., Lewandowska, M., Zakrzewska, A., Falandysz, J., & Zhang, D. (2011). Phosphorus and certain metals in Parasol Mushrooms (*Macrolepiota procera*) and soils from the Augustowska Forest and Ełk region in north-eastern Poland. *Fresenius Environmental Bulletin, 20*, 3044–3052.

Kojta, A. K., Jarzyńska, G., & Falandysz, J. (2012). Mineral composition and heavy metal accumulation capacity of Bay Bolete (*Xerocomus badius*) fruiting bodies collected near a former gold and copper mining area. *Journal of Geochemical Exploration, 121*, 76–82.

Kułdo, E., Jarzyńska, G., Gucia, M., & Falandysz, J. (2014). Mineral constituents of edible parasol mushroom *Macrolepiota procera* (Scop. ex Fr.) Sing and soils beneath its fruiting bodies collected from a rural forest area. *Chemical Papers, 68*, 484–492.

Li, T., Zhang, J., Shen, T., Shi, Y., Yang, S., Zhang, T., ... Liu, H. (2013). Mineral element content in prized matsutake mushroom (*Tricholoma matsutake*) collected in China. *Chemical Papers, 67*, 672–676.

Liu, H., Zhang, J., Li, T., Shi, Y., & Wang, Y. (2012). Mineral element levels in wild edible mushrooms from Yunnan, China. *Biological Trace Element Research, 147*, 341–345.

Maciejczyk, E., Wieczorek, D., Zwyrzykowska, A., Halama, M., Jasicka-Misiak, I., & Kafarski, P. (2015). Phosphorus profile of Basidiomycetes. *Phosphorus, Sulfur, and Silicon, 190*, 763–768.

Mallikarjuna, S. E., Ranjini, A., Haware, D. J., Haware, J., Vijayalakshmi, M. R., Shashirekha, M. N., & Rajarathnam, S. (2013). Mineral composition of four edible mushrooms. *Journal of Chemistry*, Article ID 805284, 5 pp.

Mędyk, M., Grembecka, M., Brzezicha-Cirocka, J., & Falandysz, J. (2017). Bio- and toxic elements in mushrooms from the city of Umeå and outskirts, Sweden. *Journal of Environmental Science and Health B, 52*, 577–583.

Mleczek, M., Magdziak, Z., Gąsecka, M., Niedzielski, P., Kalač, P., Siwulski, M., ... Sobieralski, K. (2016). Content of selected elements and low-molecular-weight organic acids in fruiting bodies of edible mushroom *Boletus badius* (Fr.) Fr. from unpolluted and polluted areas. *Environmental Science and Pollution Research, 23*, 20609–20618.

Mleczek, M., Siwulski, M., Mikołajczak, P., Goliński, P., Gąsecka, M., Sobieralski, K., ... Szymańczyk, M. (2015). Bioaccumulation of elements in three selected mushroom species from southwest Poland. *Journal of Environmental Science and Health B, 50*, 207–216.

Mleczek, M., Siwulski, M., Stuper-Szablewska, K., Sobieralski, K., Magdziak, Z., & Goliński, P. (2013). Accumulation of elements by edible mushroom species. II. A comparison of aluminium, barium and nutritional element contents. *Journal of Environmental Science and Health B, 48*, 308–317.

Mleczek, M., Siwulski, M., Rzymski, P., Niedzielski, P., Gąsecka, M., Jasińska, A., ... Budka, A. (2017). Multi-elemental analysis of *Lentinula edodes* mushrooms available in trade. *Journal of Environmental Science and Health B, 52*, 196–205.

Mleczek, M., Rzymski, P., Budka, A., Siwulski, M., Jasińska, A., Kalač, P., ... Niedzielski, P. (2018). Elemental characteristics of mushroom species cultivated in China and Poland. *Journal of Food Composition and Analysis, 66*, 168–178.

Nasr, M., Malloch, D. W., & Arp, P. A. (2012). Quantifying Hg within ectomycorrhizal fruiting bodies, from emergence to senescence. *Fungal Biology, 116*, 1163–1177.

Niedzielski, P., Mleczek, M., Budka, A., Rzymski, P., Siwulski, M., Jasińska, A., ... Budzyńska, S. (2017). A screening study of elemental composition in 12 marketable mushroom species accessible in Poland. *European Food Research and Technology, 243*, 1759–1771.

Proskura, N., Podlasińska, J., & Skopicz-Radkiewicz, L. (2017). Chemical composition and bioaccumulation ability of *Boletus badius* (Fr.) Fr. collected in western Poland. *Chemosphere, 168*, 106–111.

Quinche, J.-P. (1997). [Phosphorus and heavy metals in some species of fungi.]. *Revue Suisse Agriculture, 29*, 151–156. (in French).

Rossbach, M., Kümmerle, E., Schmidt, S., Gohmert, M., Stieghorst, C., Revay, Z., & Wiehl, N. (2017). Elemental analysis of *Morchella esculenta* from Germany. *Journal of Radioanalytical and Nuclear Chemistry, 313*, 273–278.

Rudawska, M., & Leski, T. (2005). Macro- and microelement contents in fruiting bodies of wild mushrooms from the Notecka forest in west-central Poland. *Food Chemistry, 92*, 499–506.

Rzymski, P., Mleczek, M., Siwulski, M., Jasińska, A., Budka, A., Niedzielski, P., ... Budzyńska, S. (2017). Multielemental analysis of fruit bodies of three cultivated commercial *Agaricus* species. *Journal of Food Composition and Analysis, 59*, 170–178.

Salvador, C., Martins, M. R., Vicente, H., & Caldeira, A. T. (2018). A data mining approach to improve inorganic characterization of *Amanita ponderosa* mushrooms. *International Journal of Analytical Chemistry*. Available from https://doi.org/10.1155/2018/5265291, Art. ID 5265291, 18 pp.

Sarikurkcu, C., Tepe, B., Solak, M. H., & Cetinkaya, S. (2012). Metal concentrations of wild edible mushrooms from Turkey. *Ecology of Food and Nutrition, 51*, 346–363.

Seeger, R. (1978). [Content of potassium in higher fungi.]. *Zeitschrift für Lebensmittel Untersuchung und Forschung, 167*, 23–31. (in German).

Seeger, R., & Beckert, M. (1979). [Magnesium content of higher fungi.]. *Zeitschrift für Lebensmittel Untersuchung und Forschung, 168*, 264–281. (in German).

Seeger, R., & Hüttner, W. (1981). [Calcium in mushrooms.]. *Deutsche Lebensmittel-Rundschau, 77*(11), 385–392. (in German).

Seeger, R., Trumpfheller, S., & Schweinshaut, P. (1983). [On the occurrence of sodium in fungi.]. *Deutsche Lebensmittel-Rundschau, 79*(3), 80–87. (in German).

Stefanović, V., Trifković, J., Djurdjić, S., Vukojević, V., Tešić, Ž., & Mutić, J. (2016). Study of silver, selenium and arsenic concentration in wild edible mushroom *Macrolepiota procera*, health benefit and risk. *Environmental Science and Pollution Research*, *23*, 22084–22098.

Stijve, T., Diserens, H., Oberson, J. M., & de Meijer, A. A. R. (1998). The natural inorganic bromide content of edible mushrooms. *Deutsche Lebensmittel-Rundschau*, *94*(4), 112–117.

Sun, L., Chang, W., Bao, C., & Zhuang, Y. (2017). Metal contents, bioaccumulation, and health risk assessment in wild edible *Boletaceae* mushrooms. *Journal of Food Science*, *82*, 1500–1508.

Szubstarska, J., Jarzyńska, G., & Falandysz, J. (2012). Trace elements in Variegated Bolete (*Suillus variegatus*) fungi. *Chemical Papers*, *66*, 1026–1031.

Tabata, T., & Ogura, T. (2003). Absorption of calcium and magnesium to the fruit body of aragekikurage (*Auricularia polytricha* (Mont.) Sacc.) from sawdust culture media supplemented with calcium and magnesium salts. *Food Science and Technology Research*, *9*, 250–253.

Tel-Çayan, G., Öztürk, M., Duru, M. E., Yabanli, M., & Türkoğlu, A. (2017). Content of minerals and trace elements determined by ICP-MS in eleven mushroom species from Anatolia, Turkey. *Chiang Mai Journal of Science*, *44*, 939–945.

Turfan, N., Pekşen, A., Kibar, B., & Ünal, S. (2018). Determination of nutritional and bioactive properties in some selected wild growing and cultivated mushrooms from Turkey. *Acta Scientiarum Polonorum Hortorum Cultus*, *17*(3), 57–72.

Vahdani, M., Rastegar, S., Rahimzadeh, M., Ahmadi, M., & Karmostaji, A. (2017). Physicochemical characteristics, phenolic profile, mineral and carbohydrate contents of two truffle species. *Journal of Agricultural Science and Technology*, *19*, 1091–1101.

Vetter, J. (2003). Data on sodium content of common edible mushrooms. *Food Chemistry*, *81*, 589–593.

Wang, X., Zhang, J., Li, T., Li, J., Wang, Y., & Liu, H. (2015a). ICP-AES determination of mineral content in *Boletus tomentipes* collected from different sites of China. *Spectroscopy and Spectral Analysis*, *35*, 1398–1403.

Wang, X., Zhang, J., Li, T., Li, J., Wang, Y., & Liu, H. (2015b). Variations in element levels accumulated in different parts of *Boletus edulis* collected from Central Yunnan Province, China. *Journal of Chemistry*, Article ID 372152, 7 pp.

Wang, X., Zhang, J., Li, T., Wang, Y., & Liu, H. (2015). Content and bioaccumulation of nine mineral elements in ten mushroom species of the genus *Boletus*. *Journal of Analytical Methods in Chemistry*, Article ID 165412, 7 pp.

Zavastin, D. E., Biliută, G., Dodi, G., Macsim, A.-M., Lisa, G., Gherman, S. P., ... Coseri, S. (2018). Metal content and crude polysaccharide characterization of selected mushrooms growing in Romania. *Journal of Food Composition and Analysis*, *67*, 149–158.

Zellner, J. (1907). *[Chemistry of mushrooms]*. Leipzig: Verlag von Wilhelm Engelmann. (in German).

Zeng, X., Suwandi, J., Fuller, J., Doronila, A., & Ng, K. (2012). Antioxidant capacity and mineral contents of edible wild Australian mushrooms. *Food Science and Technology International*, *18*, 367–379.

Zhang, D., Frankowska, A., Jarzyńska, G., Kojta, A. K., Drewnowska, M., Wydmańska, D., ... Falandysz, J. (2010). Metals of King Bolete (*Boletus edulis*) Bull.:Fr. collected at the same site over two years. *African Journal of Agricultural Research*, *5*, 3050–3055.

Zsigmond, A. R., Varga, K., Kántor, I., Urák, I., May, Z., & Héberger, K. (2018). Elemental composition of wild growing *Agaricus campestris* mushroom in urban and peri-urban regions of Transylvania (Romania). *Journal of Food Composition and Analysis*, *72*, 15–21.

Chapter 4

Trace elements

Seven major essential elements comprising quantitatively by far the greatest part of ash in mushrooms were characterized in Chapter 3, Major essential elements. Moreover, the ash contains tens of trace elements. The content of each of them is usually limited up to 50 mg kg^{-1} FM (fresh matter) [i.e., about 500 mg kg^{-1} DM (dry matter)]. Iron and zinc are sometimes classified in food chemistry as minor essential elements due to their higher contents than is usual for trace elements. Nevertheless, both these elements will be ranked among trace elements in this chapter.

Trace elements can be classified to three groups according to their physiological roles in humans:

1. *Essential* (indispensable, obligatory) elements: B, Co, Cr, Cu, F, Fe, I, Mn, Mo, Ni, Se, Si, and Zn.
2. *Detrimental* elements: Ag, As, Ba, Be, Cd, Hg, Pb, and Tl.
3. *Nonessential* elements: Al, Au, Bi, Br, Cs, Li, platinum group elements (PGEs), rare-earth elements, Rb, Sn, Sr, Te, and V; overall about 40 elements.

The third group includes trace elements for which there is limited knowledge of nutritional and health effects. Generally, the classification is not rigorous and can be changed with the progression of knowledge. Moreover, intake of an element has to be taken in mind. Even essential elements, for example, copper, iron or selenium, can be detrimental in cases of too high intake. Chemical forms (species) of an element are an additional factor. Total content of an element i.e. sum of its present chemical species, is mostly determined in foods including mushrooms until now. Some species of an element can be detrimental, whereas others can be quite safe. More information is given in Section 2.2. and in this chapter for several elements with available speciation data.

Literature data on trace elements in mushrooms were collated in several reviews (Falandysz & Borovička, 2013; Kalač, 2010; Kalač & Svoboda, 2000; Wang et al., 2014) with many references therein. Only the weightiest articles prior to 2010 will be cited in this chapter.

Mineral Composition and Radioactivity of Edible Mushrooms.
DOI: https://doi.org/10.1016/B978-0-12-817565-1.00004-2

Data since 2010 collated in tables of this chapter (except for Tables 4.1, 4.12, 4.18 and 4.19) are mean values expressed in mg kg^{-1} DM. Similarly to the discussion of major elements in Chapter 3, Major essential elements, the relative standard deviations are commonly high. Only data on at least five fruiting bodies per species, analyzed either separately or as a pooled sample, were included in the tables. Superscripts C and S are used for the contents in caps and stipes, respectively. The superscripts are given in the order of increasing contents (e.g., $X^{C,S}$ if the level of an element is higher in stipes than in caps). The elements will be arranged in alphabetical order within the three groups.

4.1 Essential trace elements

Recent average daily requirements of eight trace elements recommended by EFSA (European Food Safety Authority, 2017) are given in Table 4.1. No requirements have been approved for boron, cobalt, nickel, and silicon. Nevertheless, available data for these elements in mushrooms will be given in following sections 4.1.1–4.1.13.

Information on essential trace elements intake is limited. The upper intake is expressed as tolerable daily intake or provisional maximum tolerable daily intake. The values are 0.3, 0.5, 0.8, 0.0028, and 0.3–1.0 mg kg^{-1} bodyweight for chromium (Cr^{III}), copper, iron, nickel, and zinc, respectively.

TABLE 4.1 Average requirements (mg day^{-1}) of trace elements for adults (≥18 years) according to the European Food Safety Authority (EFSA; 2017).

Element	Males	Females
Chromium[a]	–	–
Copper	1.6	1.5
Fluorine	3.4	2.9
Iodine	0.150	0.150
Iron	11	16 Premenopausal
		11 Postmenopausal
Manganese	3.0	3.0
Molybdenum	0.065	0.065
Selenium	0.070	0.070
Zinc	9.4–16.3[b]	7.5–12.7[b]

[a]*There is no evidence of beneficial effects associated with chromium intake in healthy subjects. The setting of an adequate intake is thus not appropriate.*
[b]*According to level of phytate intake.*

4.1.1 Boron (B)

Data on boron content published during the past decade are collected in Table 4.2. The data are limited compared to several essential and toxic trace elements. The contents vary widely between <1 and >20 mg kg^{-1} DM. The highest levels occurred primarily in cultivated species. Niedzielski et al. (2017) determined 56 ± 9 and 33 mg kg^{-1} DM in cultivated *Auricularia polytricha* and *Grifola frondosa*, respectively. Similarly high content of 32 mg kg^{-1} DM was reported by Mleczek, Siwulski, Rzymski, Niedzielski, et al. (2017) in cultivated *Lentinula edodes*. Six cultivated species of genus *Pleurotus* showed a very wide range of 0.07–24.8 mg kg^{-1} DM, with a mean level of 3.65 mg kg^{-1} DM (Siwulski et al., 2017).

Similar levels to those collated in Table 4.2 were reported by Vetter (1995) in 68 edible species from Hungary. Mean boron content was 11.7 mg kg^{-1} DM; *Clitocybe nebularis* exceeded 50 mg kg^{-1} DM. Even higher contents were determined in numerous mushroom species, both edible and inedible, in the vicinity of Turkish boron mines. The highest level of 273 mg kg^{-1} DM was quantified in *Suillus collinitus* (Şen, Alli, & Çöl, 2012). Unfortunately, only one fruiting body per species was mostly analyzed. Lavola et al. (2011) observed great variability between species (medians from 0.51 mg kg^{-1} DM in *Cortinarius caperatus* to 18.4 mg kg^{-1} DM in *Suillus grevillei*) and within species (e.g., 0.41–11.26 mg kg^{-1} DM in *Boletus edulis*). There was no clear difference in boron levels between groups of saprobic and mycorrhizal species.

No data are available either on boron distribution within fruiting bodies, or on bioaccumulation/bioexclusion. Furthermore, information from Mleczek, Niedzielski, Kalač, Budka, et al. (2016), Mleczek, Magdziak, et al. (2016) on boron content in fruiting bodies of species growing on highly contaminated substrates (Table 4.2) is limited and cannot be generalized.

4.1.2 Cobalt (Co)

As data in Table 4.3 show, cobalt contents in wild-growing species range from very low levels <0.2 to 10 mg kg^{-1} DM. However, even higher levels were observed. Wang, Liu, Li, and Wang (2017) determined 25.9 and 7.2 mg kg^{-1} DM in stipes and caps of *Xerocomus spadiceous*, respectively, the respective values for *Boletus impolitus* were 12.7 and 5.2 mg kg^{-1} DM. Cobalt content of 13.9 mg kg^{-1} DM was reported in *Lycoperdon perlatum* (Sarikurkcu, Tepe, Kocak, & Uren, 2015). Great content variations within species are apparent from Table 4.3, for example, in *B. edulis*, *Pleurotus ostreatus*, or *Xerocomus badius*. Data on cobalt content for cultivated species have been virtually lacking.

Information on cobalt distribution within fruiting bodies varies. The equal contents were observed in some species, while in other higher levels in stipes

TABLE 4.2 Data on the content (mg kg^{-1} dry matter) of *boron* in fruiting bodies of wild mushrooms collected from unpolluted (X) and anthropogenically polluted (▲) sites and in cultivated species published since 2010.

Species	<1	1–2	2–3	3–4	4–5	5–10	10–20	>20	References
Wild growing									
Agaricus bitorquis	X								Durkan, Ugulu, Unver, Dogan, and Baslar (2011)
Agaricus campestris		X							Durkan et al. (2011)
Agrocyba aegerita							X		Durkan et al. (2011)
Armillariella mellea		▲		X		X			Durkan et al. (2011), Mleczek, Niedzielski, Kalač, Budka, et al. (2016), Zavastin et al. (2018)
Boletus edulis		X^m					X		Lavola, Aphalo, and Lehto (2011), Zavastin et al. (2018)
Cantharellus cibarius						▲	X		Mleczek, Niedzielski, Kalač, Budka, et al. (2016), Zavastin et al. (2018)
Cortinarius caperatus	X^m								Lavola et al. (2011)
Helvella crispa			▲						Golubkina and Mironov (2018)
Laccaria amethystina				X					Durkan et al. (2011)
Laccaria laccata				X					Durkan et al. (2011)
Laetiporus sulphureus							X		Durkan et al. (2011)

Leccinum aurantiacum					▲				Golubkina and Mironov (2018)
Leccinum scabrum	▲			X^m	▲				Golubkina and Mironov (2018), Lavola et al. (2011), Mleczek, Niedzielski, Kalač, Budka, et al. (2016)
Lepista nuda	X								Durkan et al. (2011)
Lycoperdon perlatum						X			Durkan et al. (2011)
Morchella esculenta				X		▲			Golubkina and Mironov (2018), Rossbach et al. (2017)
Pleurotus ostreatus	▲		X						Durkan et al. (2011), Mleczek, Niedzielski, Kalač, Budka, et al. (2016)
Russula aeruginea							X^m		Lavola et al. (2011)
Russula claroflava				X^m					Lavola et al. (2011)
Russula decolorans						X^m			Lavola et al. (2011)
Russula paludosa				X^m					Lavola et al. (2011)
Suillus bovinus		X, X^m			▲				Durkan et al. (2011), Lavola et al. (2011), Mleczek, Niedzielski, Kalač, Budka, et al. (2016)
Suillus granulatus							▲		Golubkina and Mironov (2018)
Suillus grevillei				X^m					Lavola et al. (2011)
Suillus luteus		X^m, ▲							Golubkina and Mironov (2018), Lavola et al. (2011)

(Continued)

TABLE 4.2 Data on the content (mg kg^{-1} dry matter) of *boron* in fruiting bodies of wild mushrooms collected from unpolluted (X) and anthropogenically polluted (▲) sites and in cultivated species published since 2010. (Continued)

Species	<1	1–2	2–3	3–4	4–5	5–10	10–20	>20	References
Suillus variegatus		X^m							Lavola et al. (2011)
Xerocomus badius	X		▲						Mleczek, Magdziak, et al. (2016)
Xerocomus chrysenteron							X		Durkan et al. (2011)
Cultivated									
Agaricus arvensis						X			Rzymski, Mleczek, Siwulski, Jasińska, et al. (2017)
Agaricus bisporus (brown)						X			Rzymski, Mleczek, Siwulski, Jasińska, et al. (2017)
A. bisporus (white)							X	X	Mleczek, Rzymski, et al. (2018), Rzymski, Mleczek, Siwulski, Jasińska, et al. (2017)
Agaricus subrufescens							X		Rzymski, Mleczek, Siwulski, Jasińska, et al. (2017)
Agrocybe cylindracea							X		Niedzielski et al. (2017)
Auricularia auricula-judae			X						Mleczek, Rzymski, et al. (2018)
Auricularia polytricha								X	Niedzielski et al. (2017)
Clitocybe maxima			X						Niedzielski et al. (2017)
Flammulina velutipes	X								Niedzielski et al. (2017)
Grifola frondosa								X	Niedzielski et al. (2017)

Hericium erinaceus						X			Niedzielski et al. (2017)
L. sulphureus		X							Niedzielski et al. (2017)
Lentinula edodes								X	Mleczek, Siwulski, Rzymski, Niedzielski, et al. (2017), Mleczek, Rzymski, et al. (2018)
Pholiota nameko								X	Niedzielski et al. (2017)
P. ostreatus				X					Mleczek, Rzymski, et al. (2018)
Trametes versicolor						X			Niedzielski et al. (2017)
Tremella fuciformis	X								Mleczek, Rzymski, et al. (2018), Niedzielski et al. (2017)
Volvariella volvacea		X							Mleczek, Rzymski, et al. (2018)

X^m, Median values.

TABLE 4.3 Data on the mean content (mg kg^{-1} dry matter) of *cobalt* in fruiting bodies of wild-growing mushrooms collected from unpolluted (X), geologically specific (●), and anthropogenically contaminated (▲) sites and in cultivated species published since 2010.

Species	<0.2	0.2–0.5	0.5–1	1–2	2–5	5–10	References
Wild growing							
Agaricus arvensis					X		Ayaz et al. (2011), Sarikurkcu, Copur, Yildiz, and Akata (2011)
Agaricus bisporus				X			Durkan et al. (2011)
Agaricus bitorquis	X						Durkan et al. (2011)
Agaricus campestris	X	X		X	●		Campos and Tejera (2011), Durkan et al. (2011), Kosanić, Ranković, Rančić, and Stanojković (2017), Severoglu, Sumer, Yalcin, Leblebici, and Aksoy (2013)
Agaricus sylvicola					●		Campos and Tejera (2011)
Agrocybe aegerita				X			Durkan et al. (2011)
Amanita caesarea					●, X		Campos and Tejera (2011), Sarikurkcu, Tepe, Semiz, and Solak (2010)
Amanita fulva	$X^{C,S}$						Falandysz, Drewnowska, Chudzińska, and Barałkiewicz (2017)
Amanita rubescens						●	Campos and Tejera (2011)
Armillariella mellea	X			X			Durkan et al. (2011), Zavastin et al. (2018)
Boletus aestivalis					$X^{C,S}$		Wang et al. (2017)

Boletus appendiculatus	$X^{C,Sm}$	X					Alaimo et al. (2018), Dimitrijevic et al. (2016)
Boletus edulis	X	X	X, $X^{S,C}$	X	X	X	Ayaz et al. (2011), Dimitrijevic et al. (2016), Kosanić et al. (2017), Mleczek, Siwulski, Stuper-Szablewska, Rissmann, et al. (2013), Mleczek, Siwulski, Mikołajczak, Goliński, et al. (2015), Turfan, Pekşen, Kibar, and Ünal (2018), Wang et al. (2015b), Zavastin et al. (2018)
Boletus griseus				X, $X^{C,S}$			Liu, Zhang, Li, Shi, and Wang (2012), Wang et al. (2017)
Boletus impolitus	X						Dimitrijevic et al. (2016)
Boletus luridus				$●^{C,S}$	X^{C}	X^{S}	Falandysz, Zhang, Wiejak, Barałkiewicz, and Hanć (2017), Wang et al. (2017)
Boletus magnificus			$●^{C,S}$				Falandysz, Zhang, Wiejak, et al. (2017)
Boletus pinophilus		X					Dospatliev and Ivanova (2017)
Boletus regius	X						Dimitrijevic et al. (2016)
Boletus speciosus			X		$X^{C,S}$		Liu et al. (2012), Wang et al. (2017)
Boletus tomentipes			X^{C}, $●^{C}$	X^{S}, $●^{S}$			Falandysz, Zhang, Wiejak, et al. (2017), Wang et al. (2015a)
Boletus umbriniporus					X^{C}	X^{S}	Wang et al. (2017)

(*Continued*)

TABLE 4.3 Data on the mean content (mg kg^{-1} dry matter) of *cobalt* in fruiting bodies of wild-growing mushrooms collected from unpolluted (X), geologically specific (●), and anthropogenically contaminated (▲) sites and in cultivated species published since 2010. (Continued)

Species	<0.2	0.2–0.5	0.5–1	1–2	2–5	5–10	References
Cantharellu cibarius	X	▲, X	X		●		Árvay et al. (2014), Ayaz et al. (2011), Campos and Tejera (2011), Drewnowska and Falandysz (2015), Falandysz and Drewnowska (2015a), Falandysz, Chudzińska, Barałkiewicz, Drewnowska, and Hanć (2017), Mleczek, Siwulski, Stuper-Szablewska, Rissmann, et al. (2013), Mleczek, Niedzielski, Kalač, Budka, et al. (2016), Zavastin et al. (2018)
Cantharellus tubaeformis	X						Ayaz et al. (2011), Falandysz et al. (2017)
Clitocybe gambosa		X					Severoglu et al. (2013)
Clitocybe geotropa		X			●		Campos and Tejera (2011), Sarikurkcu et al. (2010)
Clitocybe gibba					●		Campos and Tejera (2011)
Clitopilus prunulus		X^{m}					Alaimo et al. (2018)
Coprinus comatus	X						Severoglu et al. (2013)
Craterellus cornucopioides			X				Turfan et al. (2018)
Cyanoboletus pulverulentus		▲					Árvay et al. (2014)
Ganoderma lucidum						●	Campos and Tejera (2011)
Gomphus clavatus		X					Sarikurkcu et al. (2015)

Helvella leucopus		X					Gezer and Kaygusuz (2014)
Hydnum repandum	X	X					Ayaz et al. (2011), Severoglu et al. (2013)
Hygrophorus russula					●		Campos and Tejera (2011)
Laccaria amethystina				X			Durkan et al. (2011)
Laccaria laccata		X		X			Ayaz et al. (2011), Durkan et al. (2011)
Lactarius deliciosus		X	X	X	●		Campos and Tejera (2011), Gezer and Kaygusuz (2014), Mleczek, Siwulski, Stuper-Szablewska, Rissmann, et al. (2013), Severoglu et al. (2013), Turfan et al. (2018)
Lactarius hygrophoroides					X		Liu et al. (2012)
Lactarius salmonicolor	X, ND						Sarikurkcu et al. (2011), Severoglu et al. (2013)
Lactarius sanguifluus					●		Campos and Tejera (2011)
Laetiporus sulphureus			X	X			Durkan et al. (2011), Sarikurkcu et al. (2015), Turfan et al. (2018)
Leccinum aurantiacum			X				Mleczek, Siwulski, Stuper-Szablewska, Rissmann, et al. (2013)
Leccinum crocipodium		X					Dimitrijevic et al. (2016)
Leccinum griseum	$X^{C,S}$						Jarzyńska and Falandysz (2012b)
Leccinum rugosiceps			X^{C}		X^{S}		Wang et al. (2017)
Leccinum pseudoscabrum		X					Dimitrijevic et al. (2016)

(*Continued*)

TABLE 4.3 Data on the mean content (mg kg^{-1} dry matter) of *cobalt* in fruiting bodies of wild-growing mushrooms collected from unpolluted (X), geologically specific (●), and anthropogenically contaminated (▲) sites and in cultivated species published since 2010. (Continued)

Species	<0.2	0.2–0.5	0.5–1	1–2	2–5	5–10	References
Leccinum scabrum	▲					X	Mleczek, Siwulski, Mikołajczak, Goliński, et al. (2015), Mleczek, Niedzielski, Kalač, Budka, et al. (2016)
Lepista nuda	X			X		●	Ayaz et al. (2011), Campos and Tejera (2011), Durkan et al. (2011)
Leucoagaricus leucothites				X			Sarikurkcu et al. (2010)
Leucopaxillus giganteus			X				Liu et al. (2012)
Lycoperdon perlatum				X			Durkan et al. (2011)
Macrocybe gigantea		X					Liu et al. (2012)
Macrolepiota procera	X^{C}	$X^{S,C}$	▲, X, X^{S}		●		Árvay et al. (2014), Campos and Tejera (2011), Falandysz, Sapkota, Dryżalowska, Mędyk, and Feng (2017), Gucia et al. (2012), Kojta et al. (2011), Sarikurkcu et al. (2015), Severoglu et al. (2013)
Marasmius oreades			X		●		Campos and Tejera (2011), Turfan et al. (2018)
Melanoluca arcuata				X			Liu et al. (2012)
Morchella conica				X			
Morchella deliciosa			X				Liu et al. (2012)
Morchella esculenta		X					Gezer and Kaygusuz (2014),

Mycena haematopus				X			Liu et al. (2012)
Pleurotus ostreatus	X, ●	X	X	X			Durkan et al. (2011), Gezer and Kaygusuz (2014), Mleczek, Niedzielski, Kalač, Budka, et al. (2016), Severoglu et al. (2013), Tel-Çayan, Öztürk, Duru, Yabanli, and Türkoğlu (2017)
Polyporus squamosus	ND						Sarikurkcu et al. (2011)
Ramaria aurea	X						Severoglu et al. (2013)
Ramaria botrytis					X		Turfan et al. (2018)
Ramaria stricta	X						Severoglu et al. (2013)
Russula xerampelina		▲					Árvay et al. (2014)
Sarcodon imbricatus			$X^{S,C}$				Mędyk, Chudzińska, Barałkiewicz, and Falandysz (2017)
Sparassis crispa		X					Severoglu et al. (2013)
Suillus bovinus	X	X, ▲					Durkan et al. (2011), Mleczek, Niedzielski, Kalač, Budka, et al. (2016), Severoglu et al. (2013)
Suillus grevillei		X	▲				Árvay et al. (2014), Mleczek, Siwulski, Stuper-Szablewska, Rissmann, et al. (2013)
Suillus luteus		X					Gezer and Kaygusuz (2014)
Suillus variegatus	$X^{S,C}$						Szubstarska, Jarzyńska, and Falandysz (2012)

(*Continued*)

TABLE 4.3 Data on the mean content (mg kg^{-1} dry matter) of *cobalt* in fruiting bodies of wild-growing mushrooms collected from unpolluted (X), geologically specific (●), and anthropogenically contaminated (▲) sites and in cultivated species published since 2010. (Continued)

Species	<0.2	0.2–0.5	0.5–1	1–2	2–5	5–10	References
Tricholoma equestre					●		Campos and Tejera (2011)
Tricholoma fracticum		X					Tel-Çayan et al.(2017)
Tricholoma imbricatum	X						Sarikurkcu et al. (2011)
Tricholoma matsutake				X			Liu et al. (2012)
Tricholoma terreum		X		X			Gezer and Kaygusuz (2014), Severoglu et al. (2013), Turfan et al. (2018)
Xerocomus badius	X, ▲	X^{C}, ▲	▲	X^{S},X		X	Dimitrijevic et al. (2016), Gąsecka et al. (2017), Mleczek, Siwulski, Stuper-Szablewska, Rissmann, et al. (2013), Mleczek, Siwulski, Kaczmarek, et al. (2013), Mleczek, Siwulski, Mikołajczak, Gąsecka, Sobieralski, et al. (2015), Mleczek, Siwulski, Mikołajczak, Goliński, et al. (2015), Mleczek, Magdziak, et al. (2016), Proskura, Podlasińska, and Skopicz-Radkiewicz (2017)
Xerocomus chrysenteron	X			X			Dimitrijevic et al. (2016), Durkan et al. (2011), Sarikurkcu et al. (2011)
Xerocomus subtomentosus	X^{C}						Jarzyńska, Chojnacka, Dryżałowska, Nnorom, and Falandysz (2012)

Cultivated							
A. bisporus (unspecified)		X					Gaur, Rao, and Kushwaha (2016)
Calocybe indica		X					Gaur et al. (2016)
Hericium erinaceus					X		Turfan et al. (2018)
Lentinula edodes		X	X	X			Gaur et al. (2016), Mleczek, Siwulski, Rzymski, Niedzielski, et al. (2017), Turfan et al. (2018)
M. gigantea					X		Gaur et al. (2016)
Pleurotus eryngii	X						Rashid, Rahman, Correll, and Naidu (2018)
P. ostreatus	X			X			Rashid et al. (2018), Turfan et al. (2018)
Pleurotus sajor-caju	X						Gaur et al. (2016)

C, Caps; *ND*, below limit of detection; *S*, stipes; X^m, median value.

than in caps (Table 4.3). As results from the partial data show, cobalt is not bioaccumulated in fruiting bodies; bioconcentration factor (BCF) values are generally slightly lower than 1. Nevertheless, bioconcentration was observed in *Cantharellus cibarius* growing in podzol soils poor in mineral nutrients (Falandysz, Drewnowska, et al., 2012).

Cobalt content decreased by 75% of the initial level by blanching of *Amanita fulva* caps (Drewnowska, Falandysz, et al., 2017).

4.1.3 Copper (Cu)

Data in Table 4.4 show usual copper contents from <10 to 75 mg kg^{-1} DM in wild-growing species and lower levels up to 30 mg kg^{-1} DM in cultivated ones. Nevertheless, considerably higher contents were observed in mushrooms growing in polluted sites. Among wild-growing accumulating species *L. perlatum* is ranked with the highest copper content at 505 mg kg^{-1} DM (Svoboda, Zimmermannová, & Kalač, 2000), *Macrolepiota rhacodes* had averages of 110 ± 45 and 280 ± 101 mg kg^{-1} DM from an unpolluted site and in the vicinity of a lead smelter, respectively (Kalač, Burda, & Stašková, 1991), *Lepista nuda* had a mean level 231 mg kg^{-1} DM (Kalač, Nižnanská, Bevilaqua, & Stašková, 1996), *Macrolepiota procera* had mean values ranging between 155 and 236 mg kg^{-1} DM (Giannaccini et al., 2012; Harangozo and Stanovič, 2016; Kalač et al., 1996; Kojta et al., 2011; Kułdo, Jarzyńska, Gucia, & Falandysz, 2014; Jarzyńska, Gucia, Kojta, Rezulak, & Falandysz, 2011), and *Agaricus arvensis* had a mean content 187 mg kg^{-1} DM (Sarikurkcu et al., 2011). Surprisingly high levels (i.e., 341 ± 59 and 318 ± 101 mg kg^{-1} DM, respectively) were found in *X. badius* growing in extremely contaminated flotation tailings and soils (Mleczek, Siwulski, Mikołajczak, Gąsecka, Sobieralski, et al., 2015). Very high content of 180 mg kg^{-1} DM was reported by Bach, Helm, Bellettini, Maciel, and Haminiuk (2017) in cultivated *Agaricus subrufescens*. Great variability in copper content within a species can be seen in Table 4.4, particularly in *M. procera* and *X. badius*.

Copper is distributed within fruiting bodies evenly or with higher levels in caps than in stipes (Table 4.4 and Wang et al., 2015b). As reported by Alonso, Garcia, Pérez-López, and Melgar (2003) and Árvay et al. (2015), hymenophore had a higher copper level than the rest of the fruiting body.

Literature data on BCF values vary widely, from values around 1 to tens (e.g., Alonso et al., 2003; Árvay et al., 2015; Falandysz & Drewnowska, 2015a; Mleczek, Siwulski, Stuper-Szablewska, Rissmann, et al., 2013; Proskura et al., 2017; Vinichuk, 2013). The wide ranges do not refer to various species only, but also concern the intraspecies situation. Interesting information was reported for BCF values in 13 edible species collected from the same unpolluted sites during 3 consecutive years. The highest mean BCF values 66.3, 58.2, and 60.3 were observed in *M. procera* in the individual

TABLE 4.4 Data on the mean content (mg kg^{-1} dry matter) of *copper* in fruiting bodies of wild-growing mushrooms collected from unpolluted (X), geologically specific (●), and anthropogenically contaminated (▲) sites and in cultivated species published since 2010.

Species	<10	10–30	30–50	50–75	75–100	>100	References
Wild growing							
Agaricus arvensis				X			Ayaz et al. (2011)
Agaricus bisporus		X					Zhu et al. (2011)
Agaricus campestris	X	●	X, X^S, $▲^{S,C}$	X	X^C		Campos and Tejera (2011), Kosanić et al. (2017), Sarikurkcu, Tepe, Solak, and Cetinkaya (2012), Severoglu et al. (2013), Zsigmond et al. (2018)
Agaricus lanipes		X					Gezer et al. (2016)
Agaricus sylvicola						●	Campos and Tejera (2011)
Agrocybe aegerita		X					Zhu et al. (2011)
Agrocybe cylindracea			X				Sarikurkcu et al. (2012)
Albatrellus ovinus	$X^{C,S}$						Mędyk, Grembecka, Brzezicha-Cirocka, and Falandysz (2017)
Amanita caesarea		●	X				Campos and Tejera (2011), Sarikurkcu et al. (2010)

(*Continued*)

TABLE 4.4 Data on the mean content (mg kg^{-1} dry matter) of *copper* in fruiting bodies of wild-growing mushrooms collected from unpolluted (X), geologically specific (●), and anthropogenically contaminated (▲) sites and in cultivated species published since 2010. (Continued)

Species	<10	10–30	30–50	50–75	75–100	>100	References
Amanita fulva			X^{S}	X^{C}			Falandysz, Drewnowska, et al. (2017)
Amanita ponderosa						X	Salvador, Martins, Vicente, and Caldeira (2018)
Amanita rubescens		●					Campos and Tejera (2011)
Armillariella mellea	$X^{S,C}$	X, ▲					Georgescu et al. (2016), Radulescu, Stihi, Busuioc, Gheboianu, and Popescu (2010), Širić, Kasap, et al. (2016), Zavastin et al. (2018)
Boletus aestivalis		X, X^{S}	▲, X^{C}				Harangozo and Stanovič (2016), Širić, Kos, Bedeković, Kaić, and Kasap (2014), Širić, Kasap, et al. (2016), Wang et al. (2017)
Boletus appendiculatus		$X^{S,Cm}$	X, X^{S}	X^{C}			Alaimo et al. (2018), Dimitrijevic et al. (2016), Mleczek, Siwulski, Mikołajczak, Gąsecka, Rissmann, et al. (2015), Sun, Chang, Bao, and Zhuang (2017), Wang, Zhang, Li, Wang, and Liu (2015)
Boletus bicolor		X					Sun et al. (2017)
Boletus brunneissimus		X^{S}	X^{C}				Wang et al. (2015)

Boletus edulis		X, $X^{S,C}$	X, $X^{S,C}$	X^{C}			Ayaz et al. (2011), Brzezicha-Cirocka, Mędyk, Falandysz, and Szefer (2016), Cvetkovic, Mitic, Stankov-Jovanovic, Dimitrijevic, and Nikolic-Mandic (2015), Dimitrijevic et al. (2016), Falandysz et al. (2011), Frankowska, Ziółkowska, Bielawski, and Falandysz (2010), Georgescu et al. (2016), Giannaccini et al. (2012), Kosanić et al. (2017), Mazurkiewicz and Podlasińska (2014), Mędyk, Grembecka, et al. (2017), Mleczek, Siwulski, Stuper-Szablewska, Rissmann, et al. (2013), Mleczek, Siwulski, Mikołajczak, Gąsecka, Rissmann, et al. (2015), Mleczek, Siwulski, Mikołajczak, Goliński, et al. (2015), Širić, Kasap, et al. (2016), Sun et al. (2017), Turfan et al. (2018), Wang et al. (2015, 2015b), Zhang et al. (2010), Zavastin et al. (2018)
Boletus flammans			X				Sun et al. (2017)
Boletus griseus		X^{S}	X, X^{C}	X			Liu et al. (2012), Sun et al. (2017), Wang et al. (2015, 2017)
Boletus impolitus		X					Dimitrijevic et al. (2016)
Boletus luridus		X^{S}, $●^{S}$	X^{C}	X^{C}, $●^{C}$			Falandysz, Zhang, Wiejak, et al. (2017), Wang et al. (2015, 2017)

(*Continued*)

TABLE 4.4 Data on the mean content (mg kg^{-1} dry matter) of *copper* in fruiting bodies of wild-growing mushrooms collected from unpolluted (X), geologically specific (●), and anthropogenically contaminated (▲) sites and in cultivated species published since 2010. (Continued)

Species	<10	10–30	30–50	50–75	75–100	>100	References
Boletus magnificus		$●^{S}$	$●^{C}$				Falandysz, Zhang, Wiejak, et al. (2017)
Boletus pallidus			X^{S}		X^{C}		Wang et al. (2015)
Boletus pinophilus		X	X				Dospatliev and Ivanova (2017), Mleczek, Siwulski, Mikołajczak, Gąsecka, Rissmann, et al. (2015)
Boletus pulverulentus				▲			Árvay et al. (2014)
Boletus regius		X					Dimitrijevic et al. (2016)
Boletus rubellus			X^{S}	X^{C}			Wang et al. (2015)
Boletus sinicus			X				Sun et al. (2017)
Boletus speciosus		X,X^{S}	X,X^{S}	X^{C}			Liu et al. (2012), Sun et al. (2017), Wang et al. (2015, 2017)
Boletus tomentipes		X^{S}	X^{C}	$●^{S}$	$X^{S,C}$ $●^{C}$		Falandysz, Zhang, Wiejak, et al. (2017), Wang et al. (2015, 2015a)
Boletus umbriniporus			X^{S}	X^{C}			Wang et al. (2015, 2017)
Calocybe gambosa	X						Severoglu et al. (2013)

Cantharellus cibarius	X^C,X	X^S, ▲	X, ●	X, ▲			Árvay et al. (2014), Ayaz et al. (2011), Brzezicha-Cirocka et al. (2016), Campos and Tejera (2011), Cvetkovic et al. (2015), Drewnowska and Falandysz (2015), Falandysz and Drewnowska (2015a), Falandysz, Chudzińska, et al. (2017), Georgescu et al. (2016), Harangozo and Stanovič (2016), Mazurkiewicz and Podlasińska (2014), Mleczek, Siwulski, Stuper-Szablewska, Rissmann, et al. (2013), Mleczek, Niedzielski, Kalač, Budka, et al. (2016), Zavastin et al. (2018)
Cantharellus tubaeformis			X				Ayaz et al. (2011), Falandysz, Chudzińska, et al. (2017)
Clitocybe geotropa				●, X			Campos and Tejera (2011), Sarikurkcu et al. (2010)
Clitocybe gibba			●				Campos and Tejera (2011)
Clitocybe inversa		X					Širić, Kasap, et al. (2016)
Clitocybe nebularis		X					Širić, Kasap, et al. (2016)
Clitopilus prunulus		X^m					Alaimo et al. (2018),
Coprinus comatus	X		X				Severoglu et al. (2013), Zhu et al. (2011)
Craterellus cornucopioides						X	Turfan et al. (2018)

(Continued)

TABLE 4.4 Data on the mean content (mg kg^{-1} dry matter) of *copper* in fruiting bodies of wild-growing mushrooms collected from unpolluted (X), geologically specific (●), and anthropogenically contaminated (▲) sites and in cultivated species published since 2010. (Continued)

Species	<10	10–30	30–50	50–75	75–100	>100	References
Fistulina hepatica		▲					Radulescu et al. (2010),
Flammulina velutipes	X			X^{C}			Zeng, Suwandi, Fuller, Doronila, and Ng (2012), Zhu et al. (2011)
Ganoderma lucidum		●					Campos and Tejera (2011)
Gomphidius glutinosus	$X^{C,S}$						Mędyk, Grembecka, et al. (2017)
Gomphus clavatus			X				Sarikurkcu et al. (2015)
Helvella leucopus		X	X				Gezer and Kaygusuz (2014), Sarikurkcu et al. (2012)
Hericium erinaceus	X						Zhu et al. (2011)
Hydnum imbricatum		X					Mędyk, Chudzińska, et al. (2017)
Hydnum repandum	X	X					Ayaz et al. (2011), Jedidi, Ayoub, Philippe, and Bouzouita (2017), Severoglu et al. (2013)
Hygrophorus russula			●				Campos and Tejera (2011)
Hypsizygus marmoreus	X						Zhu et al. (2011)
Laccaria laccata				X			Ayaz et al. (2011)

Lactarius deliciosus	X, ●	X	X	X			Aloupi, Koutrotsios, Koulousaris, and Kalogeropoulos (2012), Campos and Tejera (2011), Çayir, Coşkun, and Coşkun (2010), Gezer and Kaygusuz (2014), Jedidi et al. (2017), Mleczek, Siwulski, Stuper-Szablewska, Rissmann, et al. (2013), Mleczek, Siwulski, Mikołajczak, Gąsecka, Rissmann, et al. (2015), Severoglu et al. (2013), Turfan et al. (2018)
Lactarius deterrimus	X						Širić, Kasap, et al. (2016)
Lactarius hygrophoroides		X					Liu et al. (2012)
Lactarius piperatus			X				Cvetkovic et al. (2015)
Lactarius salmonicolor	X	X, $X^{S,C}$					Chowaniak, Niemiec, and Paluch (2017), Sarikurkcu et al. (2011), Severoglu et al. (2013)
Lactarius sanguifluus	●						Aloupi et al. (2012), Campos and Tejera (2011)
Lactarius semisanguifllus	●						Aloupi et al. (2012)
Laetiporus sulphureus	X	X					Brzezicha-Cirocka et al. (2016), Sarikurkcu et al. (2015), Turfan et al. (2018)
Leccinum aurantiacum		X	X				Mleczek, Siwulski, Stuper-Szablewska, Rissmann, et al. (2013), Mleczek, Siwulski, Mikołajczak, Gąsecka, Rissmann, et al. (2015)

(*Continued*)

TABLE 4.4 Data on the mean content (mg kg^{-1} dry matter) of *copper* in fruiting bodies of wild-growing mushrooms collected from unpolluted (X), geologically specific (●), and anthropogenically contaminated (▲) sites and in cultivated species published since 2010. (Continued)

Species	<10	10–30	30–50	50–75	75–100	>100	References
Leccinum crocipodium		C	X				Dimitrijevic et al. (2016), Sun et al. (2017)
Leccinum duriusculum	X^S	X^C					Jarzyńska and Falandysz (2012a)
Leccinum griseum		$X^{S,C}$					Jarzyńska and Falandysz (2012b)
Leccinum pseudoscabrum		X					Dimitrijevic et al. (2016)
Leccinum rugosiceps		X^S	X^C				Wang et al. (2017)
Leccinum scabrum		X, ●	▲	X			Harangozo and Stanovič (2016), Mleczek, Siwulski, Mikołajczak, Gąsecka, Rissmann, et al. (2015), Mleczek, Siwulski, Mikołajczak, Goliński, et al. (2015), Mleczek, Niedzielski, Kalač, Budka, et al. (2016), Mędyk, Grembecka, et al. (2017)
Leccinum versipelle			X				Mędyk, Grembecka, et al. (2017)
Lentinus cladopus	X						Mallikarjuna et al. (2013)
Lentinula edodes	X						Zhu et al. (2011)
Lepista nuda				●, X			Ayaz et al. (2011), Campos and Tejera (2011)
Lepista sordida	X						Zhu et al. (2011)
Leucoagaricus leucothites			X				Sarikurkcu et al. (2010)

Leucopaxillus giganteus			X				Liu et al. (2012)
Lycoperdon perlatum		▲		X	X	X	Brzezicha-Cirocka et al. (2016), Mędyk, Grembecka, et al. (2017), Radulescu et al. (2010), Sarikurkcu et al. (2015)
Macrocybe gigantea		X					Liu et al. (2012)
Macrolepiota excoriata			$X^{S,C}$			X^{S}	Georgescu et al. (2016)
Macrolepiota procera		X,X^{S}	▲, X^{C}	X	$X^{C,S}$	X, $X^{S,C}$	Árvay et al. (2014), Campos and Tejera (2011), Falandysz, Sapkota, Dryżalowska et al. (2017), Georgescu et al. (2016), Gucia et al. (2012), Jarzyńska et al. (2011), Kojta et al. (2011), Kułdo et al. (2014), Mazurkiewicz and Podlasińska (2014), Mleczek, Siwulski, Mikołajczak, Gąsecka, Rissmann, et al. (2015), Sarikurkcu et al. (2015), Severoglu et al. (2013), Širić, Kasap, et al. (2016)
Marasmius oreades				X,●		X	Campos and Tejera (2011), Cvetkovic et al. (2015), Turfan et al. (2018)
Melanoleuca arcuata		X					Liu et al. (2012)
Morchella conica					X		Turfan et al. (2018)
Morchella deliciosa				X			Liu et al. (2012)

(*Continued*)

TABLE 4.4 Data on the mean content (mg kg^{-1} dry matter) of *copper* in fruiting bodies of wild-growing mushrooms collected from unpolluted (X), geologically specific (●), and anthropogenically contaminated (▲) sites and in cultivated species published since 2010. (Continued)

Species	<10	10–30	30–50	50–75	75–100	>100	References
Morchella elata		X^{C}					Zeng et al. (2012)
Morchella esculenta		X	X				Gezer and Kaygusuz (2014), Rossbach et al. (2017), Sarikurkcu et al. (2012)
Mycena haematopus		X					Liu et al. (2012)
Pleurotus djamor		X					Mallikarjuna et al. (2013)
Pleurotus eryngii	X^{C},X						Zeng et al. (2012), Zhu et al. (2011)
Pleurotus nebrodensis	X						Zhu et al. (2011)
Pleurotus ostreatus	X, $X^{S,C}$, ▲	X, ▲					Georgescu et al. (2016), Gezer and Kaygusuz (2014), Mleczek, Niedzielski, Kalač, Budka, et al. (2016), Radulescu et al. (2010), Severoglu et al. (2013), Tel-Çayan et al.(2017), Zhu et al. (2011)
Polyporus squamosus		X					Sarikurkcu et al. (2011)
Ramaria aurea	X						Severoglu et al. (2013)
Ramaria botrytis						X	Turfan et al. (2018)
Ramaria stricta	X						Severoglu et al. (2013)
Russula aeruginea		$X^{C,S}$					Elekes and Busuioc (2013)
Russula alutacea		$X^{C,S}$					Elekes and Busuioc (2013), Georgescu et al. (2016)

Russula cyanoxantha	X^S	X^C, $X^{S,C}$					Elekes and Busuioc (2013), Georgescu et al. (2016)
Russula delica		●					Aloupi et al. (2012)
Russula lepida	X^C	X^S					Elekes and Busuioc (2013)
Russula olivacea			▲				Harangozo and Stanovič (2016)
Russula vesca		$X^{C,S}$					Elekes and Busuioc (2013)
Russula virescens	$X^{S,C}$						Elekes and Busuioc (2013)
Russula xerampelina				▲			Árvay et al. (2014), Harangozo and Stanovič (2016)
Sparassis crispa	X						Severoglu et al. (2013)
Suillus bellinii	●						
Suillus bovinus	X,X^S	X, X^C					Mleczek, Siwulski, Mikołajczak, Gąsecka, Rissmann, et al. (2015), Mędyk, Grembecka, et al. (2017), Severoglu et al. (2013)
Suillus granulatus							
Suillus grevillei		X	▲			▲	Árvay et al. (2014), Harangozo and Stanovič (2016), Mleczek, Siwulski, Mikołajczak, Gąsecka, Rissmann, et al. (2015)

(*Continued*)

TABLE 4.4 Data on the mean content (mg kg^{-1} dry matter) of *copper* in fruiting bodies of wild-growing mushrooms collected from unpolluted (X), geologically specific (●), and anthropogenically contaminated (▲) sites and in cultivated species published since 2010. (Continued)

Species	<10	10–30	30–50	50–75	75–100	>100	References
Suillus luteus	X^S, X^C	X, X^C					Gezer and Kaygusuz (2014), Mleczek, Siwulski, Stuper-Szablewska, Rissmann, et al. (2013), Mleczek, Siwulski, Mikołajczak, Gąsecka, Rissmann, et al. (2015), Mędyk, Grembecka, et al. (2017), Zeng et al. (2012)
Suillus variegatus	X^S	X, X^C					Szubstarska et al. (2012), Severoglu et al. (2013)
Terfezia claveryi		X	X				Kivrak (2015), Vahdani, Rastegar, Rahimzadeh, Ahmadi, and Karmostaji (2017)
Terfezia olbiensis			X				Kivrak (2015)
Tirmania nivea		X					Vahdani et al. (2017)
Tirmania pinoyi				X			Bouatia et al. (2018)
Tricholoma equestre	X		●				Campos and Tejera (2011), Jedidi et al. (2017)
Tricholoma fracticum	X						Tel-Çayan et al.(2017)
Tricholoma imbricatum	X						Sarikurkcu et al. (2011)
Tricholoma matsutake		X					Li et al. (2013), Liu et al. (2012)
Tricholoma portentosum		X					Širić, Kasap, et al. (2016)

Tricholoma terreum	X	X			X		Gezer and Kaygusuz (2014), Severoglu et al. (2013), Širić, Kasap, et al. (2016), Turfan et al. (2018)
Volvariella volvacea		X					Zhu et al. (2011)
Xerocomus badius	X	X^S, X, $▲^S$	▲	X, X^C, ▲, $▲^C$	X^C		Dimitrijevic et al. (2016), Gąsecka et al. (2017), Harangozo and Stanovič (2016), Kojta, Jarzyńska, and Falandysz (2012), Mleczek, Siwulski, Stuper-Szablewska, Rissmann, et al. (2013), Mleczek, Siwulski, Kaczmarek, et al. (2013), Mleczek, Siwulski, Mikołajczak, Gąsecka, Rissmann, et al. (2015), Mleczek, Siwulski, Mikołajczak, Goliński, et al. (2015), Mleczek, Magdziak, et al. (2016), Podlasińska, Proskura, and Szymańska (2015), Proskura et al. (2017)
Xerocomus chrysenteron	X	X					Dimitrijevic et al. (2016), Sarikurkcu et al. (2011)
Xerocomus spadiceus		$X^{S,C}$					Wang et al. (2017)
Xerocomus subtomentosus		X, X^S	X^C				Jarzyńska et al. (2012), Mleczek, Siwulski, Mikołajczak, Gąsecka, Rissmann, et al. (2015), Mędyk, Grembecka, et al. (2017)

(Continued)

TABLE 4.4 Data on the mean content (mg kg^{-1} dry matter) of *copper* in fruiting bodies of wild-growing mushrooms collected from unpolluted (X), geologically specific (●), and anthropogenically contaminated (▲) sites and in cultivated species published since 2010. (Continued)

Species	<10	10–30	30–50	50–75	75–100	>100	References
Cultivated							
A. arvensis			X				Rzymski, Mleczek, Siwulski, Jasińska, et al. (2017)
A. bisporus (unspecified)					X		Gaur et al. (2016)
A. bisporus (brown)			X	X			Bach et al. (2017), Rzymski, Mleczek, Siwulski, Jasińska, et al. (2017)
A. bisporus (white)		X	X				Bach et al. (2017), Jedidi et al. (2017), Mleczek, Rzymski, et al. (2018), Rzymski, Mleczek, Siwulski, Jasińska, et al. (2017)
Agaricus subrufescens					X		Rzymski, Mleczek, Siwulski, Jasińska, et al. (2017)
A. cylindracea		X					Niedzielski et al. (2017)
Auricularia auricula-judae	X						Mleczek, Rzymski, et al. (2018)
Auricularia polytricha		X					Niedzielski et al. (2017)
Auricularia thailandica	X						Bandara et al. (2017)
Calocybe indica		X					Gaur et al. (2016)
Clitocybe maxima		X					Niedzielski et al. (2017)
F. velutipes	X						Bach et al. (2017), Niedzielski et al. (2017)
Grifola frondosa			X				Niedzielski et al. (2017)

H. erinaceus		X	X				Niedzielski et al. (2017), Turfan et al. (2018)
L. sulphureus	X						Niedzielski et al. (2017)
L. edodes	X	X					Bach et al. (2017), Gaur et al. (2016), Gonçalves, de Souza, Rocha, Medeiros, and do Couto Jacob (2014), Mallikarjuna et al. (2013), Mleczek, Siwulski, Rzymski, Niedzielski, et al. (2017), Mleczek, Rzymski, et al. (2018), Turfan et al. (2018)
M. gigantea						X	Gaur et al. (2016)
Pholiota nameko		X					Niedzielski et al. (2017)
P. djamor		X					Bach et al. (2017)
P. eryngii	X	X					Bach et al. (2017), Gonçalves et al. (2014), Rashid et al. (2018)
Pleurotus floridanus	X	X					Khani, Moudi, and Khojech (2017), Mallikarjuna et al. (2013)
P. ostreatus		X					Bach et al. (2017), Gonçalves et al. (2014), Mleczek, Rzymski, et al. (2018), Rashid et al. (2018), Turfan et al. (2018)
Pleurotus sajor-caju					X		Gaur et al. (2016)
Trametes versicolor		X					Niedzielski et al. (2017)
Tremella fuciformis	X		X				Mleczek, Rzymski, et al. (2018), Niedzielski et al. (2017)
V. volvacea			X				Mleczek, Rzymski, et al. (2018)

C, Caps; *S*, stipes; X^m, median value.

years, respectively. In contrast, the respective values for *Leccinum scabrum* were 11.9, 7.7 and 11.4 (Mleczek, Siwulski, Mikołajczak, Gąsecka, Rissmann, et al., 2015). Extremely low BCF values of 0.1 and 0.2 were found in *X. badius* growing in two heavily contaminated substrates (Mleczek, Siwulski, Mikołajczak, Gąsecka, Sobieralski, et al., 2015).

Copper contents were effectively elevated in fruiting bodies of *Agaricus bisporus* (Rzymski, Mleczek, Niedzielski, Siwulski, & Gąsecka, 2017), *P. ostreatus*, and *Pleurotus eryngii* (Poniedziałek et al., 2017) cultivated in substrates fortified with a combination of selenium and copper salts. For more information see Section 4.1.11.

The copper content decreased by 68% of the initial level by blanching of *A. fulva* caps (Drewnowska, Hanć, Barałkiewicz, & Falandysz, 2017).

Collin-Hansen, Yttri, Andersen, Berthelsen, and Steinnes (2002) detected copper-binding metallothionein-like proteins in 72% of 44 tested mushroom samples, the proportion being lower than that for such proteins binding cadmium or zinc. Shimaoka, Kodama, Nishino, and Itokawa (1993) isolated from inedible *G. frondosa* an acidic peptide possessing specific properties to bind copper or to maintain copper in the soluble state at physiological pH. The peptide most probably enhances copper absorption in the small intestine.

Testing of true copper absorption from mushroom soup using extrinsically added stable isotope ^{65}Cu was 35% ± 11%. The observed rate of the absorption was comparable with concurrently analyzed extrinsically labeled sunflower seeds, lower than from red wine and in particular than from a reference dose, but higher than from both extrinsically and intrinsically labeled soy beans (Harvey et al., 2005). Unfortunately, mushroom species were not given.

4.1.4 Chromium (Cr)

Chromium is considered as an essential mineral by the US Institute of Medicine, but not by the European Food Safety Authority, which make decisions for the European Union (Table 4.1).

Usual content of total chromium in mushrooms ranges between 0.5 and 10 mg kg^{-1} DM. Great ranges are apparent in *C. cibarius* and *M. procera* (Table 4.5). Surprisingly, the contents above 20 mg kg^{-1} DM occur in several cultivated species.

Elevated levels were reported in wild mushrooms growing on quartzite acidic soils (Campos & Tejera, 2011) and polymetallic soils (Falandysz, Zhang, Wiejak, et al., 2017). High levels were determined by Zhu et al. (2011) in all of the 14 analyzed edible species. The lowest mean content 10.7 mg kg^{-1} DM was observed in *Coprinus comatus*, while the highest level was 42.7 mg kg^{-1} DM in *Russula albida*. Unfortunately, from the article is not clear whether the tested samples originated from polymetallic soils

TABLE 4.5 Data on the mean content (mg kg^{-1} dry matter) of *chromium* in fruiting bodies of wild-growing mushrooms collected from unpolluted (X), geologically specific (●), and anthropogenically contaminated (▲) sites and in cultivated species published since 2010.

Species	<0.5	0.5–1	1–2	2–5	5–10	10–20	>20	References
Wild growing								
Agaricus arvensis			X		X			Ayaz et al. (2011), Sarikurkcu et al. (2011)
Agaricus bisporus							X	Zhu et al. (2011)
Agaricus campestris			X	X	●			Campos and Tejera (2011), Kosanić et al. (2017), Širić, Humar, et al. (2016), Severoglu et al. (2013)
Agaricus sylvicola				●				Campos and Tejera (2011)
Agrocybe aegerita							X	Zhu et al. (2011)
Amanita caesarea					●	X		Campos and Tejera (2011), Sarikurkcu et al. (2010)
Amanita fulva	$X^{C,S}$							Falandysz, Drewnowska, et al. (2017)
Amanita ponderosa			X					Salvador et al. (2018)
Amanita rubescens					●			Campos and Tejera (2011)
Armillariella mellea			▲	X				Radulescu et al. (2010), Širić, Humar, et al. (2016)
Boletus aestivalis				X				Širić et al. (2014), Širić, Humar, et al. (2016)
Boletus appendiculatus	X, $X^{S,Cm}$							Alaimo et al. (2018), Dimitrijevic et al. (2016)

(Continued)

TABLE 4.5 Data on the mean content (mg kg^{-1} dry matter) of *chromium* in fruiting bodies of wild-growing mushrooms collected from unpolluted (X), geologically specific (●), and anthropogenically contaminated (▲) sites and in cultivated species published since 2010. (Continued)

Species	<0.5	0.5–1	1–2	2–5	5–10	10–20	>20	References
Boletus edulis	$X^{C,S}$	X	X	X				Ayaz et al. (2011), Cvetkovic et al. (2015), Dimitrijevic et al. (2016), Giannaccini et al. (2012), Kosanić et al. (2017), Mazurkiewicz and Podlasińska (2014), Mleczek, Siwulski, Mikołajczak, Goliński, et al. (2015), Širić, Humar, et al. (2016), Turfan et al. (2018)
Boletus griseus				X				Liu et al. (2012)
Boletus impolitus	X							Dimitrijevic et al. (2016)
Boletus luridus					$●^{S,C}$			Falandysz, Zhang, Wiejak, et al. (2017)
Boletus magnificus					$●^{S,C}$			Falandysz, Zhang, Wiejak, et al. (2017)
Boletus regius	X							Dimitrijevic et al. (2016)
Boletus speciosus	X							Liu et al. (2012)
Boletus tomentipes				$●^{S,C}$		X^{C}	X^{S}	Falandysz, Zhang, Wiejak, et al. (2017), Wang et al. (2015a),
Calocybe gambosa				X				Severoglu et al. (2013)
Cantharellus cibarius	X, ●	▲	X	X	X, ●			Árvay et al. (2014), Ayaz et al. (2011), Campos and Tejera (2011), Cvetkovic et al. (2015), Drewnowska and Falandysz (2015), Falandysz and Drewnowska (2015a), Falandysz, Chudzińska, et al. (2017), Mazurkiewicz and Podlasińska (2014), Mleczek, Niedzielski, Kalač, Budka, et al. (2016)

Cantharellus tubaeformis	X		X					Ayaz et al. (2011), Falandysz, Chudzińska, et al. (2017)
Clitocybe geotropa					●, X			Campos and Tejera (2011), Sarikurkcu et al. (2010)
Clitocybe gibba					●			Campos and Tejera (2011)
Clitocybe inversa				X				Širić, Humar, et al. (2016)
Clitocybe nebularis		X						Širić, Humar, et al. (2016)
Clitopilus prunulus			X[m]					Alaimo et al. (2018)
Collybia velutipes						X		Zhu et al. (2011)
Coprinus comatus			X			X		Severoglu et al. (2013), Zhu et al. (2011)
Craterellus cornucopioides						X		Turfan et al. (2018)
Cyanoboletus pulverulentus			▲					Árvay et al. (2014)
Fistulina hepatica			▲					Radulescu et al. (2010)
Ganoderma lucidum				●				Campos and Tejera (2011)
Gomphus clavatus						X		Sarikurkcu et al. (2015)
Helvella leucopus		X						Gezer and Kaygusuz (2014),
Hericium erinaceus							X	Zhu et al. (2011)
Hydnum repandum		X		X				Ayaz et al. (2011), Severoglu et al. (2013)
Hygrophorus russula					●			Campos and Tejera (2011)
Hypsizygus marmoreus						X		Zhu et al. (2011)
Laccaria laccata		X						Ayaz et al. (2011)

(*Continued*)

TABLE 4.5 Data on the mean content (mg kg^{-1} dry matter) of *chromium* in fruiting bodies of wild-growing mushrooms collected from unpolluted (X), geologically specific (●), and anthropogenically contaminated (▲) sites and in cultivated species published since 2010. (Continued)

Species	<0.5	0.5–1	1–2	2–5	5–10	10–20	>20	References
Lactarius deliciosus	X, ●	X				●		Aloupi et al. (2012), Campos and Tejera (2011), Çayir et al. (2010), Gezer and Kaygusuz (2014), Severoglu et al. (2013), Turfan et al. (2018)
Lactarius deterrimus			X					Širić, Humar, et al. (2016)
Lactarius hygrophoroides			X					Liu et al. (2012)
Lactarius piperatus				X				Cvetkovic et al. (2015)
Lactarius salmonicolor			X				X	Sarikurkcu et al. (2011), Severoglu et al. (2013)
Lactarius sanguifluus	●					●		Aloupi et al. (2012), Campos and Tejera (2011)
Lactarius semisanguifluus				▲				Aloupi et al. (2012)
Laetiporus sulphureus				X				Sarikurkcu et al. (2015), Turfan et al. (2018)
Leccinum crocipodium	X							Dimitrijevic et al. (2016)
Leccinum duriusculum	$X^{S,C}$							Jarzyńska and Falandysz (2012a)
Leccinum griseum	$X^{S,C}$							Jarzyńska and Falandysz (2012b)
Leccinum pseudoscabrum			X					Dimitrijevic et al. (2016)
Leccinum scabrum	▲		X					Mleczek, Siwulski, Mikołajczak, Goliński, et al. (2015), Mleczek, Niedzielski, Kalač, Budka, et al. (2016)

Lentinula edodes						X		Zhu et al. (2011)
Lepista nuda			X		●			Ayaz et al. (2011), Campos and Tejera (2011)
Lepista sordida							X	Zhu et al. (2011)
Leucoagaricus leucothites				X				Sarikurkcu et al. (2010)
Leucopaxillus giganteus					X			Liu et al. (2012)
Lycoperdon perlatum			▲				X	Radulescu et al. (2010), Sarikurkcu et al. (2015)
Macrocybe gigantea		X						Liu et al. (2012)
Macrolepiota procera	$X^{C,S}$	▲	X, X^{C}	X	●			Árvay et al. (2014), Campos and Tejera (2011), Giannaccini et al. (2012), Gucia et al. (2012), Kojta et al. (2011), Mazurkiewicz and Podlasińska (2014), Sarikurkcu et al. (2015), Severoglu et al. (2013), Širić, Humar, et al. (2016)
Marasmius oreades					●, X	X		Campos and Tejera (2011), Cvetkovic et al. (2015), Turfan et al. (2018)
Melanoleuca arcuata				X				Liu et al. (2012)
Morchella conica					X			Turfan et al. (2018)
Morchella deliciosa					X			Liu et al. (2012)
Morchella esculenta		X						Gezer and Kaygusuz (2014)
Mycena haematopus			X					Liu et al. (2012)
Pleurotus eryngii							X	Zhu et al. (2011)
Pleurotus nebrodensis							X	Zhu et al. (2011)

(Continued)

TABLE 4.5 Data on the mean content (mg kg^{-1} dry matter) of *chromium* in fruiting bodies of wild-growing mushrooms collected from unpolluted (X), geologically specific (●), and anthropogenically contaminated (▲) sites and in cultivated species published since 2010. (Continued)

Species	<0.5	0.5–1	1–2	2–5	5–10	10–20	>20	References
Pleurotus ostreatus	▲	X	X, ▲			X		Gezer and Kaygusuz (2014), Mleczek, Niedzielski, Kalač, Budka, et al. (2016), Radulescu et al. (2010), Severoglu et al. (2013), Tel-Çayan et al.(2017), Zhu et al. (2011)
Polyporus squamosus					X			Sarikurkcu et al. (2011)
Ramaria aurea			X					Severoglu et al. (2013)
Ramaria botrytis					X			Turfan et al. (2018)
Ramaria stricta	X							Severoglu et al. (2013)
Russula delica		●						Aloupi et al. (2012)
Russula xerampelina		▲						Árvay et al. (2014)
Sarcodon imbricatus	$X^{C,S}$							Mędyk, Chudzińska, et al. (2017)
Sparassis crispa	X							Severoglu et al. (2013)
Suillus bovinus	▲	X						Mleczek, Niedzielski, Kalač, Budka, et al. (2016), Severoglu et al. (2013)
Suillus bellinii	●							Aloupi et al. (2012)
Suillus grevillei				▲				Árvay et al. (2014)
Suillus luteus		X						Gezer and Kaygusuz (2014)
Suillus variegatus	$X^{S,C}$							Szubstarska et al. (2012)
Terfezia claveryi				X				Kivrak (2015)
Terfezia olbiensis			X					Kivrak (2015)

Tricholoma equestre						●		Campos and Tejera (2011)
Tricholoma fracticum	X							Tel-Çayan et al.(2017)
Tricholoma imbricatum	X							Sarikurkcu et al. (2011)
Tricholoma matsutake				X				Liu et al. (2012)
Tricholoma portentosum		X						Širić, Humar, et al. (2016)
Tricholoma terreum	X	X			X			Gezer and Kaygusuz (2014), Severoglu et al. (2013), Širić, Humar, et al. (2016), Turfan et al. (2018)
Volvariella volvacea							X	Zhu et al. (2011)
Xerocomus badius	X, ▲	▲, ▲^{C,S}		X, X^{C,S}	▲			Dimitrijevic et al. (2016), Gąsecka et al. (2017), Kojta et al. (2012), Mleczek, Siwulski, Mikołajczak, Gąsecka, Sobieralski, et al. (2015), Mleczek, Siwulski, Mikołajczak, Goliński, et al. (2015), Mleczek, Magdziak, et al. (2016), Proskura et al. (2017)
Xerocomus chrysenteron	ND	X						Dimitrijevic et al. (2016), Sarikurkcu et al. (2011)
Xerocomus subtomentosus	X^{C}							Jarzyńska et al. (2012)
Cultivated								
A. arvensis	X							Rzymski, Mleczek, Siwulski, Jasińska, et al. (2017)
A. bisporus (unspecified)						X		Gaur et al. (2016)
A. bisporus (brown)	X							Rzymski, Mleczek, Siwulski, Jasińska, et al. (2017)

(*Continued*)

TABLE 4.5 Data on the mean content (mg kg^{-1} dry matter) of *chromium* in fruiting bodies of wild-growing mushrooms collected from unpolluted (X), geologically specific (●), and anthropogenically contaminated (▲) sites and in cultivated species published since 2010. (Continued)

Species	<0.5	0.5–1	1–2	2–5	5–10	10–20	>20	References
A. bisporus (white)	X						X	Mleczek, Rzymski, et al. (2018), Rzymski, Mleczek, Siwulski, Jasińska, et al. (2017)
Agaricus subrufescens	X							Rzymski, Mleczek, Siwulski, Jasińska, et al. (2017)
Auricularia auricula-judae	X							Mleczek, Rzymski, et al. (2018)
Auricularia thailandica				X				Bandara et al. (2017)
Calocybe indica				X				Gaur et al. (2016)
H. erinaceus							X	Turfan et al. (2018)
L. edodes	X	X		X	X		X	Gaur et al. (2016), Gonçalves et al. (2014), Mleczek, Siwulski, Rzymski, Niedzielski, et al. (2017), Mleczek, Rzymski, et al. (2018), Turfan et al. (2018)
M. gigantea					X			Gaur et al. (2016)
P. eryngii	X							Gonçalves et al. (2014), Rashid et al. (2018), Turfan et al. (2018)
P. ostreatus	X	X			X		X	Gonçalves et al. (2014), Mleczek, Rzymski, et al. (2018), Rashid et al. (2018)
Tremella fuciformis						X		Mleczek, Rzymski, et al. (2018)
V. volvacea							X	Mleczek, Rzymski, et al. (2018)

C, Caps; *ND*, below limit of detection; *S*, stipes; X^m, median value.

in Yunnan Province, China. Very high content (42.2 mg kg^{-1} DM) was observed in *L. perlatum* (Sarikurkcu et al., 2015).

Chromium is distributed evenly within caps and stipes. As was observed in several wild-growing species, chromium is not bioaccumulated in fruiting bodies. The determined BCF values were mostly below 0.5; somewhat higher levels were reported for stipes than for caps (Falandysz & Drewnowska, 2015a; Kułdo et al., 2014; Proskura et al., 2017; Širić, Humar, et al., 2016). Similar values were determined by Sithole, Mugivhisa, Amoo, and Olowoyo (2017) in *A. bisporus* (white and crimini varieties) cultivated in polluted soils.

Previous data refer to the total chromium content in mushrooms. However, although trivalent chromium Cr^{III} is necessary for the normal metabolism of cholesterol, fat, and glucose, hexavalent chromium Cr^{VI} is toxic. Figueiredo, Soares, Baptista, Castro, and Bastos (2007) determined mean contents of total chromium 1.14 and 1.11 mg kg^{-1} DM and those of hexavalent chromium 0.10 and 0.14 mg kg^{-1} DM in caps and stipes, respectively, of 15 species. The BCFs were always <1, whereas for Cr^{VI} these were 10 times higher than for total chromium. Unfortunately, further information on the proportion of Cr^{VI} in mushrooms is lacking.

Chromium content decreased by 40% of the initial level by blanching of *A. fulva* caps (Drewnowska, Falandysz, et al., 2017).

4.1.5 Fluorine

In a singular short communication, Lasota and Florczak (1983) reported fluorine contents of 1–9 mg kg^{-1} DM in 14 edible species from Poland.

4.1.6 Iodine (I)

Data on inorganic iodine content were reported by Vetter (2010). The mean content in 49 samples of wild-growing species was 0.28 ± 0.21 mg kg^{-1} DM. The highest values of 0.56 and 0.49 mg kg^{-1} DM were observed in *M. procera* and *C. nebularis*, respectively. The levels in wood-decaying species were significantly lower than in mycorrhizal and saprobic ones. Mean values for cultivated *A. bisporus*, *P. ostreatus*, and *L. edodes* were 0.17, 0.19, and 0.15 mg kg^{-1} DM, respectively.

Overall, mushrooms seem to be a very limited source of dietary iodine. Nevertheless, this data originated from inland Hungary. It would be useful to obtain information from coastal sites with elevated iodine content in soils and in precipitation.

4.1.7 Iron (Fe)

Iron is one the most frequently determined trace elements in mushrooms (Table 4.6). The extent of usual iron contents in wild species is very wide,

TABLE 4.6 Data on the mean content (mg kg^{-1} dry matter) of *iron* in fruiting bodies of wild-growing mushrooms collected from unpolluted (X), geologically specific (●), and anthropogenically contaminated (▲) sites and in cultivated species published since 2010.

Species	<50	50–100	100–200	200–300	300–400	400–500	500–1000	>1000	References
Wild growing									
Agaricus arvensis				X				X	Ayaz et al. (2011), Sarikurkcu et al. (2011)
Agaricus bisporus			X						Zhu et al. (2011)
Agaricus campestris	X, $X^{C,S}$		X, $▲^{C,S}$	X					Kosanić et al. (2017), Sarikurkcu et al. (2012), Severoglu et al. (2013), Širić, Kasap, et al. (2016), Zsigmond et al. (2018)
Agaricus lanipes			X						Gezer et al. (2016)
Agrocybe aegerita			X						Zhu et al. (2011)
Agrocybe cylindracea		X							Sarikurkcu et al. (2012)
Albatrellus ovinus	$X^{S,C}$								Mędyk, Grembecka, et al. (2017)
Amanita caesarea								X	Sarikurkcu et al. (2010)
Amanita fulva	$X^{C,S}$								Falandysz, Drewnowska, et al. (2017)
Amanita ponderosa		X							Salvador et al. (2018)
Armillariella mellea		X		X		$X^{C,S}$	▲		Georgescu et al. (2016), Radulescu et al. (2010), Širić, Kasap, et al. (2016), Zavastin et al. (2018)

Boletus aestivalis		X					$X^{S,C}$		Širić et al. (2014), Širić, Kasap, et al. (2016), Wang et al. (2017)
Boletus appendiculatus		X, X^{Sm}	X^{Cm}				X^{C}	X^{S}	Alaimo et al. (2018), Dimitrijevic et al. (2016), Sun et al. (2017), Wang et al. (2015)
Boletus bicolor			X						Sun et al. (2017)
Boletus brunneissimus							$X^{S,C}$		Wang et al. (2015)
Boletus crocipodium			X						Sun et al. (2017)
Boletus edulis	X, X^{C}	X, $X^{S,C}$	X, X^{S}				X^{S}	X^{C}	Ayaz et al. (2011), Cvetkovic et al. (2015), Dimitrijevic et al. (2016), Falandysz et al. (2011), Frankowska et al. (2010), Georgescu et al. (2016), Kosanić et al. (2017), Mędyk, Grembecka, et al. (2017), Mleczek, Siwulski, Stuper-Szablewska, Sobieralski, et al. (2013), Mleczek, Siwulski, Mikołajczak, Goliński, et al. (2015), Sarikurkcu et al. (2015), Širić, Kasap, et al. (2016), Sun et al. (2017), Turfan et al. (2018), Wang et al. (2015), Zhang et al. (2010), Zavastin et al. (2018)

(*Continued*)

TABLE 4.6 Data on the mean content (mg kg^{-1} dry matter) of *iron* in fruiting bodies of wild-growing mushrooms collected from unpolluted (X), geologically specific (●), and anthropogenically contaminated (▲) sites and in cultivated species published since 2010. (Continued)

Species	<50	50–100	100–200	200–300	300–400	400–500	500–1000	>1000	References
Boletus flammans			X						Sun et al. (2017)
Boletus griseus	X		X			X^{C}	X^{S}	$X^{C,S}$	Liu et al. (2012), Sun et al. (2017), Wang et al. (2015, 2017)
Boletus impolitus	X						X^{C}	X^{S}	Dimitrijevic et al. (2016), Wang et al. (2017)
Boletus luridus								$X^{S,C}$	Wang et al. (2015)
Boletus pallidus								$X^{S,C}$	Wang et al. (2015)
Boletus pulverulentus			▲						Árvay et al. (2014)
Boletus regius	X								Dimitrijevic et al. (2016)
Boletus rubellus								$X^{S,C}$	Wang et al. (2015)
Boletus sinicus			X						Sun et al. (2017)
Boletus speciosus		X					$X^{C,S}$	X^{C}	Liu et al. (2012), Sun et al. (2017), Wang et al. (2015, 2017)
Boletus tomentipes					X^{S}		X^{C}	$X^{C,S}$	Wang et al. (2015, 2015a)
Boletus umbriniporus					X^{S}		$X^{S,C}$		Wang et al. (2015, 2017)
Calocybe gambosa	X								Severoglu et al. (2013)

Cantharellus cibarius	X^{C}, ▲	X, ▲	X,X^{S}		X				Árvay et al. (2014), Ayaz et al. (2011), Brzezicha-Cirocka et al. (2016), Cvetkovic et al. (2015), Drewnowska and Falandysz (2015), Falandysz and Drewnowska (2015a), Georgescu et al. (2016), Mleczek, Siwulski, Stuper-Szablewska, Sobieralski, et al. (2013), Mleczek, Niedzielski, Kalač, Budka, et al. (2016), Zavastin et al. (2018)
Cantharellus tubaeformis			X						Ayaz et al. (2011)
Clitocybe geotropa							X		Sarikurkcu et al. (2010)
Clitocybe inversa		X							Širić, Kasap, et al. (2016)
Clitocybe nebularis		X							Širić, Kasap, et al. (2016)
Clitopilus prunulus				X^{m}					Alaimo et al. (2018)
Collybia velutipes			X						Zhu et al. (2011)
Coprinus comatus		X	X						Severoglu et al. (2013), Zhu et al. (2011)
Craterellus cornucopioides							X		Turfan et al. (2018)
Fistulina hepatica					▲				Radulescu et al. (2010),

(*Continued*)

TABLE 4.6 Data on the mean content (mg kg^{-1} dry matter) of *iron* in fruiting bodies of wild-growing mushrooms collected from unpolluted (X), geologically specific (●), and anthropogenically contaminated (▲) sites and in cultivated species published since 2010. (Continued)

Species	<50	50–100	100–200	200–300	300–400	400–500	500–1000	>1000	References
Gomphidius glutinosus		X^S	X^C						Mędyk, Grembecka, et al. (2017)
Gomphus clavatus								X	Sarikurkcu et al. (2015)
Helvella leucopus			X	X					Gezer and Kaygusuz (2014), Sarikurkcu et al. (2012)
Hericium erinaceus			X						Zhu et al. (2011)
Hydnum repandum	X	X	X						Ayaz et al. (2011), Jedidi et al. (2017), Severoglu et al. (2013)
Hypsizygus marmoreus		X							Zhu et al. (2011)
Laccaria laccata					X			▲	Ayaz et al. (2011), Baumann, Arnold, and Haferburg (2014)
Lactarius deliciosus	X, ●		X	X					Aloupi et al. (2012), Gezer and Kaygusuz (2014), Jedidi et al. (2017), Mleczek, Siwulski, Stuper-Szablewska, Sobieralski, et al. (2013), Severoglu et al. (2013), Turfan et al. (2018)
Lactarius deterrimus	X								Širić, Kasap, et al. (2016)
Lactarius hygrophoroides	X								Liu et al. (2012)

Lactarius piperatus		X							Cvetkovic et al. (2015)
Lactarius salmonicolor		X		X					Sarikurkcu et al. (2011), Severoglu et al. (2013)
Lactarius sanguifluus	●								Aloupi et al. (2012)
Lactarius semisanguifluus	●								Aloupi et al. (2012)
Laetiporus sulphureus		X	X						Severoglu et al. (2013), Turfan et al. (2018)
Leccinum aurantiacum			X	X					Brzezicha-Cirocka et al. (2016), Mleczek, Siwulski, Stuper-Szablewska, Sobieralski, et al. (2013)
Leccinum crocipodium	X		X						Dimitrijevic et al. (2016), Sun et al. (2017)
Leccinum duriusculum	$X^{S,C}$								Jarzyńska and Falandysz (2012a)
Leccinum griseum	X^{S}	X^{C}							Jarzyńska and Falandysz (2012b)
Leccinum pseudoscabrum	X								Dimitrijevic et al. (2016)
Leccinum scabrum	X, ▲	X					▲		Baumann et al. (2014), Mędyk, Grembecka, et al. (2017), Mleczek, Siwulski, Mikołajczak, Goliński, et al. (2015), Mleczek, Niedzielski, Kalač, Budka, et al. (2016)

(Continued)

TABLE 4.6 Data on the mean content (mg kg^{-1} dry matter) of *iron* in fruiting bodies of wild-growing mushrooms collected from unpolluted (X), geologically specific (●), and anthropogenically contaminated (▲) sites and in cultivated species published since 2010. (Continued)

Species	<50	50–100	100–200	200–300	300–400	400–500	500–1000	>1000	References
Leccinum versipelle		X			▲				Baumann et al. (2014), Mędyk, Grembecka, et al. (2017)
Leccinum rugosiceps					X^S	X^C			Wang et al. (2017)
Lentinula edodes		X							Zhu et al. (2011)
Lentinus cladopus					X				Mallikarjuna et al. (2013)
Lepista nuda			X						Ayaz et al. (2011)
Lepista sordida							X		Zhu et al. (2011)
Leucoagaricus leucothites							X		Sarikurkcu et al. (2010)
Leucopaxillus giganteus							X		Liu et al. (2012)
Lycoperdon perlatum			X			X	▲	X	Brzezicha-Cirocka et al. (2016), Mędyk, Grembecka, et al. (2017), Radulescu et al. (2010), Sarikurkcu et al. (2015)
Macrocybe gigantea		X							Liu et al. (2012)
Macrolepiota excoriata			X^C				X^S		Georgescu et al. (2016)

Macrolepiota procera	X, X^C		▲, X, $X^{C,S}$				X^S	X	Árvay et al. (2014), Georgescu et al. (2016), Gucia et al. (2012), Kojta et al. (2011), Kułdo et al. (2014), Sarikurkcu et al. (2015), Severoglu et al. (2013), Širić, Kasap, et al. (2016)
Marasmius oreades					X		X		Cvetkovic et al. (2015), Turfan et al. (2018)
Melanoleuca arcuata	X								Liu et al. (2012)
Morchella conica					X				Turfan et al. (2018)
Morchella deliciosa	X								Liu et al. (2012)
Morchella esculenta	X		X						Gezer and Kaygusuz (2014), Sarikurkcu et al. (2012)
Mycena haematopus			X						Liu et al. (2012)
Pleurotus djamor			X						Mallikarjuna et al. (2013)
Pleurotus eryngii				X					Zhu et al. (2011)
Pleurotus nebrodensis			X						Zhu et al. (2011)
Pleurotus ostreatus	$X^{S,C}$, X, ▲	X			X, ▲				Georgescu et al. (2016), Gezer and Kaygusuz (2014), Mleczek, Niedzielski, Kalač, Budka, et al. (2016), Radulescu et al. (2010), Severoglu et al. (2013), Širić, Kasap, et al. (2016), Tel-Çayan et al. (2017), Zhu et al. (2011)

(*Continued*)

TABLE 4.6 Data on the mean content (mg kg^{-1} dry matter) of *iron* in fruiting bodies of wild-growing mushrooms collected from unpolluted (X), geologically specific (●), and anthropogenically contaminated (▲) sites and in cultivated species published since 2010. (Continued)

Species	<50	50–100	100–200	200–300	300–400	400–500	500–1000	>1000	References
Polyporus squamosus			X						Sarikurkcu et al. (2011)
Ramaria aurea	X								Severoglu et al. (2013)
Ramaria botrytis				X					Turfan et al. (2018)
Ramaria stricta	X								Severoglu et al. (2013)
Russula aeruginea				X^{C}	X^{S}				Elekes and Busuioc (2013)
Russula alutacea		X^{S}	$X^{C,S}$				X^{C}		Elekes and Busuioc (2013), Georgescu et al. (2016)
Russula cyanoxantha	X^{S}		$X^{C,S}$		X^{C}				Elekes and Busuioc (2013), Georgescu et al. (2016)
Russula delica	●								Aloupi et al. (2012)
Russula lepida					X^{S}		X^{C}		Elekes and Busuioc (2013)
Russula vesca			$X^{S,C}$						Elekes and Busuioc (2013)
Russula virescens	X^{S}	X^{C}							Elekes and Busuioc (2013)
Russula xerampelina					▲				Árvay et al. (2014)
Sparassis crispa	X								Severoglu et al. (2013)
Suillus bellinii	●								Aloupi et al. (2012)
Suillus bovinus	X	$X^{C,S}$							Mędyk, Grembecka, et al. (2017), Severoglu et al. (2013)
Suillus grevillei							▲		Árvay et al. (2014)

Suillus luteus		X	$X^{S,C}$, X						Gezer and Kaygusuz (2014), Mędyk, Grembecka, et al. (2017), Mleczek, Siwulski, Stuper-Szablewska, Sobieralski, et al. (2013)
Suillus variegatus							X^{S}	X^{C}	Szubstarska et al. (2012)
Terfezia claveryi	X							X	Kivrak (2015), Vahdani et al. (2017)
Terfezia olbiensis		X							Kivrak (2015)
Tirmania nivea								X	Vahdani et al. (2017)
Tricholoma equestre	X								Jedidi et al. (2017)
Tricholoma fracticum				X					Tel-Çayan et al. (2017)
Tricholoma imbricatum							X		Sarikurkcu et al. (2011)
Tricholoma matsutake	X								Li et al. (2013), Liu et al. (2012)
Tricholoma portentosum			X						Širić, Kasap, et al. (2016)
Tricholoma terreum	X	X	X				X		Gezer and Kaygusuz (2014), Severoglu et al. (2013), Širić, Kasap, et al. (2016), Turfan et al. (2018)
Volvariella volvacea		X							Zhu et al. (2011)

(*Continued*)

TABLE 4.6 Data on the mean content (mg kg^{-1} dry matter) of *iron* in fruiting bodies of wild-growing mushrooms collected from unpolluted (X), geologically specific (●), and anthropogenically contaminated (▲) sites and in cultivated species published since 2010. (Continued)

Species	<50	50–100	100–200	200–300	300–400	400–500	500–1000	>1000	References
Xerocomus badius	X, ▲, $▲^{S,C}$	$X^{C,S}$, ▲	X^{C},X	X					Dimitrijevic et al. (2016), Gąsecka et al. (2017), Kojta et al. (2012), Mleczek, Siwulski, Stuper-Szablewska, Sobieralski, et al. (2013), Mleczek, Siwulski, Kaczmarek, et al. (2013), Mleczek, Siwulski, Mikołajczak, Gąsecka, Sobieralski, et al. (2015), Mleczek, Siwulski, Mikołajczak, Goliński, et al. (2015), Mleczek, Magdziak, et al. (2016), Podlasińska et al. (2015), Proskura et al. (2017)
Xerocomus chrysenteron	X		X						Dimitrijevic et al. (2016), Sarikurkcu et al. (2011)
Xerocomus spadiceus								$X^{C,S}$	Wang et al. (2017)
Xerocomus subtomentosus	$X^{S,C}$	X^{C}							Jarzyńska et al. (2012), Mędyk, Grembecka, et al. (2017)

Cultivated									
A. arvensis		X							Rzymski, Mleczek, Siwulski, Jasińska, et al. (2017)
A. bisporus (unspecified)						X			Gaur et al. (2016)
A. bisporus (brown)	X	X							Bach et al. (2017), Rzymski, Mleczek, Siwulski, Jasińska, et al. (2017)
A. bisporus (white)	X	X	X						Bach et al. (2017), Huang, Jia, Wan, Li, and Jiang (2015), Jedidi et al. (2017), Mleczek, Rzymski, et al. (2018), Rzymski, Mleczek, Siwulski, Jasińska, et al. (2017)
Agaricus subrufescens		X	X						Bach et al. (2017), Rzymski, Mleczek, Siwulski, Jasińska, et al. (2017)
Agrocybe chaxinggu				X					Huang et al. (2015)
A. cylindracea		X							Niedzielski et al. (2017)
A. mellea							X		Huang et al. (2015)
Auricularia auricula-judae					X	X			Huang et al. (2015), Mleczek, Rzymski, et al. (2018)
Auricularia polytricha		X							Niedzielski et al. (2017)
Auricularia thailandica		X							Bandara et al. (2017)

(*Continued*)

TABLE 4.6 Data on the mean content (mg kg^{-1} dry matter) of *iron* in fruiting bodies of wild-growing mushrooms collected from unpolluted (X), geologically specific (●), and anthropogenically contaminated (▲) sites and in cultivated species published since 2010. (Continued)

Species	<50	50–100	100–200	200–300	300–400	400–500	500–1000	>1000	References
Calocybe indica			X						Gaur et al. (2016)
Clitocybe maxima	X								Niedzielski et al. (2017)
Flammulina velutipes			X						Bach et al. (2017), Huang et al. (2015), Niedzielski et al. (2017)
Grifola frondosa				X					Niedzielski et al. (2017)
H. erinaceus		X							Niedzielski et al. (2017), Turfan et al. (2018)
L. sulphureus			X						Niedzielski et al. (2017)
L. edodes	X	X	X	X					Bach et al. (2017), Gaur et al. (2016), Gonçalves et al. (2014), Huang et al. (2015), Mallikarjuna et al. (2013), Mleczek, Siwulski, Rzymski, Niedzielski, et al. (2017), MMleczek, Rzymski, et al. (2018), Turfan et al. (2018)
M. gigantea			X						Gaur et al. (2016)
Pholiota nameko			X		X				Huang et al. (2015), Niedzielski et al. (2017)

P. djamor			X						Bach et al. (2017)
P. eryngii			X	X					Bach et al. (2017), Gonçalves et al. (2014)
Pleurotus floridanus		X							Mallikarjuna et al. (2013)
P. ostreatus		X	X	X					Bach et al. (2017), Gonçalves et al. (2014), Huang et al. (2015), Mleczek, Rzymski, et al. (2018), Turfan et al. (2018)
Pleurotus sajor-caju			X						Gaur et al. (2016)
Trametes versicolor			X						Niedzielski et al. (2017)
Tremella fuciformis	X	X	X						Huang et al. (2015), Mleczek, Rzymski, et al. (2018), Niedzielski et al. (2017)
V. volvacea				X					Mleczek, Rzymski, et al. (2018)

C, Caps; *S*, stipes; X^m, median value.

between <50 and 1000 mg kg^{-1} DM. Content above 1000 mg kg^{-1} DM often occur in *Boletus* spp. These levels are higher than those reported until 2010 (Kalač, 2010). Usual levels in cultivated species are lower, <50–300 mg kg^{-1} DM. *Suillus variegatus* was known for decades as a highly accumulating species. Extreme levels 24,600, 6760, 4660, and 4200 mg kg^{-1} DM were observed in *L. perlatum* (Sarikurkcu et al., 2015), in stipes of *X. spadiceous* (Wang et al., 2017), in caps of *B. edulis* (Wang et al., 2015), and in *Amanita caesarea* (Sarikurkcu et al., 2010), respectively.

Distribution of iron within fruiting bodies seems to be even in many species, although the content in some is higher in caps than in stipes. The peel of caps had significantly higher levels of iron than caps in white, brown, and portobello varieties of cultivated *A. bisporus* (Muszyńska et al., 2017).

The reported BCF values were very low, below 0.1 (e.g., Falandysz & Drewnowska, 2015a; Kułdo et al., 2014; Proskura et al., 2017). Iron, thus, belongs among trace elements bioexcluded by mushrooms.

According to the WHO data, dietary iron shortage is the most prevalent nutritional deficiency worldwide and affects more than two billion people, particularly young children and women of reproductive age living in developing countries. Foods of animal origin are the main sources of dietary iron, particularly in its heminic form (Fe^{II}). Therefore initial investigations to fortify cultivated *P. ostreatus* with iron have been undertaken. Fruiting bodies growing on coffee husks enriched with a solution of ferrous sulfate at level of 0.8 mg Fe kg^{-1} contained 149 mg kg^{-1} DM of iron in comparison with the content 112 mg kg^{-1} DM in those produced in the control unsupplemented variant (Vieira et al., 2013). Yokota et al. (2016) tested considerably higher doses of iron, up to 1500 mg Fe kg^{-1} applying ferrous sulfate solution to a substrate consisting of sugarcane bagasse and soybean fiber. Substrate naturally contained 22 mg Fe kg^{-1}. Fruiting bodies occurred only on the substrates with iron levels up to 500 mg kg^{-1} DM. Nevertheless, the yields decreased with increasing supplementation of the substrate. Biological efficiency, a ratio between FM of produced mushrooms to DM of the substrate expressed in percent, decreased from 36.5% in the control variant to 19.2% and 2.1% in the substrate variants with 200 and 500 mg Fe kg^{-1}, respectively. The respective iron contents in fruiting bodies were 108, 262, and 479 mg kg^{-1} DM and its in vitro determined bioavailability was 64.8%, 60.8%, and 61.4%. The bioaccumulation of iron was higher in the mycelium than in the fruiting bodies.

4.1.8 Manganese (Mn)

Data on manganese content in edible mushrooms have grown considerably during the past decade (Table 4.7). Usual contents range between <25 − 75 and <25 mg kg^{-1} DM in wild-growing and cultivated fruiting bodies, respectively. However, highly elevated levels were reported. The highest

TABLE 4.7 Data on the mean content (mg kg^{-1} dry matter) of *manganese* in fruiting bodies of wild-growing mushrooms collected from unpolluted (X), geologically specific (●), and anthropogenically contaminated (▲) sites and in cultivated species published since 2010.

Species	<25	25–50	50–75	75–100	>100	References
Wild growing						
Agaricus arvensis		X	X			Ayaz et al. (2011), Sarikurkcu et al. (2011)
Agaricus bisporus		X				Zhu et al. (2011)
Agaricus campestris	X, $X^{S,C}$, $▲^{S,C}$					Kosanić et al. (2017), Sarikurkcu et al. (2012), Zsigmond et al. (2018)
Agaricus lanipes		X				Gezer et al. (2016)
Agrocybe aegerita	X					Zhu et al. (2011)
Agrocybe cylindracea	X					Sarikurkcu et al. (2012)
Albatrellus ovinus	$X^{C,S}$					Mędyk, Grembecka, et al. (2017)
Armillariella mellea	▲	X, $X^{C,S}$				Georgescu et al. (2016), Radulescu et al. (2010), Zavastin et al. (2018)
Amanita fulva	$X^{C,S}$					Falandysz, Drewnowska, et al. (2017)
Amanita ponderosa			X			Salvador et al. (2018)
Boletus aestivalis		$X^{C,S}$				Wang et al. (2017)
Boletus appendiculatus	X, $X^{S,Cm}$	X^{C}		X^{S}		Alaimo et al. (2018), Falandysz, Chudzińska, et al. (2017), Wang et al. (2015)

(*Continued*)

TABLE 4.7 Data on the mean content (mg kg^{-1} dry matter) of *manganese* in fruiting bodies of wild-growing mushrooms collected from unpolluted (X), geologically specific (●), and anthropogenically contaminated (▲) sites and in cultivated species published since 2010. (Continued)

Species	<25	25–50	50–75	75–100	>100	References
Boletus brunneissimus		$X^{C,S}$				Wang et al. (2015)
Boletus edulis	X, $X^{C,S}$	X, $X^{C,S}$	X, X^{S}		X^{S}	Ayaz et al. (2011), Brzezicha-Cirocka et al. (2016), Cvetkovic et al. (2015), Dimitrijevic et al. (2016), Falandysz et al. (2011); Falandysz, Chudzińska, et al. (2017), Frankowska et al. (2010), Georgescu et al. (2016), Giannaccini et al. (2012), Kosanić et al. (2017), Mazurkiewicz and Podlasińska (2014), Mędyk, Grembecka, et al. (2017), Mleczek, Siwulski, Stuper-Szablewska, Sobieralski, et al. (2013), Mleczek, Siwulski, Mikołajczak, Goliński, et al. (2015), Turfan et al. (2018), Wang et al. (2015), Zhang et al. (2010), Zavastin et al. (2018)
Boletus griseus	$X^{C,S}$	X^{C}	X,X^{S}			Liu et al. (2012), Wang et al. (2015, 2017)
Boletus impolitus	X, X^{C}	X^{S}				Dimitrijevic et al. (2016), Wang et al. (2017)
Boletus luridus	$X^{C,S}$	●^{C,S}	X^{C}	X^{S}		Falandysz, Zhang, Wiejak, et al. (2017), Wang et al. (2015, 2017)
Boletus magnificus	●^{C,S}					Falandysz, Zhang, Wiejak, et al. (2017)
Boletus pallidus		$X^{C,S}$				Wang et al. (2015)
Boletus pinophilus	X					Dospatliev and Ivanova (2017)

Boletus pulverulentus	▲					Árvay et al. (2014)
Boletus regius	X					Dimitrijevic et al. (2016)
Boletus rubellus		X^{C}	X^{S}			Wang et al. (2015)
Boletus speciosus	X, $X^{C,S}$	X^{S}				Liu et al. (2012), Wang et al. (2015, 2017)
Boletus tomentipes	X^{C}, $●^{C}$	X^{S}, $●^{S}$				Falandysz, Zhang, Wiejak, et al. (2017), Wang et al. (2015)
Boletus umbriniporus	X^{C}	$X^{C,S}$				Wang et al. (2015, 2017)
Cantharellus cibarius	X, $X^{C,S}$, ▲	X, ▲				Árvay et al. (2014), Ayaz et al. (2011), Brzezicha-Cirocka et al. (2016), Cvetkovic et al. (2015), Drewnowska and Falandysz (2015), Falandysz and Drewnowska (2015a), Falandysz, Chudzińska, et al. (2017), Georgescu et al. (2016), Mazurkiewicz and Podlasińska (2014), Mleczek, Siwulski, Stuper-Szablewska, Sobieralski, et al. (2013), Mleczek, Niedzielski, Kalač, Budka, et al. (2016), Zavastin et al. (2018)
Cantharellus tubaeformis		X				Ayaz et al. (2011), Falandysz, Chudzińska, et al. (2017)
Clitocybe geotropa		X				Sarikurkcu et al. (2010)
Clitopilus prunulus		X^{m}				Alaimo et al. (2018)
Collybia velutipes		X				Zhu et al. (2011)
Coprinus comatus		X				Zhu et al. (2011)
Craterellus cornucopioides					X	Turfan et al. (2018)

(*Continued*)

TABLE 4.7 Data on the mean content (mg kg^{-1} dry matter) of *manganese* in fruiting bodies of wild-growing mushrooms collected from unpolluted (X), geologically specific (●), and anthropogenically contaminated (▲) sites and in cultivated species published since 2010. (Continued)

Species	<25	25–50	50–75	75–100	>100	References
Fistulina hepatica	▲					Radulescu et al. (2010)
Gomphidius glutinosus	$X^{S,C}$					Mędyk, Grembecka, et al. (2017)
Gomphus clavatus		X				Sarikurkcu et al. (2015)
Helvella leucopus	X					Gezer and Kaygusuz (2014), Sarikurkcu et al. (2012)
Hericium erinaceus	X					Zhu et al. (2011)
Hydnum imbricatum	$X^{S,C}$					Mędyk, Chudzińska, et al. (2017)
Hydnum repandum	X					Ayaz et al. (2011)
Hypsizygus marmoreus				X		Zhu et al. (2011)
Laccaria laccata		X	▲			Ayaz et al. (2011), Baumann et al. (2014)
Lactarius deliciosus	●	X	X			Aloupi et al. (2012), Gezer and Kaygusuz (2014), Mleczek, Siwulski, Stuper-Szablewska, Sobieralski, et al. (2013), Turfan et al. (2018)
Lactarius hygrophoroides	X					Liu et al. (2012)
Lactarius piperatus	X					Cvetkovic et al. (2015)
Lactarius salmonicolor	X					Sarikurkcu et al. (2011)
Lactarius sanguifluus	●					Aloupi et al. (2012)
Lactarius semesanguifluus	V					Aloupi et al. (2012)

Laetiporus sulphureus	X			X		Sarikurkcu et al. (2015), Turfan et al. (2018)
Leccinum aurantiacum	X					Brzezicha-Cirocka et al. (2016), Mleczek, Siwulski, Stuper-Szablewska, Sobieralski, et al. (2013)
Leccinum crocipodium	X					Dimitrijevic et al. (2016)
Leccinum duriusculum	$X^{S,C}$					Jarzyńska and Falandysz (2012a)
Leccinum griseum	$X^{S,C}$					Jarzyńska and Falandysz (2012b)
Leccinum pseudoscabrum	X					Dimitrijevic et al. (2016)
Leccinum rugosiceps	$X^{C,S}$					Wang et al. (2017)
Leccinum scabrum	X, ▲		▲			Baumann et al. (2014), Mędyk, Grembecka, et al. (2017), Mleczek, Siwulski, Mikołajczak, Goliński, et al. (2015), Mleczek, Niedzielski, Kalač, Budka, et al. (2016)
Leccinum versipelle	X, ▲					Baumann et al. (2014), Mędyk, Grembecka, et al. (2017)
Lentinula edodes		X				Zhu et al. (2011)
Lentinus cladopus	X					Mallikarjuna et al. (2013)
Lepista nuda			X			Ayaz et al. (2011)
Lepista sordida			X			Zhu et al. (2011)
Leucoagaricus leucothites		X				Sarikurkcu et al. (2010)
Leucopaxillus giganteus			X			Liu et al. (2012)
Lycoperdon perlatum	X,▲	X				Brzezicha-Cirocka et al. (2016), Mędyk, Grembecka, et al. (2017), Radulescu et al. (2010)

(*Continued*)

TABLE 4.7 Data on the mean content (mg kg^{-1} dry matter) of *manganese* in fruiting bodies of wild-growing mushrooms collected from unpolluted (X), geologically specific (●), and anthropogenically contaminated (▲) sites and in cultivated species published since 2010. (Continued)

Species	<25	25–50	50–75	75–100	>100	References
Macrocybe gigantea	X					Liu et al. (2012)
Macrolepiota excoriata		X^{C}		X^{S}		Georgescu et al. (2016)
Macrolepiota procera	$X^{C,S}$, X	$X^{S,C}$, ▲	X, X^{S}	X^{S}		Árvay et al. (2014), Georgescu et al. (2016), Giannaccini et al. (2012), Gucia et al. (2012), Jarzyńska et al. (2011), Kojta et al. (2011), Kułdo et al. (2014), Mazurkiewicz and Podlasińska (2014), Sarikurkcu et al. (2015)
Marasmius oreades		X		X		Cvetkovic et al. (2015), Turfan et al. (2018)
Melanoleuca arcuata	X					Liu et al. (2012)
Morchella conica					X	Turfan et al. (2018),
Morchella deliciosa			X			Liu et al. (2012)
Morchella esculenta	X	X				Gezer and Kaygusuz (2014), Rossbach et al. (2017), Sarikurkcu et al. (2012)
Mycena haematopus	X					Liu et al. (2012)
Pleurotus djamor	X					Mallikarjuna et al. (2013)
Pleurotus eryngii	X					Zhu et al. (2011)
Pleurotus nebrodensis		X				Zhu et al. (2011)
Pleurotus ostreatus	X, ▲, $X^{S,C}$	X				Georgescu et al. (2016), Gezer and Kaygusuz (2014), Mleczek, Niedzielski, Kalač, Budka, et al. (2016), Radulescu et al. (2010), Tel-Çayan et al.(2017), Zhu et al. (2011)

Polyporus squamosus	X					Sarikurkcu et al. (2011)
Ramaria botrytis					X	Turfan et al. (2018)
Russula aeruginea			$X^{S,C}$			Elekes and Busuioc (2013)
Russula alutacea	X^{S}	X^{C}				Georgescu et al. (2016)
Russula cyanoxantha	X^{S}	X^{C}				Elekes and Busuioc (2013), Georgescu et al. (2016)
Russula delica	●					Aloupi et al. (2012)
Russula lepida				X^{S}		Elekes and Busuioc (2013)
Russula vesca	$X^{C,S}$					Elekes and Busuioc (2013)
Russula virescens	$X^{C,S}$					Elekes and Busuioc (2013)
Russula xerampelina	▲					Árvay et al. (2014)
Suillus bellinii	●					Aloupi et al. (2012)
Suillus bovinus	$X^{C,S}$					Mędyk, Grembecka, et al. (2017)
Suillus grevillei				▲		Árvay et al. (2014)
Suillus luteus	$X^{S,C}$, X		X			Gezer and Kaygusuz (2014), Mędyk, Grembecka, et al. (2017), Mleczek, Siwulski, Stuper-Szablewska, Sobieralski, et al. (2013)
Suillus variegatus	X^{C}	X^{S}				Szubstarska et al. (2012)
Terfezia claveryi		X		X		Kivrak (2015), Vahdani et al. (2017)
Tirmania nivea		X				Vahdani et al. (2017)
Tricholoma fracticum	X					Tel-Çayan et al.(2017)

(*Continued*)

TABLE 4.7 Data on the mean content (mg kg^{-1} dry matter) of *manganese* in fruiting bodies of wild-growing mushrooms collected from unpolluted (X), geologically specific (●), and anthropogenically contaminated (▲) sites and in cultivated species published since 2010. (Continued)

Species	<25	25–50	50–75	75–100	>100	References
Tricholoma imbricatum		X				Sarikurkcu et al. (2011)
Tricholoma matsutake	X					Li et al. (2013), Liu et al. (2012)
Tricholoma terreum		X				Gezer and Kaygusuz (2014), Turfan et al. (2018)
Volvariella volvacea	X					Zhu et al. (2011)
Xerocomus badius	▲, $X^{C,S}$, X, X^{C}, $▲^{C}$	▲, $▲^{S}$, X^{S}		▲		Dimitrijevic et al. (2016), Gąsecka et al. (2017), Kojta et al. (2012), Kojta and Falandysz (2016a), Mleczek, Siwulski, Stuper-Szablewska, Sobieralski, et al. (2013), Mleczek, Siwulski, Kaczmarek, et al. (2013), Mleczek, Siwulski, Mikołajczak, Gąsecka, Sobieralski, et al. (2015), Mleczek, Siwulski, Mikołajczak, Goliński, et al. (2015), Mleczek, Magdziak, et al. (2016), Podlasińska et al. (2015), Proskura et al. (2017)
Xerocomus chrysenteron	X	X				Dimitrijevic et al. (2016), Sarikurkcu et al. (2011)
Xerocomus spadiceous		X^{C}			X^{S}	Wang et al. (2017)
Xerocomus subtomentosus	$X^{C,S}$					Jarzyńska et al. (2012), Mędyk, Grembecka, et al. (2017)

Cultivated						
A. arvensis	X					Rzymski, Mleczek, Siwulski, Jasińska, et al. (2017)
A. bisporus (unspecified)		X				Gaur et al. (2016)
A. bisporus (brown)	X					Bach et al. (2017), Rzymski, Mleczek, Siwulski, Jasińska, et al. (2017)
A. bisporus (white)	X					Bach et al. (2017), Mleczek, Rzymski, et al. (2018), Rzymski, Mleczek, Siwulski, Jasińska, et al. (2017)
Agaricus subrufescens	X					Bach et al. (2017), Rzymski, Mleczek, Siwulski, Jasińska, et al. (2017)
A. cylindracea	X					Niedzielski et al. (2017)
Auricularia auricula-judae	X					Mleczek, Rzymski, et al. (2018)
Auricularia polytricha	X					Niedzielski et al. (2017)
Auricularia thailandica	X					Bandara et al. (2017)
Calocybe indica	X					Gaur et al. (2016)
Clitocybe maxima	X					Niedzielski et al. (2017)
Flammulina velutipes	X					Bach et al. (2017), Niedzielski et al. (2017)
Grifola frondosa		X				Niedzielski et al. (2017)
H. erinaceus	X	X				Niedzielski et al. (2017), Turfan et al. (2018)
L. sulphureus	X					Niedzielski et al. (2017)

(*Continued*)

TABLE 4.7 Data on the mean content (mg kg^{-1} dry matter) of *manganese* in fruiting bodies of wild-growing mushrooms collected from unpolluted (X), geologically specific (●), and anthropogenically contaminated (▲) sites and in cultivated species published since 2010. (Continued)

Species	<25	25–50	50–75	75–100	>100	References
L. edodes	X	X	X			Bach et al. (2017), Gaur et al. (2016), Gonçalves et al. (2014), Mallikarjuna et al. (2013), Mleczek, Siwulski, Rzymski, Niedzielski, et al. (2017), Mleczek, Rzymski, et al. (2018), Turfan et al. (2018)
M. gigantea	X					Gaur et al. (2016)
Pholiota nameko	X					Niedzielski et al. (2017)
P. djamor	X					Bach et al. (2017)
P. eryngii	X					Bach et al. (2017), Gonçalves et al. (2014), Rashid et al. (2018)
Pleurotus floridanus	X					Mallikarjuna et al. (2013)
P. ostreatus	X	X				Bach et al. (2017), Gonçalves et al. (2014), Mleczek, Rzymski, et al. (2018), Rashid et al. (2018), Turfan et al. (2018)
Pleurotus sajor-caju		X				Gaur et al. (2016)
Trametes versicolor		X				Niedzielski et al. (2017)
Tremella fuciformis	X	X				Mleczek, Rzymski, et al. (2018), Niedzielski et al. (2017)
V. volvacea	X					Mleczek, Rzymski, et al. (2018)

C, Caps; *S*, stipes; X^m, median value.

content of 514 mg kg^{-1} DM was observed in *L. perlatum* (Sarikurkcu et al., 2015). Elekes and Busuioc (2013) found 219 ± 310 and 183 ± 259 mg kg^{-1} DM in caps and stipes, respectively, of *Russula alutacea* and 210 ± 76 mg kg^{-1} DM in caps of *Russula lepida*. Also, the mean contents 178 and 167 mg kg^{-1} DM in *Terfezia olbiensis* (Kivrak, 2015) and *A. caesarea* (Sarikurkcu et al., 2010), respectively, are considerably high.

Manganese was distributed evenly in a part of the tested species, whereas in the rest the reported contents were higher in stipes than in caps. The difference is great in some species, for example, in white and crimini *A. bisporus* (Sithole et al., 2017). Values of BCF are commonly <0.5, and only rarely over 1.0 (Falandysz & Drewnowska, 2015a; Kułdo et al., 2014; Mleczek, Siwulski, Stuper-Szablewska, Sobieralski, et al., 2013; Proskura et al., 2017; Sithole et al., 2017). Manganese is, thus, bioexcluded.

Manganese content decreased by 79% and 97% of the initial level by blanching and following pickling, respectively, of *A. fulva* caps (Drewnowska, Falandysz, et al., 2017). A lower loss of 45% during blanching of *A. bisporus* for 15 min observed Coşkuner and Özdemir (1997).

4.1.9 Molybdenum (Mo)

Data on molybdenum content (Table 4.8) are limited in comparison with many essential trace elements, apparently due to some difficulties linked with the determination of molybdenum using atomic absorption spectroscopy belong probably among reasons of such state. Usual contents vary from undetectable levels to 1 mg kg^{-1} DM in wild and cultivated species. Higher observed contents of up to 3 mg kg^{-1} DM occur, however, this was often reported by only one laboratory. Information on both molybdenum distribution within fruiting bodies and bioaccumulation from substrates has been lacking.

Overall, molybdenum seems to be ranked among elements with very low levels and its nutritional asset from mushrooms appears to be marginal.

4.1.10 Nickel (Ni)

As results from data collated in Table 4.9 show, contents of nickel in mushrooms vary widely from levels below 0.5 mg kg^{-1} DM, occurring particularly in cultivated fruiting bodies, to more than 20 mg kg^{-1} DM. The most frequent content seems to be within the range 0.5–5 mg kg^{-1} DM. Nevertheless, the content can vary widely within a species as may be seen, for example, in *C. cibarius* or *X. badius*. Extremely high levels at 58.6 and 55.0 mg kg^{-1} DM were observed in *C. comatus* (Yamaç, Yildiz, Sarikürkcü, Çelikkollu, & Solak, 2007) and in *L. perlatum* (Sarikurkcu et al., 2015), respectively. Even higher nickel contents in all six species collected around the city of Denizli, Turkey, were reported by Gezer and Kaygusuz (2014).

TABLE 4.8 Data on the content (mg kg^{-1} dry matter) of *molybdenum* in fruiting bodies of wild-growing mushrooms collected from unpolluted (X) and anthropogenically polluted (▲) sites and cultivated species published since 2010.

Species	<0.5	0.5–1	1–1.5	1.5–2	2–3	>3	References
Wild growing							
Agaricus arvensis	X						Ayaz et al. (2011)
Boletus appendiculatus	$X^{S,Cm}$						Alaimo et al. (2018)
Boletus edulis	X		X			X	Ayaz et al. (2011), Cvetkovic et al. (2015), Turfan et al. (2018)
Cantharellus cibarius	ND			X			Ayaz et al. (2011), Cvetkovic et al. (2015)
Cantharellus tubaeformis	ND						Ayaz et al. (2011)
Clitopilus prunulus	X^{m}						Alaimo et al. (2018)
Craterellus cornucopioides		X					Turfan et al. (2018)
Hydnum repandum	ND						Ayaz et al. (2011)
Laccaria laccata	X						Ayaz et al. (2011)
Lactarius deliciosus			X				Turfan et al. (2018)
Laetiporus sulphureus		X					Turfan et al. (2018)
Lepista nuda				X			Ayaz et al. (2011)
Macrolepiota procera		X^{C}					Falandysz, Sapkota, Dryżałowska et al. (2017)
Marasmius oreades			X		X		Cvetkovic et al. (2015), Turfan et al. (2018)
Morchella conica		X					Turfan et al. (2018)
Ramaria botrytis		X					Turfan et al. (2018)
Tricholoma terreum	X						Turfan et al. (2018)
Xerocomus badius	X, ▲	▲					Mleczek, Siwulski, Mikołajczak, Gąsecka, Sobieralski, et al. (2015), Mleczek, Magdziak, et al. (2016)

Cultivated							
Agaricus bisporus (white)			X				Mleczek, Rzymski, et al. (2018)
Agrocybe cylindracea	X						Niedzielski et al. (2017)
Auricularia auricula-judae		X					Mleczek, Rzymski, et al. (2018)
Auricularia polytricha	X						Niedzielski et al. (2017)
Clitocybe maxima	X						Niedzielski et al. (2017)
Flammulina velutipes	ND						Niedzielski et al. (2017)
Grifola frondosa		X					Niedzielski et al. (2017)
Hericium erinaceus	X						Turfan et al. (2018)
L. sulphureus	X						Niedzielski et al. (2017)
Lentinula edodes	X			X			Gonçalves et al. (2014), Mleczek, Siwulski, Rzymski, Niedzielski, et al. (2017), Mleczek, Rzymski, et al. (2018), Turfan et al. (2018)
Pholiota nameko	ND						Niedzielski et al. (2017)
Pleurotus eryngii	X						Gonçalves et al. (2014)
Pleurotus ostreatus	X	X	X				Gonçalves et al. (2014), Mleczek, Rzymski, et al. (2018), Turfan et al. (2018)
Trametes versicolor	X						Niedzielski et al. (2017)
Tremella fuciformis	ND	X					Mleczek, Rzymski, et al. (2018), Niedzielski et al. (2017)
Volvariella volvacea					X		Mleczek, Rzymski, et al. (2018)

C, Caps; *ND*, below limit of detection; X^m, median value.

TABLE 4.9 Data on the mean content (mg kg^{-1} dry matter) of *nickel* in fruiting bodies of wild-growing mushrooms collected from unpolluted (X), geologically specific (●), and anthropogenically contaminated (▲) sites and in cultivated species published since 2010.

Species	<0.25	0.25–0.5	0.5–1	1–2	2–5	5–10	10–20	>20	References
Wild growing									
Agaricus arvensis			X			X			Ayaz et al. (2011), Sarikurkcu et al. (2011)
Agaricus bisporus			X						Zhu et al. (2011)
Agaricus campestris				X	X, ●				Campos and Tejera (2011), Kosanić et al. (2017), Sarikurkcu et al. (2012), Severoglu et al. (2013), Širić, Humar, et al. (2016)
Agaricus sylvicola				●					Campos and Tejera (2011)
Agrocybe aegerita					X				Zhu et al. (2011)
Agrocybe cylindracea				X					Sarikurkcu et al. (2012)
Amanita caesarea					●		X		Campos and Tejera (2011), Sarikurkcu et al. (2010)
Amanita fulva	X	X							Falandysz, Drewnowska, et al. (2017)
Amanita rubescens					●				Campos and Tejera (2011)
Armillariella mellea			X	▲	X				Radulescu et al. (2010), Širić, Humar, et al. (2016), Zavastin et al. (2018)
Boletus aestivalis					X			$X^{C,S}$	Širić et al. (2014), Širić, Humar, et al. (2016), Wang et al. (2017)

Boletus appendiculatus			X	$X^{S,Cm}$					Alaimo et al. (2018), Dimitrijevic et al. (2016)
Boletus edulis				X, X^{S}	X, X^{C}	X	X		Ayaz et al. (2011), Cvetkovic et al. (2015), Dimitrijevic et al. (2016), Giannaccini et al. (2012), Kosanić et al. (2017), Mazurkiewicz and Podlasińska (2014), Mleczek, Siwulski, Stuper-Szablewska, Rissmann, et al. (2013), Mleczek, Siwulski, Mikołajczak, Goliński, et al. (2015), Širić, Humar, et al. (2016), Turfan et al. (2018), Wang et al. (2015b), Zavastin et al. (2018)
Boletus griseus								$X^{S,C}$	Wang et al. (2017)
Boletus impolitus			X			X^{C}	X^{S}		Dimitrijevic et al. (2016), Wang et al. (2017)
Boletus luridus					●^{C}	X^{C}, ●^{S}		X^{S}	Falandysz, Zhang, Wiejak, et al. (2017), Wang et al. (2017)
Boletus magnificus			●^{S,C}						Falandysz, Zhang, Wiejak, et al. (2017)
Boletus pulverulentus			▲						Árvay et al. (2014)
Boletus regius				X					Dimitrijevic et al. (2016)
Boletus speciosus								$X^{S,C}$	Wang et al. (2017)
Boletus tomentipes				●^{C,S}	$X^{C,S}$				Falandysz, Zhang, Wiejak, et al. (2017), Wang et al. (2015a)

(*Continued*)

TABLE 4.9 Data on the mean content (mg kg^{-1} dry matter) of *nickel* in fruiting bodies of wild-growing mushrooms collected from unpolluted (X), geologically specific (●), and anthropogenically contaminated (▲) sites and in cultivated species published since 2010. (Continued)

Species	<0.25	0.25–0.5	0.5–1	1–2	2–5	5–10	10–20	>20	References
Boletus umbriniporus								$X^{S,C}$	Wang et al. (2017)
Calocybe gambosa				X					Severoglu et al. (2013)
Cantharellus cibarius		X	▲	X, ▲	X	●			Árvay et al. (2014), Ayaz et al. (2011), Campos and Tejera (2011), Cvetkovic et al. (2015), Drewnowska and Falandysz (2015), Falandysz and Drewnowska (2015a), Falandysz, Chudzińska, et al. (2017), Mazurkiewicz and Podlasińska (2014), Mleczek, Siwulski, Stuper-Szablewska, Rissmann, et al. (2013), Mleczek, Niedzielski, Kalač, Budka, et al. (2016), Zavastin et al. (2018)
Cantharellus tubaeformis		X	X						Ayaz et al. (2011), Falandysz, Chudzińska, et al. (2017)
Clitocybe geotropa					●, X				Campos and Tejera (2011), Sarikurkcu et al. (2010)
Clitocybe gibba					●				Campos and Tejera (2011)
Clitocybe inversa					X				Širić, Humar, et al. (2016)
Clitocybe nebularis					X				Širić, Humar, et al. (2016)
Clitopilus prunulus			X^{m}						Alaimo et al. (2018)

Coprinus comatus			X		X				Severoglu et al. (2013), Zhu et al. (2011)
Craterellus cornucopioides							X		Turfan et al. (2018)
Fistulina hepatica				▲					Radulescu et al. (2010)
Flammulina velutipes				X					Zhu et al. (2011)
Ganoderma lucidum					●				Campos and Tejera (2011)
Gomphus clavatus						X			Sarikurkcu et al. (2015)
Helvella leucopus					X				Sarikurkcu et al. (2012)
Hericium erinaceus					X				Zhu et al. (2011)
Hydnum imbricatum			$X^{S,C}$						Mędyk, Chudzińska, et al. (2017)
Hydnum repandum			X		X				Ayaz et al. (2011), Severoglu et al. (2013)
Hygrophorus russula					●				Campos and Tejera (2011)
Hypsizygus marmoreus				X					Zhu et al. (2011)
Laccaria laccata			X						Ayaz et al. (2011)
Lactarius deliciosus	●		X				X, ●		Aloupi et al. (2012), Campos and Tejera (2011), Mleczek, Siwulski, Stuper-Szablewska, Rissmann, et al. (2013), Severoglu et al. (2013), Turfan et al. (2018)
Lactarius deterrimus					X				Širić, Humar, et al. (2016)
Lactarius piperatus					X				Cvetkovic et al. (2015)

(*Continued*)

TABLE 4.9 Data on the mean content (mg kg^{-1} dry matter) of *nickel* in fruiting bodies of wild-growing mushrooms collected from unpolluted (X), geologically specific (●), and anthropogenically contaminated (▲) sites and in cultivated species published since 2010. (Continued)

Species	<0.25	0.25–0.5	0.5–1	1–2	2–5	5–10	10–20	>20	References
Lactarius salmonicolor				X	X				Sarikurkcu et al. (2011), Severoglu et al. (2013)
Lactarius sanguifluus			●			●			Aloupi et al. (2012), Campos and Tejera (2011),
Lactarius semisanguifluus					●				Aloupi et al. (2012)
Laetiporus sulphureus				X		X			Sarikurkcu et al. (2015), Turfan et al. (2018)
Leccinum aurantiacum				X					Mleczek, Siwulski, Stuper-Szablewska, Rissmann, et al. (2013),
Leccinum crocipodium		X							Dimitrijevic et al. (2016)
Leccinum duriusculum			$X^{S,C}$						Jarzyńska and Falandysz (2012a)
Leccinum griseum	$X^{S,C}$								Jarzyńska and Falandysz (2012b)
Leccinum pseudoscabrum				X					Dimitrijevic et al. (2016)
Leccinum rugosiceps						X^{S}		X^{C}	Wang et al. (2017)
Leccinum scabrum	▲					X			Mleczek, Siwulski, Mikołajczak, Goliński, et al. (2015), Mleczek, Niedzielski, Kalač, Budka, et al. (2016)
Lentinula edodes				X					Zhu et al. (2011)
Lentinus cladopus			X						Mallikarjuna et al. (2013)

Lepista nuda				X	●				Ayaz et al. (2011), Campos and Tejera (2011)
Lepista sordida					X				Zhu et al. (2011)
Leucoagaricus leucothites							X		Sarikurkcu et al. (2010)
Lycoperdon perlatum				▲				X	Radulescu et al. (2010), Sarikurkcu et al. (2015)
Macrolepiota procera		$X^{C,S}$	▲	X, $X^{S,C}$	X, ●	X			Árvay et al. (2014), Campos and Tejera (2011), Falandysz, Sapkota, Dryżalowska et al. (2017), Giannaccini et al. (2012), Gucia et al. (2012), Mazurkiewicz and Podlasińska (2014), Sarikurkcu et al. (2015), Severoglu et al. (2013), Širić, Humar, et al. (2016)
Marasmius oreades					●	X			Campos and Tejera (2011), Cvetkovic et al. (2015), Turfan et al. (2018)
Morchella conica							X		Turfan et al. (2018)
Morchella esculenta						X			Sarikurkcu et al. (2012)
Pleurotus djamor				X					Mallikarjuna et al. (2013)
Pleurotus eryngii			X						Zhu et al. (2011)
Pleurotus nebrodensis			X						Zhu et al. (2011)
Pleurotus ostreatus	▲			X, ▲	X	X			Mleczek, Niedzielski, Kalač, Budka, et al. (2016), Radulescu et al. (2010), Severoglu et al. (2013), Tel-Çayan et al. (2017), Zhu et al. (2011)

(*Continued*)

TABLE 4.9 Data on the mean content (mg kg^{-1} dry matter) of *nickel* in fruiting bodies of wild-growing mushrooms collected from unpolluted (X), geologically specific (●), and anthropogenically contaminated (▲) sites and in cultivated species published since 2010. (Continued)

Species	<0.25	0.25–0.5	0.5–1	1–2	2–5	5–10	10–20	>20	References
Polyporus squamosus					X				Sarikurkcu et al. (2011)
Ramaria aurea		X							Severoglu et al. (2013)
Ramaria botrytis								X	Turfan et al. (2018)
Ramaria stricta				X					Severoglu et al. (2013)
Russula aeruginea				$X^{C,S}$					Elekes and Busuioc (2013)
Russula alutacea				X^{C}	X^{S}				Elekes and Busuioc (2013)
Russula cyanoxantha				X^{S}	X^{C}				Elekes and Busuioc (2013)
Russula delica					●				Aloupi et al. (2012)
Russula lepida				$X^{C,S}$					Elekes and Busuioc (2013)
Russula vesca				$X^{S,C}$					Elekes and Busuioc (2013)
Russula virescens		$X^{S,C}$							Elekes and Busuioc (2013)
Russula xerampelina			▲						Árvay et al. (2014)
Sparassis crispa					X				Severoglu et al. (2013)
Suillus bellinii					●				Aloupi et al. (2012)
Suillus bovinus		X							Severoglu et al. (2013)
Suillus grevillei					▲				Árvay et al. (2014)
Suillus luteus				X					Mleczek, Siwulski, Stuper-Szablewska, Rissmann, et al. (2013)

Suillus variegatus		X^{S}	X^{C}						Szubstarska et al. (2012)
Terfezia claveryi				X					Kivrak (2015)
Terfezia olbiensis					X				Kivrak (2015)
Tricholoma equestre							●		Campos and Tejera (2011)
Tricholoma fracticum				X					Tel-Çayan et al.(2017)
Tricholoma imbricatum			X						Sarikurkcu et al. (2011)
Tricholoma portentosum					X	X			Širić, Humar, et al. (2016), Tel-Çayan et al.(2017)
Tricholoma terreum					X		X		Severoglu et al. (2013), Širić, Humar, et al. (2016), Turfan et al. (2018)
Volvariella volvacea				X					Zhu et al. (2011)
Xerocomus badius		▲,X, ▲^{S,C}	X	X,▲	$X^{C,S}$		X, ▲		Dimitrijevic et al. (2016), Gąsecka et al. (2017), Kojta et al. (2012), Mleczek, Siwulski, Stuper-Szablewska, Rissmann, et al. (2013), Mleczek, Siwulski, Kaczmarek, et al. (2013), Mleczek, Siwulski, Mikołajczak, Gąsecka, Sobieralski, et al. (2015), Mleczek, Siwulski, Mikołajczak, Goliński, et al. (2015), Mleczek, Magdziak, et al. (2016), Proskura et al. (2017)
Xerocomus chrysenteron		X		X					Dimitrijevic et al. (2016), Sarikurkcu et al. (2011)

(*Continued*)

TABLE 4.9 Data on the mean content (mg kg^{-1} dry matter) of *nickel* in fruiting bodies of wild-growing mushrooms collected from unpolluted (X), geologically specific (●), and anthropogenically contaminated (▲) sites and in cultivated species published since 2010. (Continued)

Species	<0.25	0.25–0.5	0.5–1	1–2	2–5	5–10	10–20	>20	References
Xerocomus spadiceus								$X^{C,S}$	Wang et al. (2017)
Xerocomus subtomentosus			X^{C}						Jarzyńska et al. (2012)
Cultivated									
A. arvensis				X					Rzymski, Mleczek, Siwulski, Jasińska, et al. (2017)
A. bisporus (brown)				X					Rzymski, Mleczek, Siwulski, Jasińska, et al. (2017)
A. bisporus (white)				X			X		Mleczek, Rzymski, et al. (2018), Rzymski, Mleczek, Siwulski, Jasińska, et al. (2017)
Agaricus subrufescens					X				Rzymski, Mleczek, Siwulski, Jasińska, et al. (2017)
A. cylindracea	X								Niedzielski et al. (2017)
Auricularia auricula-judae			X						Mleczek, Rzymski, et al. (2018)
Auricularia polytricha		X							Niedzielski et al. (2017)
Auricularia thailandica						X			Bandara et al. (2017)
Clitocybe maxima	X								Niedzielski et al. (2017)
F. velutipes	ND								Niedzielski et al. (2017)

Grifola frondosa			X						Niedzielski et al. (2017)
H. erinaceus	X						X		Niedzielski et al. (2017), Turfan et al. (2018)
L. sulphureus	X								Niedzielski et al. (2017)
L. edodes		X		X		X			Gonçalves et al. (2014), Mallikarjuna et al. (2013), Mleczek, Siwulski, Rzymski, Niedzielski, et al. (2017), Mleczek, Rzymski, et al. (2018), Turfan et al. (2018)
Pholiota nameko	X								Niedzielski et al. (2017)
P. eryngii		X			X				Gonçalves et al. (2014), Rashid et al. (2018)
Pleurotus floridanus			X						Mallikarjuna et al. (2013)
P. ostreatus		X			X		X		Gonçalves et al. (2014), Mleczek, Rzymski, et al. (2018), Rashid et al. (2018), Turfan et al. (2018)
Trametes versicolor	X								Niedzielski et al. (2017)
Tremella fuciformis	X	X							Mleczek, Rzymski, et al. (2018), Niedzielski et al. (2017)
V. volvacea							X		Mleczek, Rzymski, et al. (2018)

C, Caps; *ND*, below limit of detection; *S*, stipes; X^{m}, median value.

The contents varied between 53.8 and 132 mg kg^{-1} DM in *Morchella esculenta* and *P. ostreatus*, respectively. Nickel levels in underlying substrates varied from 77.2 to 421 mg kg^{-1} DM.

According to the data in Table 4.9, distribution of nickel within fruiting bodies of various species differs. The contents are similar in caps and stipes in a part of species, while different in others. A general conclusion, thus, seems to be impossible.

BCFs <1 were observed by Mleczek, Siwulski, Stuper-Szablewska, Rissmann, et al. (2013), Širić, Humar, et al. (2016), and Sithole et al. (2017), and values slightly >1 were reported by Falandysz and Drewnowska (2015a) and Proskura et al. (2017). Therefore nickel does not belong among elements bioaccumulated in mushroom fruiting bodies.

Nickel content decreased by 57% of the initial level by blanching of *A. fulva* caps (Drewnowska, Falandysz, et al., 2017).

4.1.11 Selenium (Se)

Selenium is a hugely important essential metalloid generally occurring in about 30 mammalian selenoenzymes and selenoproteins involved in the Se–antioxidant defense system. It is insufficient in food chains in many world regions. Numerous mushroom species seem to be a promising source of dietary selenium. Moreover, production of several cultivated species highly enriched with the element is feasible. Comprehensive reviews on selenium in edible mushrooms have been published (Falandysz, 2008; Tsivileva & Perfileva, 2017) and, thereafter a review dealing with analytical methods for the element determination in mushrooms (Falandysz, 2013) drawing attention to excessive selenium values reported in some articles due to using improper analytical methods.

Values of recommended daily allowance (RDA) of selenium vary between 55 and 70 μg for adults, being somewhat higher for men than for women. Nevertheless, daily selenium consumption of about 400 μg is considered to be the upper limit as increased intake could cause some ailments. However, food chains in Europe, Australia, New Zealand, Brazil, and some regions of China are deficient in selenium. Even very moderate insufficiency can detrimentally affect health in various modes.

4.1.11.1 Level and bioconcentration in fruiting bodies

As results from data in Table 4.10 show as well as data published until 2010 (Falandysz, 2008; Kalač, 2010), usual selenium contents in both cultivated and wild-growing mushrooms range between <0.5 and 5 mg kg^{-1} DM. However, higher contents are not rare, in particular among some species of the genus *Boletus*, especially "true" boletes *B. edulis, B. pinophilus*, and *B. aestivalis*, and in genus *Agaricus*, namely *A. bisporus*, *A. bitorquis*,

TABLE 4.10 Data on the mean content (mg kg^{-1} dry matter) of total *selenium* in fruiting bodies of wild-growing mushrooms collected from unpolluted (X) or anthropogenically contaminated (▲) sites and in cultivated species published since 2010.

Species	<0.5	0.5–1	1–2	2–5	5–10	10–20	>20	References
Wild growing								
Agaricus lanipes					X			Gezer et al. (2016)
Armillariella mellea		X				▲		Radulescu et al. (2010), Zavastin et al. (2018)
Boletus appendiculatus		X				X^{Sm}	X^{Cm}	Alaimo et al. (2018), Dimitrijevic et al. (2016)
Boletus edulis				X			X	Dimitrijevic et al. (2016), Giannaccini et al. (2012), Turfan et al. (2018), Zavastin et al. (2018)
Boletus impolitus	X							Dimitrijevic et al. (2016)
Boletus regius			X					Dimitrijevic et al. (2016)
Cantharellus cibarius	X							Zavastin et al. (2018)
Clitopilus prunulus					X^{m}			Alaimo et al. (2018)
Fistulina hepatica				▲				Radulescu et al. (2010)
Lactarius deliciosus					X			Turfan et al. (2018)
Laetiporus sulphureus			X					Turfan et al. (2018)
Leccinum crocipodium		X						Dimitrijevic et al. (2016)
Leccinum pseudoscabrum	X							Dimitrijevic et al. (2016)
Lentinus cladopus			X					Mallikarjuna et al. (2013)
Lycoperdon perlatum							▲	Radulescu et al. (2010)
Macrolepiota procera		$X^{S,C}$		X				Giannaccini et al. (2012), Stefanović et al. (2016)
Marasmius oreades						X		Turfan et al. (2018)
Morchella conica	X							Turfan et al. (2018)
Pleurotus djamor			X					Mallikarjuna et al. (2013)
Pleurotus ostreatus	X			▲				Radulescu et al. (2010), Tel-Çayan et al.(2017)

(Continued)

TABLE 4.10 Data on the mean content (mg kg^{-1} dry matter) of total *selenium* in fruiting bodies of wild-growing mushrooms collected from unpolluted (X) or anthropogenically contaminated (▲) sites and in cultivated species published since 2010. (Continued)

Species	<0.5	0.5–1	1–2	2–5	5–10	10–20	>20	References
Ramaria botrytis							X	Turfan et al. (2018)
Terfezia claveryi				X				Kivrak (2015)
Terfezia olbiensis				X				Kivrak (2015)
Tirmania pinoyi							X	Bouatia et al. (2018)
Tricholoma fracticum	X							Tel-Çayan et al.(2017)
Xerocomus badius	X		▲	▲				Dimitrijevic et al. (2016), Gąsecka et al. (2017), Mleczek, Magdziak, et al. (2016)
Xerocomus chrysenteron	X							Dimitrijevic et al. (2016)
Cultivated								
Agaricus arvensis				X				Rzymski, Mleczek, Siwulski, Jasińska, et al. (2017)
Agaricus bisporus (brown)				X				Rzymski, Mleczek, Siwulski, Jasińska, et al. (2017)
A. bisporus (white)				X				Rzymski, Mleczek, Siwulski, Jasińska, et al. (2017)
Agaricus subrufescens				X				Rzymski, Mleczek, Siwulski, Jasińska, et al. (2017)
Agrocybe aegerita				X				Gąsecka, Mleczek, Siwulski, Niedzielski, and Kozak (2016)
Hericium erinaceus			X			X		Gąsecka et al. (2016), Turfan et al. (2018)
Lentinula edodes	X		X					Gonçalves et al. (2014), Mallikarjuna et al. (2013), Mleczek, Siwulski, Rzymski, Niedzielski, et al. (2017), Turfan et al. (2018)
Pholiota nameko				X				Niedzielski et al. (2015)
Pleurotus eryngii	X				X			Gonçalves et al. (2014), Niedzielski et al. (2015)
Pleurotus floridanus	X							Mallikarjuna et al. (2013)
P. ostreatus	X			X				Gonçalves et al. (2014), Niedzielski et al. (2015)

C, Caps; *S*, stipes; X^m, median value.

A. macrosporus, and *A. sylvaticus*. Very high content 48.6 ± 17.0 mg kg^{-1} DM was observed in *B. edulis* collected in Tuscany, Italy (Giannaccini et al., 2012), and an even higher level of 115 mg kg^{-1} DM was reported from Turkey (Turfan et al., 2018). Extremely high levels between 42 and 367 mg kg^{-1} DM were reported for *Albatrellus pes-caprae*, popular in Italy but rarely consumed elsewhere, and in related *Albatrellus ellisii*. Other tested *Albatrellus* species had only moderate to low selenium levels (Stijve, Noorloos, Byrne, Šlejkovec, & Goessler, 1998).

Reports on selenium distribution within fruiting bodies vary. Even contents in caps and stipes were observed in some species, whereas in others the levels were higher in caps than in stipes. For instance, Stijve (1977) observed 16.3, 7.65, and 6.35 mg kg^{-1} DM in tubes and the fleshy parts of caps and stipes, respectively, in *B. edulis*.

Information on BCFs varies widely. For instance, Stijve and Besson (1976) reported for *A. bitorquis* (syn. *A. edulis*) BCF 75–150, while Komárek, Chrastný, and Štíchová (2007) for *B. edulis* only 8–10. It seems that some *Boletus* and *Agaricus* species bioaccumulate selenium, whereas some species related to boletes, for example, *X. badius* and *Xerocomus chrysenteron*, are bioexcluders (Komárek et al., 2007).

4.1.11.2 Speciation of selenocompounds

Some data on selenium species in mushrooms are available. Selenites $Me^{I}_2Se^{IV}O_3$ are the main inorganic forms. Amino acids selenocysteine, Se–methyl-selenocysteine, selenocystine, and selenomethionine (Fig. 4.1) occur and are usually bound in selenoproteins. For instance, Maseko et al. (2013) observed in *A. bisporus* much higher levels of selenocystine compared

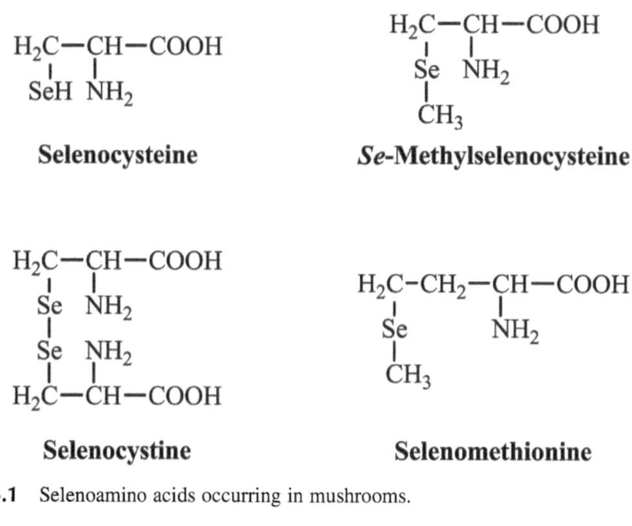

FIGURE 4.1 Selenoamino acids occurring in mushrooms.

to selenomethionine and Se–methyl-selenocysteine. Fang et al. (2018) found in *P. eryngii* the highest proportion of selenium, about 33% of the total element, in albumin fraction, followed by glutelin, globulin, and gliadin fractions. Selenomethione was the main detected Se–species. Its proportion increased during the growing stage while that of selenocysteine decreased. Egressy-Molnar, Ouerdane, Györfi, and Dernovics (2016) identified in *Hericium erinaceus* three Se–adenosyl compounds, two of which were previously linked only to selenium metabolism of yeast.

There exists consensus that organic selenium highly prevails to inorganic forms in mushrooms. For instance, Niedzielski et al. (2015) determined in cultivated species *Pholiota nameko*, *P. eryngii*, and *P. ostreatus* 96%, 97%, and 88% organic selenium of total content of the element, respectively. Within inorganic selenium, Se^{VI} compounds prevailed to Se^{IV} salts. Selenates (Se^{VI}) and particularly selenites (Se^{IV}) show detrimental effects, probably due to their prooxidant properties.

4.1.11.3 Biofortification

Mushrooms accumulate more selenium than biofortified yeast. The processes of mushroom enrichment with selenium have two directions. First, biofortification of mushroom mycelia seems to be very effective because mycelial selenium content could be several times higher than that in fruiting bodies. For detailed data and numerous references see the review by Tsivileva and Perfileva (2017).

Klimaszewska, Górska, Dawidowski, Podsadni, and Turło (2016) observed increased levels of Se–methyl-selenocysteine in mycelium of *L. edodes* from an undetectable value in the unfortified (control) culture medium to 120 mg kg^{-1} DM, and concurrently contents of Se–methionine from an undetectable level to 672 mg kg^{-1} DM in the medium variant containing 20 mg L^{-1} selenium applied as sodium selenite. However, mycelium mass in this variant decreased to about 63% of the yield in the unfortified medium. Among eight tested mushroom species, mycelium of *P. ostreatus* showed very high potential to bioaccumulate selenium during submerged cultivation in a medium enriched with sodium selenite (Milovanović et al., 2013). The content of selenium in the mycelium was 20.3 mg kg^{-1} DM, that is, 62.5% of the element level 0.37 mg L^{-1} in the medium. Also in these experiments mycelium biomass decreased, below 50% weight of that in the unfortified medium. Wang, Wang, Zhang, and Wu (2016) observed growth inhibition of *Flammulina velutipes* mycelium in a liquid medium already at 0.1 mM addition of Na_2SeO_3, complete growth inhibition occurred at level 3 mM of the supplemented salt. These results indicate that a minor portion of selenite uptake was metabolism dependent, whereas carrier-facilitated passive transport may be crucial. A selenite concentration of 0.03–0.1 mM was recommended to maintain the balance between mycelium production and selenium enrichment. Mycelium of *F. velutipes* was capable of reducing selenite to elemental selenium (Se^0), including Se^0 nanoparticles.

However, since the aim of this book is to provide information on the mineral composition of fruiting bodies, the second direction of research on biofortification with selenium will be given in more detail. An effort to biofortify some cultivated and medicinal mushroom species started in the 1990s. One method is based on the cultivation of mushrooms on naturally selenium-rich growing substrates, however, these are limited by their accessibility. The most common experimentally tested procedure is supplementation of growing substrates with sodium selenite, sodium selenate, or selenized yeast. Another variant is irrigation of the substrate with selenite solutions after the appearance of fruiting bodies.

Kaur, Kalia, and Sodhi (2018) were successful in biofortification of *Pleurotus* spp. cultivated in selenium-rich wheat straw originating from a seleniferous region of Punjab, India. Total selenium contents were 184, 182, and 191 mg kg^{-1} DM in *Pleurotus florida*, *P. ostreatus*, and *Pleurotus sajor-caju*, respectively, cultivated in selenium-rich straw, whereas the respective contents in the control variants were only 1.5, 2.8, and 4.6 mg kg^{-1} DM. Another recent paper from the same country (Solovyev et al., 2018) reports similar results. *Pleurotus citrinopileatus*, *P. ostreatus*, *P. sajor-caju*, and *A. bisporus* were cultivated on Se–rich wheat straw, *Volvariella volvacea* on paddy (rice) straw, both the substrates originating from a seleniferous region. Substrates from nonseleniferous area were used for control variants. The respective mean total selenium contents in fruiting bodies were 306, 405, 399, 1396, and 231 mg kg^{-1} DM, while only 17.1, 28.5, 77.6, 46.8, and 3.77 mg kg^{-1} DM were reported in the control variants. The highest enrichment factor of 61.3 was found in *V. volvacea* and the lowest of 5.1 in *P. sajor-caju*. The observed yield data were comparable in both the variants for all tested mushroom species.

Most of following data on the applied doses of selenium compounds are expressed in milimoles (mM). For sodium selenite Na_2SeO_3, 1 mM is 173 mg, which is equivalent to 79 mg of selenium. The respective values are 189 and 79 mg for sodium selenate Na_2SeO_4.

In an experiment by Maseko et al. (2013), white *A. bisporus* was cultivated in a compost. The young fruiting bodies were irrigated with solutions of sodium selenite containing 0, 10, 20, or 40 mg Se L^{-1}.The irrigation was carried out twice a day until the fruit bodies reached harvesting maturity. Unfortunately, information on total applied selenium is lacking. Selenium content in caps increased in a quadratic fashion from 12.2 mg kg^{-1} DM in the control variant irrigated with deionized water to a maximum of 347 mg kg^{-1} DM at 20 mg Se L^{-1} of the irrigation solution. Even higher bioaccumulation was observed in stipes. The contents of selenium increased linearly from 9.6 to 415 mg kg^{-1} DM in the control variant and in that irrigated with 40 mg Se L^{-1} solution, respectively.

An efficient fortification was reached also in *Calocybe indica* cultivated in wheat straw enriched with various levels of supplementation with sodium selenite (Rathore, Sharma, Prasad, & Sharma, 2018). Selenium in fruiting bodies was integrated mainly into proteins and polysaccharides.

Rzymski, Mleczek, Niedzielski, et al. (2017) investigated, for the first time, whether *A. bisporus* may be cultivated on substrates supplemented with selenium in combination with copper and/or zinc. The substrate composed of wheat straw, chicken manure, and gypsum was used as a control variant or it was supplemented with five tested concentrations 0.1, 0.2, 0.4, 0.6, and 0.8 mM L^{-1} of each element. Sodium selenite, sodium selenate, $copper^{II}$ selenate, and zinc nitrate were used. The accumulation of the elements in fruiting bodies from the first flush and their growth were observed in five variants: (1) no supplementation, control, (2) Se addition, (3) Se + Cu addition, (4) Se + Zn addition, and (5) Se + Cu + Zn addition. Substrate supplementation did not affect the yield of the biomass up to the element concentration of 0.6 mM L^{-1} regardless the experimental variant. The maximum element contents were observed at 0.6 mM L^{-1} in the variants Se + Zn and Se + Cu + Zn and at 0.8 mM L^{-1} in the variants Se and Se + Cu. The organically bound selenium constituted the greatest proportion from total selenium.

Savic et al. (2012) reported a double effect reached by supplementation of *A. bisporus, P. ostreatus*, and *Pleurotus cornucopiae* growing substrates with selenized yeast. The most suitable dose of the yeast showed to be 70–100 mg of selenium per kg DM of the substrates. Selenium contents in fruiting bodies were about 100 and 200 mg kg^{-1} DM in both *Pleurotus* spp. and *A. bisporus*, respectively. The additional effect was inhibition of the growth of mycopathogenic molds.

An experimental model similar to that of Rzymski, Mleczek, Niedzielski, et al. (2017), used Poniedziałek et al. (2017) for cultivation of *P. ostreatus* and *P. eryngii*. The substrate for *P. ostreatus* was prepared from wheat straw, that for *P. eryngii* from a mixture of beech sawdust, flax shives, wheat brans, and corn flour. Salts of selenium, copper, and zinc were dissolved in water and applied to both the substrates to obtain concentrations 0.1, 0.3, 0.6, 0.9, and 1.2 mM for all of the elements in the substrate. Five experimental variants were prepared: (1) no supplementation (control), (2) Se, (3) Se + Cu, (4) Se + Zn, and (5) Se + Cu + Zn. The biomass of *P. eryngii* was even in all the variants, whereas yield of *P. ostreatus* decreased with increasing concentration of the elements in the substrate. The yield was satisfactory up to 0.9 mM of Se, Se + Cu, and Se + Zn. The combination of all three elements yielded low biomass in 0.9 and 1.2 mM. The addition of selenium to the growth substrates increased its bioaccumulation in the fruiting bodies of both species in a concentration-dependent manner. Higher contents were observed in *P. ostreatus* than in *P. eryngii*. The mean contents of organic selenium in fruiting bodies increased from 0.6 to 90 mg kg^{-1} DM in *P. ostreatus* and from 1.1 to 21 mg kg^{-1} DM in *P. eryngii* in the controls and variants enriched with 0.9 mM Se, respectively. Selenium was predominantly bioaccumulated as its organic compounds.

In a work by Silva et al. (2012), *P. ostreatus* was cultivated in coffee husks enriched with sodium selenite at seven levels from 3.2 to 102 mg Se kg^{-1}. In the substrates with Se concentrations above 12.8 mg kg^{-1}, fruiting bodies possessed larger stipes and smaller caps than in the substrates with lower Se concentrations or in the control (unsupplemented) variant. Moreover, an unpleasant smell was observed in mushrooms cultivated in substrates with Se concentrations above 25.4 mg kg^{-1}. Times for fruiting bodies formation prolonged during the first flush at added Se levels 25.4 mg kg^{-1} and higher as compared with the levels 0–12.8 mg kg^{-1}. The highest biological efficiency (expressed as ratio of FM of the fruiting bodies to DM of the substrate × 100) was observed at Se level 12.8 mg kg^{-1} in both first and second flushes. Selenium contents in fruiting bodies increased considerably, for example, from 0.12 to 0.96 mg kg^{-1} DM in the control variant to 57.6 mg kg^{-1} DM at the lowest enrichment with 3.2 mg Se kg^{-1}. Selenium addition to the substrate did not affect content of 10 determined elements in the fruiting bodies. Overall, addition of 12.8 mg Se kg^{-1} substrate showed maximum biological efficiency and selenium accumulation into *P. ostreatus* fruiting bodies.

Milovanovic et al. (2019) determined in *Pleurotus pulmonarius* cultivated in a substrate based on wheat straw supplemented with sodium selenite 23.1 mg kg^{-1} DM of total selenium. Most of selenomethionine (84%), the major Se–compound, was found to occur in free form in the fruiting bodies.

Fortification with selenium is possible also for *L. edodes*. Nunes et al. (2012) cultivated shii-take on logs composed of eucalyptus sawdust. Fruiting induction was carried out by a cold shock of the logs in water containing sodium selenite at six concentrations of 0.08–1.28 mM and in pure water (control variant). No fruiting bodies grew in the variants with 0.96 or 1.28 mM Na_2SeO_3. The major productivity (expressed as ratio fruit bodies DM to substrate DM × 100) occurred at concentrations of 0.16 and 0.32 mM. Selenium contents were observed in fruiting bodies in the variant with 0.64 mM Na_2SeO_3. Selenium accumulation did not affect color, moisture, and protein content of the fruiting bodies. Zhou et al. (2018) fortified substrate based on wood chips and wheat bran containing 0.17 mg Se kg^{-1} with 0.5–5 mg Se kg^{-1} as selenite, selenate or selenized yeast. The efficiency of selenium utilization decreased in order selenite > selenate > Se–yeast. Selenomethionine predominated among selenocompounds determined in the fruiting bodies.

Niedzielski et al. (2014) used the same substrate as later Poniedzialek et al. (2017) (see above) for cultivation of *Agrocybe aegerita* and *H. erinaceus* (Niedzielski et al., 2014). The substrate was supplemented with sodium selenite or sodium selenate at concentrations of 0–1.5 mM. Both the species grew under Se additions 0 – 0.6 mM. There was no significant decrease in biomass up to 0.4 mM in *A. aegerita* and up to 0.2 mM in *H. erinaceus*. Concentrations exceeding 0.4 mM caused a diminution of fruiting bodies or even their total absence. Moreover, color changes of fruiting bodies occurred. Proportion of organic selenium was higher in *A. aegerita* than in *H. erinaceus*. Accumulation of inorganic Se^{IV} in fruiting bodies of both species was significantly higher than that of Se^{VI}. Total selenium contents were 4.6 and 23 mg kg^{-1} DM in *A. aegerita* in control and in the variant 0.4 mM, respectively. The respective values in *H. erinaceus* were 14.3 and 30 mg kg^{-1} DM (Gąsecka et al., 2016). It seems that both species bioaccumulate selenium at a lower extent than above given species.

Recently commercially cultivated *Pleurotus tuoliensis*, known under its Chinese name as Bai Ling Gu, was identified as an extensive selenium bioaccumulator (Zou, Du, Zhang, & Hu, 2018). At application of 20 mg sodium selenite per kilogram of substrate, contents of selenocysteine were 31.5 and 42.2 mg kg^{-1} DM and those of selenomethionine 49.2 and 41.5 mg kg^{-1} DM in caps and stipes, respectively. The respective levels in fruiting bodies growing in the unsupplemented substrate were 0.65 and 0.64 mg kg^{-1} DM for selenocysteine, and 0.25 and 0.55 mg kg^{-1} DM for selenomethionine. At the supplementation above 20 mg kg^{-1} the growth and development of the fruiting bodies were damaged.

4.1.11.4 Bioavailability

It has been repeatedly demonstrated for various foods that selenium is much more bioavailable both to humans and animals in its organic compounds compared to inorganic salts. Moreover, the former compounds have higher threshold level for toxicity compared to the latter. Unfortunately, information on bioavailability of selenium from mushrooms has remained limited and contradictory. Apart from the chemical species of selenium, chitin content should also be taken into consideration. This construction polysaccharide is known to limit the bioavailability of some mushroom components.

Chansler, Mutanen, Morris, and Levander (1986) used an animal model based on the restoration of glutathione peroxidase activity in Se–dependent rats. They compared sodium selenite, a Brazil nut meal (*Bertholetia excelsa*), and powders of dried *B. edulis* and cultivated *A. bisporus*. While selenium from the selenite and nut meal was fully available, the availability from both the mushrooms was very poor. In a follow-up experiment, Mutanen (1986) tested bioavailability of selenium by young Finnish women during intake of 150 μg Se daily for 4 weeks from *B. edulis*. The selenium level in erythrocytes increased significantly, while only slight enhancement was found in plasma selenium and in plasma or platelet glutathione peroxidase activity. The results indicated the metabolism of *B. edulis* selenium was different from that of concurrently tested wheat selenium or sodium selenate. The bioavailability of *B. edulis* selenium, thus, showed to be reasonably low.

Contrary results were reported by Silva et al. (2010) who tested in vivo selenium bioavailability using Wistar rats. Four of eight different diets tested *P. ostreatus*, namely nonenriched with selenium or containing 0.15, 0.30, and 0.45 mg Se kg^{-1} produced in a substrate fortified with sodium selenite. The highest Se concentration in plasma was observed in a peptide of low-molecular weight (8 kDa). Selenium concentration was significantly higher in the plasma of rats fed with three diets containing Se-enriched fruiting bodies than in other variants including sodium selenite. Selenium from *P. ostreatus* enriched via fortification of growing substrate was, thus, well bioavailable.

Powders of dried fruiting bodies fortified with selenium are recommended as a supplement to various foods for improving the nutritional and health status of consumers. Cremades et al. (2012) tested a different approach by developing a dried enzymatic extract (DM about 93%) with a mean selenium concentration 52 mg kg^{-1} from white *A. bisporus*. The used button mushrooms were produced using irrigation water supplemented with a selenite. More than 86% of selenium occurred in organic forms. Around 1 g of the product can achieve an RDA of 55 μg.

Overall, information on selenium bioavailability from unfortified and variously fortified mushrooms is ambiguous. Further research of the topic is, thus, needed.

4.1.12 Silicon (Si)

Data on silicon in mushrooms have been very scarce. Difficult determination of the element by the common methods of trace element analysis has been one of reasons. Cvetkovic et al. (2015) determined 132, 130, and 217 mg kg^{-1} DM in *B. edulis*, *C. cibarius*, and *Marasmius oreades*, respectively. A wide range between 35.7 and 1830 mg kg^{-1} DM was found in eight wild and three cultivated species with the minimum in *Laetiporus sulphureus* and maximum in *Craterellus cornucopioides*. Usual values were in tens and hundreds mg kg^{-1} DM (Turfan et al., 2018). Such contents are comparable with numerous vegetables.

Contents in the order of tens mg kg^{-1} DM were reported also for six species growing in the vicinity of a contaminated phosphogypsum storage site (Golubkina & Mironov, 2018).

4.1.13 Zinc (Zn)

Zinc belongs among the most reported elements in mushrooms. Comprehensive data published since 2010 are collated in Table 4.11. The contents range widely from levels below 25 to more than 200 mg kg^{-1} DM in wild-growing and cultivated species. The most common levels vary between <25 and 125 mg kg^{-1} DM; however, higher contents are not rare. Moreover, wide ranges within

TABLE 4.11 Data on the mean content (mg kg^{-1} dry matter) of *zinc* in fruiting bodies of wild-growing mushrooms collected from unpolluted (X), geologically specific (●), and anthropogenically contaminated (▲) sites and in cultivated species published since 2010.

Species	<25	25–50	50–75	75–100	100–125	125–150	150–200	>200	References
Wild growing									
Agaricus arvensis				X	X				Ayaz et al. (2011), Sarikurkcu et al. (2011)
Agaricus bisporus				X					Zhu et al. (2011)
Agaricus campestris	X	X	X, ●	X, X^{S}, $▲^{S,C}$		X^{C}			Campos and Tejera (2011), Kosanić et al. (2017), Sarikurkcu et al. (2012), Severoglu et al. (2013), Širić, Kasap, et al. (2016), Zsigmond et al. (2018)
Agaricus lanipes			X						Gezer et al. (2016)
Agaricus sylvicola			●						Campos and Tejera (2011)
Agrocybe aegerita			X						Zhu et al. (2011)
Agrocybe cylindracea					X				Sarikurkcu et al. (2012)
Albatrellus ovinus		$X^{C,S}$							Mędyk, Grembecka, et al. (2017)
Amanita caesarea			●		X				Campos and Tejera (2011), Sarikurkcu et al. (2010)
Amanita fulva						X^{S}	X^{C}		Falandysz, Drewnowska, et al. (2017)
Amanita ponderosa			X						Salvador et al. (2018)
Amanita rubescens				●					Campos and Tejera (2011)

Armillariella mellea	$X^{S,C}$	X,		X			▲		Georgescu et al. (2016), Radulescu et al. (2010), Širić, Kasap, et al. (2016), Zavastin et al. (2018)
Boletus aestivalis	X^{S}	X^{S}		X			▲		Harangozo and Stanovič (2016), Širić et al. (2014), Širić, Kasap, et al. (2016), Wang et al. (2017)
Boletus appendiculatus			X^{S}, X^{Sm}		X, X^{Cm}		X, X^{C}		Alaimo et al. (2018), Dimitrijevic et al. (2016), Sun et al. (2017), Wang et al. (2015)
Boletus bicolor							X		Sun et al. (2017)
Boletus brunneissimus				X^{S}			X^{C}		Wang et al. (2015)
Boletus edulis	X, X^{S}	X, $X^{S,C}$	X, X^{S}	X, $X^{S,C}$	X, X^{C}	X, X^{C}	X, X^{C}	X	Ayaz et al. (2011), Brzezicha-Cirocka et al. (2016), Cvetkovic et al. (2015), Dimitrijevic et al. (2016), Falandysz et al. (2011), Frankowska et al. (2010), Georgescu et al. (2016), Giannaccini et al. (2012), Kosanić et al. (2017), Mazurkiewicz and Podlasińska (2014), Mędyk, Grembecka, et al. (2017), Mleczek, Siwulski, Stuper-Szablewska, Rissmann, et al. (2013), Mleczek, Siwulski, Mikołajczak, Goliński, et al. (2015), Širić, Kasap, et al. (2016), Sun et al. (2017), Turfan et al. (2018), Wang et al. (2015, 2015b), Zavastin et al. (2018), Zhang et al. (2010)

(*Continued*)

TABLE 4.11 Data on the mean content (mg kg^{-1} dry matter) of *zinc* in fruiting bodies of wild-growing mushrooms collected from unpolluted (X), geologically specific (●), and anthropogenically contaminated (▲) sites and in cultivated species published since 2010. (Continued)

Species	<25	25–50	50–75	75–100	100–125	125–150	150–200	>200	References
Boletus flammans						X			Sun et al. (2017)
Boletus griseus				X,X^S	X, X^C,X^S			X^C	Liu et al. (2012), Sun et al. (2017), Wang et al. (2015, 2017)
Boletus impolitus		X^S		X^C			X		Dimitrijevic et al. (2016), Wang et al. (2017)
Boletus luridus			X^S	$●^S$	X^S	X^C	$●^C$		Falandysz, Zhang, Wiejak, et al. (2017), Wang et al. (2015, 2017)
Boletus magnificus			$●^S$			$●^C$			Falandysz, Zhang, Wiejak, et al. (2017)
Boletus pallidus		$X^{S,C}$							Wang et al. (2015)
Boletus pinophilus			X						Dospatliev and Ivanova (2017)
Boletus pulverulentus				▲					Árvay et al. (2014)
Boletus regius				X					Dimitrijevic et al. (2016)
Boletus rubellus						X^S		X^C	Wang et al. (2015)
Boletus sinicus						X			Sun et al. (2017)
Boletus speciosus		X	X^S	X	X^S	X^C	X^C		Liu et al. (2012), Sun et al. (2017), Wang et al. (2015, 2017)

Boletus tomentipes				X^S, ●^{S}	X^C	●^{C}			Falandysz, Zhang, Wiejak, et al. (2017), Wang et al. (2015, 2015a)
Boletus umbriniporus		X^S	X^S	X^C			X^C		Wang et al. (2015, 2017)
Calocybe gambosa	X								Severoglu et al. (2013)
Cantharellus cibarius	X^C	X^S,X	X	X, ▲	▲		X		Árvay et al. (2014), Ayaz et al. (2011), Brzezicha-Cirocka et al. (2016), Campos and Tejera (2011), Cvetkovic et al. (2015), Drewnowska and Falandysz (2015), Falandysz and Drewnowska (2015a), Falandysz, Chudzińska, et al. (2017), Georgescu et al. (2016), Harangozo and Stanovič (2016), Mazurkiewicz and Podlasińska (2014), Mleczek, Siwulski, Stuper-Szablewska, Rissmann, et al. (2013), Zavastin et al. (2018)
Cantharellus tubaeformis			X	X					Ayaz et al. (2011), Falandysz, Chudzińska, et al. (2017), Vinichuk (2013)
Clitocybe geotropa				●		X			Campos and Tejera (2011), Sarikurkcu et al. (2010)
Clitocybe gibba				●					Campos and Tejera (2011)

(*Continued*)

TABLE 4.11 Data on the mean content (mg kg^{-1} dry matter) of *zinc* in fruiting bodies of wild-growing mushrooms collected from unpolluted (X), geologically specific (●), and anthropogenically contaminated (▲) sites and in cultivated species published since 2010. (Continued)

Species	<25	25–50	50–75	75–100	100–125	125–150	150–200	>200	References
Clitocybe inversa			X						Širić, Kasap, et al. (2016)
Clitocybe nebularis			X						Širić, Kasap, et al. (2016)
Clitopilus prunulus				X^m					Alaimo et al. (2018)
Coprinus comatus	X		X						Severoglu et al. (2013), Zhu et al. (2011)
Craterellus cornucopioides								X	Turfan et al. (2018)
Fistulina hepatica		▲							Radulescu et al. (2010),
Flammulina velutipes		X							Zeng et al. (2012), Zhu et al. (2011)
Ganoderma lucidum				●					Campos and Tejera (2011)
Gomphidius glutinosus	X^S	X^C							Mędyk, Grembecka, et al. (2017)
Gomphus clavatus					X				Sarikurkcu et al. (2015)
Helvella leucopus		X						X	Gezer and Kaygusuz (2014), Sarikurkcu et al. (2012)
Hericium erinaceus		X							Zhu et al. (2011)
Hydnum imbricatum				X^S			X, X^C		Mędyk, Chudzińska, et al. (2017), Vinichuk (2013)

Hydnum repandum	X	X							Ayaz et al. (2011), Jedidi et al. (2017), Severoglu et al. (2013)
Hygrophorus russula					●				Campos and Tejera (2011)
Hypsizygus marmoreus				X					Zhu et al. (2011)
Laccaria laccata								X	Ayaz et al. (2011)
Lactarius deliciosus	X			X, ●		X		X	Aloupi et al. (2012), Campos and Tejera (2011), Çayir et al. (2010), Gezer and Kaygusuz (2014), Jedidi et al. (2017), Mleczek, Siwulski, Stuper-Szablewska, Rissmann, et al. (2013), Severoglu et al. (2013), Turfan et al. (2018)
Lactarius deterrimus			X	X					Vinichuk (2013), Širić, Kasap, et al. (2016)
Lactarius hygrophoroides	X								Liu et al. (2012)
Lactarius piperatus		X							Cvetkovic et al. (2015)
Lactarius salmonicolor	X		$X^{S,C}$	X					Chowaniak et al. (2017), Sarikurkcu et al. (2011), Severoglu et al. (2013)
Lactarius sanguifluus				●	●				Aloupi et al. (2012), Campos and Tejera (2011)
Lactarius semisanguifluus					●				Aloupi et al. (2012)
Laetiporus sulphureus			X		X				Sarikurkcu et al. (2015), Turfan et al. (2018)

(*Continued*)

TABLE 4.11 Data on the mean content (mg kg^{-1} dry matter) of *zinc* in fruiting bodies of wild-growing mushrooms collected from unpolluted (X), geologically specific (●), and anthropogenically contaminated (▲) sites and in cultivated species published since 2010. (Continued)

Species	<25	25–50	50–75	75–100	100–125	125–150	150–200	>200	References
Leccinum aurantiacum			X						Mleczek, Siwulski, Stuper-Szablewska, Rissmann, et al. (2013)
Leccinum crocipodium			X						Dimitrijevic et al. (2016)
Leccinum duriusculum			X^S			X^C			Jarzyńska and Falandysz (2012a)
Leccinum griseum					X^S			X^C	Jarzyńska and Falandysz (2012b)
Leccinum pseudoscabrum						X			Dimitrijevic et al. (2016)
Leccinum rugosiceps			X^S	X^C					Wang et al. (2017)
Leccinum scabrum		X		X, ▲	X				Brzezicha-Cirocka et al. (2016), Harangozo and Stanovič (2016), Mędyk, Grembecka, et al. (2017), Mleczek, Siwulski, Mikołajczak, Goliński, et al. (2015)
Leccinum versipelle				X					Mędyk, Grembecka, et al. (2017)
Lentinula edodes			X						Zhu et al. (2011)
Lentinus cladopus	X								Mallikarjuna et al. (2013)

Lepista nuda				X, ●					Ayaz et al. (2011), Campos and Tejera (2011)
Lepista sordida			X						Zhu et al. (2011)
Leucoagaricus leucothites						X			Sarikurkcu et al. (2010)
Leucopaxillus giganteus				X					Liu et al. (2012)
Lycoperdon perlatum						▲	X	X	Brzezicha-Cirocka et al. (2016), Mędyk, Grembecka, et al. (2017), Radulescu et al. (2010), Sarikurkcu et al. (2015)
Macrocybe gigantea							X		Liu et al. (2012)
Macrolepiota excoriata	$X^{S,C}$								Georgescu et al. (2016)
Macrolepiota procera	X, $X^{S,C}$	X, X^{S}	$X^{S,C}$, ●, ▲	▲, X, X^{C}	X^{C}	X			Árvay et al. (2014), Campos and Tejera (2011), Falandysz, Sapkota, Dryżałowska et al. (2017), Georgescu et al. (2016), Giannaccini et al. (2012), Gucia et al. (2012), Harangozo and Stanovič (2016), Jarzyńska et al. (2011), Kojta et al. (2011), Kułdo et al. (2014), Mazurkiewicz and Podlasińska (2014), Sarikurkcu et al. (2015), Severoglu et al. (2013), Širić, Kasap, et al. (2016)

(Continued)

TABLE 4.11 Data on the mean content (mg kg^{-1} dry matter) of *zinc* in fruiting bodies of wild-growing mushrooms collected from unpolluted (X), geologically specific (●), and anthropogenically contaminated (▲) sites and in cultivated species published since 2010. (Continued)

Species	<25	25–50	50–75	75–100	100–125	125–150	150–200	>200	References
Marasmius oreades				●	X			X	Campos and Tejera (2011), Cvetkovic et al. (2015), Turfan et al. (2018)
Melanoleuca arcuata		X							Liu et al. (2012)
Morchella conica								X	Turfan et al. (2018)
Morchella deliciosa			X						Liu et al. (2012)
Morchella elata							X^C		Zeng et al. (2012)
Morchella esculenta	X		X			X			Gezer and Kaygusuz (2014), Rossbach et al. (2017), Sarikurkcu et al. (2012)
Mycena haematopus			X						Liu et al. (2012)
Pleurotus djamor				X					Mallikarjuna et al. (2013)
Pleurotus eryngii		X^C	X						Zeng et al. (2012), Zhu et al. (2011)
Pleurotus nebrodensis			X						Zhu et al. (2011)
Pleurotus ostreatus	X, X^S	X, X^C, ▲							Georgescu et al. (2016), Gezer and Kaygusuz (2014), Radulescu et al. (2010), Severoglu et al. (2013), Tel-Çayan et al.(2017), Zhu et al. (2011)

Polyporus squamosus			X						Sarikurkcu et al. (2011)
Ramaria aurea	X								Severoglu et al. (2013)
Ramaria botrytis								X	Turfan et al. (2018)
Ramaria stricta	X								Severoglu et al. (2013)
Russula aeruginea				$X^{C,S}$					Elekes and Busuioc (2013)
Russula alutacea	$X^{S,C}$				X^{S}	X^{C}			Elekes and Busuioc (2013), Georgescu et al. (2016)
Russula cyanoxantha		$X^{S,C}$		X^{S}	X^{C}				Elekes and Busuioc (2013), Georgescu et al. (2016)
Russula delica		●							Aloupi et al. (2012)
Russula lepida			$X^{C,S}$						Elekes and Busuioc (2013)
Russula olivacea				▲					Harangozo and Stanovič (2016)
Russula vesca				X^{C}	X^{S}				Elekes and Busuioc (2013)
Russula virescens		X^{S}	X^{C}						Elekes and Busuioc (2013)
Russula xerampelina			▲		▲				Árvay et al. (2014), Harangozo and Stanovič (2016)
Sparassis crispa	X								Severoglu et al. (2013)
Suillus bellinii			●						Aloupi et al. (2012)
Suillus bovinus	X		$X^{S,C}$						Mędyk, Grembecka, et al. (2017), Severoglu et al. (2013)
Suillus granulatus		X							Vinichuk (2013)

(*Continued*)

TABLE 4.11 Data on the mean content (mg kg^{-1} dry matter) of *zinc* in fruiting bodies of wild-growing mushrooms collected from unpolluted (X), geologically specific (●), and anthropogenically contaminated (▲) sites and in cultivated species published since 2010. (Continued)

Species	<25	25–50	50–75	75–100	100–125	125–150	150–200	>200	References
Suillus grevillei					▲	▲			Árvay et al. (2014), Harangozo and Stanovič (2016)
Suillus luteus	X	X	X^S, X^C	X^C					Gezer and Kaygusuz (2014), Mędyk, Grembecka, et al. (2017), Mleczek, Siwulski, Stuper-Szablewska, Rissmann, et al. (2013), Zeng et al. (2012)
Suillus variegatus			X^S	X^C					
Terfezia claveryi		X							Kivrak (2015), Vahdani et al. (2017)
Terfezia olbiensis				X					Kivrak (2015)
Tirmania nivea		X							Vahdani et al. (2017)
Tirmania pinoyi		X							Bouatia et al. (2018)
Tricholoma equestre		X				●		X	Campos and Tejera (2011), Jedidi et al. (2017), Vinichuk (2013)
Tricholoma fracticum		X							Tel-Çayan et al.(2017)
Tricholoma imbricatum				X					Sarikurkcu et al. (2011)
Tricholoma matsutake			X						Li et al. (2013), Liu et al. (2012)
Tricholoma portentosum				X					Širić, Kasap, et al. (2016)

Tricholoma terreum	X	X		X				X	Gezer and Kaygusuz (2014), Severoglu et al. (2013), Širić, Kasap, et al. (2016), Turfan et al. (2018)
Volvariella volvacea			X						Zhu et al. (2011)
Xerocomus badius	X	X	X	▲	X^S, ▲	X, X^S, ▲, $▲^S$	X^C, $▲^C$	▲, X^C	Dimitrijevic et al. (2016), Harangozo and Stanovič (2016), Kojta et al. (2012), Kojta and Falandysz (2016a), Mleczek, Siwulski, Stuper-Szablewska, Rissmann, et al. (2013), Mleczek, Siwulski, Kaczmarek, et al. (2013), Mleczek, Siwulski, Mikołajczak, Gąsecka, Sobieralski, et al. (2015), Mleczek, Siwulski, Mikołajczak, Goliński, et al. (2015), Mleczek, Magdziak, et al. (2016), Podlasińska et al. (2015), Proskura et al. (2017)
Xerocomus chrysenteron	X				X				Dimitrijevic et al. (2016), Sarikurkcu et al. (2011)
Xerocomus spadiceus		X^C		X^S					Wang et al. (2017)
Xerocomus subtomentosus			$X^{S,C}$			X^S	X^C		Jarzyńska et al. (2012), Mędyk, Grembecka, et al. (2017)

(Continued)

TABLE 4.11 Data on the mean content (mg kg^{-1} dry matter) of *zinc* in fruiting bodies of wild-growing mushrooms collected from unpolluted (X), geologically specific (●), and anthropogenically contaminated (▲) sites and in cultivated species published since 2010. (Continued)

Species	<25	25–50	50–75	75–100	100–125	125–150	150–200	>200	References
Cultivated									
A. arvensis						X			Rzymski, Mleczek, Siwulski, Jasińska, et al. (2017)
A. bisporus (unspecified)								X	Gaur et al. (2016)
A. bisporus (brown)			X	X					Bach et al. (2017), Rzymski, Mleczek, Siwulski, Jasińska, et al. (2017)
A. bisporus (white)	X		X						Bach et al. (2017), Huang et al. (2015), Jedidi et al. (2017), Mleczek, Rzymski, et al. (2018), Rzymski, Mleczek, Siwulski, Jasińska, et al. (2017)
Agaricus subrufescens				X				X	Bach et al. (2017), Rzymski, Mleczek, Siwulski, Jasińska, et al. (2017)
Agrocybe chaxinggu			X						Huang et al. (2015)
A. cylindracea					X				Niedzielski et al. (2017)
A. mellea			X						Huang et al. (2015)
Auricularia auricula-judae	X	X							Huang et al. (2015), Mleczek, Rzymski, et al. (2018)

Auricularia polytricha				X					Niedzielski et al. (2017)
Auricularia thailandica		X							Bandara et al. (2017)
Calocybe indica				X					Gaur et al. (2016)
Clitocybe maxima				X					Niedzielski et al. (2017)
F. velutipes			X	X					Bach et al. (2017), Huang et al. (2015), Niedzielski et al. (2017)
Grifola frondosa								X	Niedzielski et al. (2017)
H. erinaceus					X		X		Niedzielski et al. (2017), Turfan et al. (2018)
L. sulphureus				X					Niedzielski et al. (2017)
L. edodes				X	X			X	Bach et al. (2017), Gaur et al. (2016), Gonçalves et al. (2014), Huang et al. (2015), Mallikarjuna et al. (2013), Mleczek, Siwulski, Rzymski, Niedzielski, et al. (2017), Mleczek, Rzymski, et al. (2018), Turfan et al. (2018)
M. gigantea						X			Gaur et al. (2016)
Pholiota nameko			X		X				Huang et al. (2015), Niedzielski et al. (2017)

(*Continued*)

TABLE 4.11 Data on the mean content (mg kg^{-1} dry matter) of *zinc* in fruiting bodies of wild-growing mushrooms collected from unpolluted (X), geologically specific (●), and anthropogenically contaminated (▲) sites and in cultivated species published since 2010. (Continued)

Species	<25	25–50	50–75	75–100	100–125	125–150	150–200	>200	References
P. djamor							X		Bach et al. (2017)
P. eryngii			X	X					Bach et al. (2017), Gonçalves et al. (2014), Rashid et al. (2018)
Pleurotus floridanus			X						Mallikarjuna et al. (2013)
P. ostreatus			X	X	X			X	Bach et al. (2017), Gonçalves et al. (2014), Huang et al. (2015), Mleczek, Rzymski, et al. (2018), Rashid et al. (2018), Turfan et al. (2018)
Pleurotus sajor-caju							X		Gaur et al. (2016)
Trametes versicolor					X				Niedzielski et al. (2017)
Tremella fuciformis		X	X		X				Huang et al. (2015), Mleczek, Rzymski, et al. (2018), Niedzielski et al. (2017)
V. volvacea				X					Mleczek, Rzymski, et al. (2018)

C, Caps; *S*, stipes; X^m, median value.

species with numerous available data may be seen from Table 4.11, for example, in *B. edulis*, *M. procera*, or *X. badius*. Caps usually have a somewhat higher zinc level than stipes and the spore-forming part has significantly higher content than the rest of fruiting body (Alonso et al., 2003). The peel of caps and caps of white, brown, and portobello varieties of *A. bisporus* have similar levels of zinc (Muszyńska et al., 2017).

Very high zinc content of 410 mg kg^{-1} DM was reported by Vinichuk (2013) in *Tricholoma equestre*. Rzymski, Mleczek, Siwulski, Jasińska, et al. (2017) determined in cultivated *A. subrufescens* a mean content 239 mg kg^{-1} DM and maximum level no fewer than 681 mg kg^{-1} DM. The respective contents in *X. badius* growing on highly contaminated soils were 471 and 681 mg kg^{-1} DM (Mleczek, Siwulski, Mikołajczak, Gąsecka, Sobieralski, et al., 2015). Considerably elevated zinc contents were observed in mushrooms in the vicinity of a zinc smelter (Collin-Hansen et al., 2002).

BCF for zinc is mostly <10 (e.g., Alonso et al., 2003; Kułdo et al., 2014; Mleczek, Siwulski, Stuper-Szablewska, Rissmann, et al., 2013; Proskura et al., 2017). Nevertheless, wide variations occur even within a species. For instance, Falandysz and Drewnowska (2015a) reported BCF values from 12 ± 6 to 39 ± 9 for *C. cibarius* collected from various sites. Even higher variability between 2 and 25 was observed in *Amanita ponderosa* from 24 sampling sites (Salvador et al., 2018).

Zinc ranks among essential trace elements often deficient in human nutrition. The possibility of enriching fruiting bodies of cultivated species has been tested only in a limited extent until now. Vieira et al. (2013) supplemented coffee husks as a substrate for *P. ostreatus* with a zinc carbonate at level 2.13 mg of zinc per kilogram. Zinc content in fruiting bodies grown on the supplemented substrate increased insignificantly to 62.6 mg kg^{-1} DM compared with nonsupplemented (control) mushrooms containing 57.7 mg kg^{-1} DM. Nevertheless, supplementation with zinc significantly decreased iron content in the fruiting bodies to 106 mg kg^{-1} DM, whereas a level of 149 mg kg^{-1} DM was observed in the control mushrooms. In an attempt to fortify white *A. bisporus* with three essential trace elements, selenium, copper, and zinc together, Rzymski, Mleczek, Niedzielski, et al. (2017) were successful in using combinations of Se + Zn and Se + Cu + Zn fortification up to 0.6 mM L^{-1} of the individual element's concentration. Zinc was applied as zinc nitrate hexahydrate. In the combination Se + Zn, the zinc level in fruiting bodies was 41.7 mg kg^{-1} DM at the supplementation level of 0.6 mM L^{-1}, while in fruiting bodies produced in the nonsupplemented substrate it was only 5.7 mg kg^{-1} DM.

Zinc is known as an efficient antiinflammatory agent. Gdula-Argasińska, Grzywacz, Krakowska, Opoka, and Muszyńska (2018) tested the possibility to enrich *C. cibarius* cultivated in vitro in a liquid medium supplemented with 20 mg L^{-1} of zinc in inorganic (zinc sulfate) or organic (zinc hydroxyaspartate) forms. Both variants contained significantly higher levels of zinc than the in vitro control and than fruiting bodies. The obtained biomass enables the precise application of zinc compounds at known concentrations.

Loss of 23% of the initial content of zinc was observed during blanching of *A. bisporus* for 15 min (Coşkuner & Özdemir, 1997). Blanching of *A. fulva* caps for 15 min and following pickling caused zinc leaching at rates of 39% and 87%, respectively (Drewnowska, Falandysz, et al., 2017).

The initial research on bioavailability of zinc from mushrooms reports a nutritional asset. The amount of Zn^{2+} ions released from freeze-dried fruiting bodies of *A. bisporus*, *X. badius*, and *C. cibarius* to artificial saliva within 1 min ranged from 0.3 to 11.4 mg kg^{-1} DM. Higher amounts were released to artificial digestive juices imitating the human gastrointestinal tract. The total mean amount of the released zinc was 41.3, 32.9, and 22.3 mg kg^{-1} DM from *X. badius*, *C. cibarius*, and *A. bisporus*, respectively. Bioavailability was thus assessed as being high (Zajac, Muszynska, Kala, Sikora, & Opoka, 2015). In a further report from the same laboratory (Muszyńska, Zając, Kała, Rojowski, & Opoka, 2016), release of zinc from six freeze-dried, powdered, mushroom species into artificial digestive juice was tested before and after boiling in a water suspension at 100°C for 60 min, which imitates the common culinary treatment of mushrooms. Thermal processing of *X. badius*, *B. edulis*, and *C. cibarius* resulted in the release of significantly higher amounts of zinc into the artificial digestive juice as compared with the level before boiling. The release of zinc from *P. ostreatus* and, in particular, from *Suillus bovinus* and *L. scabrum* was limited in comparison with the above given species. These boiled species remain an effective source of zinc.

4.1.14 Conclusion

Of the 13 trace elements commonly classified as essential for human nutrition, information on fluorine, iodine, and silicon in edible mushrooms is virtually lacking. Data on usual contents of 10 essential trace elements in wild-growing and cultivated mushrooms are given in Table 4.12. Most research has focused particularly on selenium and zinc, the elements deficient in the nutrition of a great part of the world's population. Various ways of cultivated mushroom biofortification seem to be feasible. Nevertheless, much more information is needed on the bioavailability of the elements from mushroom meals or from food supplements based on biofortified species.

Due to largely low consumption of both wild and cultivated species, mushrooms can be evaluated as only one of various dietary sources for essential trace elements, and are comparable with various vegetables usually consumed at higher amounts.

TABLE 4.12 Usual contents (mg kg^{-1} dry matter) of the essential trace elements in wild-growing and cultivated mushrooms.

Element	Wild-growing species	Cultivated species	Both groups
Boron	–	–	<1–>20
Cobalt	–	–	<0.2 – 10
Copper	< 10 – 75	Up to 30	–
Chromium	–	–	0.5 – 10
Iron	< 50 – 1000	< 50–300	–
Manganese	<25 – 75	<25	–
Molybdenum	–	–	Up to 1
Nickel	–	–	0.5–5
Selenium	–	–	<0.5 – 5
Zinc	–	–	<25 – 125

Data on fluorine, iodine, and silicon are virtually lacking.

4.2 Trace elements with detrimental health effects

Pieces of knowledge on the bioaccumulation of several detrimental trace elements in some mushroom species started to emerge during the late 1970s. Researchers initially focused on cadmium, mercury, and lead, and later included a further five elements, arsenic, barium, beryllium, silver and thallium, in this group. The contents observed early in some species have been considerably higher than levels in vegetables and other food items of plant origin. This engaged laboratories from various countries in further research.

Information on some potentially toxic elements in mushrooms, such as antimony, bismuth, or vanadium, has been very limited or they have been reported only low contents. Such elements are therefore classed in Section 4.3.

4.2.1 Arsenic (As)

There was a comprehensive review by Falandysz and Rizal (2016) on metalloid arsenic and its compounds in mushrooms, which also contains many references.

4.2.1.1 Level in fruiting bodies

Data on total arsenic content published since 2010 are given in Table 4.13. The usual levels range from undetectable to 2 mg kg^{-1} DM. Nevertheless, considerably higher, and even extremely high contents were repeatedly

TABLE 4.13 Data on the mean content (mg kg^{-1} dry matter) of total *arsenic* in fruiting bodies of wild-growing mushrooms collected from unpolluted (X), geologically specific (●), and anthropogenically contaminated (▲) sites and in cultivated species published since 2010.

Species	<0.5	0.5–1	1–2	2–5	5–10	10–50	50–100	References
Wild growing								
Agaricus arvensis				X				Ayaz et al. (2011)
Agaricus campestris				X^{S}	X^{C}			Zsigmond et al. (2018)
Albatrellus cristatus	X							Zhang, Liu, Li, Wang, and Li (2015)
Amanita fulva		X^{c}	X^{S}					Falandysz, Drewnowska, et al. (2017)
Armillariella mellea	X							Zavastin et al. (2018)
Auricularia auricula-judae	X							Zhang, Liu, et al. (2015)
Boletus appendiculatus	X, X^{Sm}	X^{Cm}	X					Alaimo et al. (2018), Dimitrijevic et al. (2016), Zhang, Liu, et al. (2015)
Boletus auripes	X							Zhang, Liu, et al. (2015)
Boletus edulis	ND,X	X	X	X				Ayaz et al. (2011), Dimitrijevic et al. (2016), Giannaccini et al. (2012), Mleczek, Siwulski, Mikołajczak, Goliński, et al. (2015), Turfan et al. (2018), Zavastin et al. (2018), Zhang, Liu, et al. (2015)
Boletus ferrugineus	X							Zhang, Liu, et al. (2015)
Boletus impolitus	X		X					Dimitrijevic et al. (2016), Zhang, Liu, et al. (2015)

Boletus luridus						●[S]	●[C]	Falandysz, Zhang, Wiejak, et al. (2017)
Boletus magnificus	X	●[S]		●[C]				Falandysz, Zhang, Wiejak, et al. (2017), Zhang, Liu, et al. (2015)
Boletus pallidus		X						Zhang, Liu, et al. (2015)
Boletus regius			X					Dimitrijevic et al. (2016)
Boletus speciosus	X							Zhang, Liu, et al. (2015)
Boletus tomentipes	X	●[C,S]		X[C,S]				Falandysz, Zhang, Wiejak, et al. (2017), Wang et al. (2015a), Zhang, Liu, et al. (2015)
Cantharellus cibarius	ND, X	▲						Ayaz et al. (2011), Falandysz, Chudzińska, et al. (2017), Melgar, Alonso, and García (2014), Mleczek, Niedzielski, Kalač, Budka, et al. (2016), Zavastin et al. (2018)
Cantharellus tubaeformis	ND,X							Ayaz et al. (2011), Falandysz, Chudzińska, et al. (2017), Melgar et al. (2014)
Clitopilus prunulus			X[m]					Alaimo et al. (2018)
Craterellus cornucopioides					X			Turfan et al. (2018)
Hydnum imbricatum		X[S]	X[C]					Mędyk, Chudzińska, et al. (2017)
Hydnum repandum	ND, X							Ayaz et al. (2011), Melgar et al. (2014)
Lactarius chichuensis	X							Zhang, Liu, et al. (2015)
Lactarius deliciosus						X		Turfan et al. (2018)
Lactarius volemus			X					Zhang, Liu, et al. (2015)

(*Continued*)

TABLE 4.13 Data on the mean content (mg kg^{-1} dry matter) of total *arsenic* in fruiting bodies of wild-growing mushrooms collected from unpolluted (X), geologically specific (●), and anthropogenically contaminated (▲) sites and in cultivated species published since 2010. (Continued)

Species	<0.5	0.5–1	1–2	2–5	5–10	10–50	50–100	References
Laetiporus sulphureus				X				Turfan et al. (2018)
Leccinum crocipodium	X							Dimitrijevic et al. (2016)
Leccinum pseudoscabrum		X						Dimitrijevic et al. (2016)
Leccinum rugosiceps	X							Zhang, Liu, et al. (2015)
Leccinum scabrum		▲	X					Mleczek, Siwulski, Mikołajczak, Goliński, et al. (2015), Mleczek, Niedzielski, Kalač, Budka, et al. (2016)
Lentinula edodes	X							Zhang, Liu, et al. (2015)
Lepista nuda	ND	X						Ayaz et al. (2011), Zhang, Liu, et al. (2015)
Macrolepiota procera		X, $X^{S,C}$	X^{C}					Falandysz, Sapkota, Dryżalowska et al. (2017), Giannaccini et al. (2012), Stefanović et al. (2016)
Marasmius oreades						X		Turfan et al. (2018)
Morchella conica					X			Turfan et al. (2018)
Morchella esculenta	X							Rossbach et al. (2017)
Pleurotus ostreatus	X, ▲							Mleczek, Niedzielski, Kalač, Budka, et al. (2016), Tel-Çayan et al. (2017), Zhang, Liu, et al. (2015)
Ramaria botrytis							X	Turfan et al. (2018)

Ramaria formosa			X					Zhang, Liu, et al. (2015)
Russula virescens		X						Zhang, Liu, et al. (2015)
Scleroderma citrinum			X					Zhang, Liu, et al. (2015)
Shiraia bambusicola	X							Zhang, Liu, et al. (2015)
Suillus bovinus			▲					Mleczek, Niedzielski, Kalač, Budka, et al. (2016)
Suillus pictus	X							Zhang, Liu, et al. (2015)
Terfezia claveryi		X						Vahdani et al. (2017)
Termitomyces globulus			X					Zhang, Liu, et al. (2015)
Tirmania nivea	X							Vahdani et al. (2017)
Tricholoma fracticum	X							Tel-Çayan et al.(2017)
Tricholoma pessundatum	X							Zhang, Liu, et al. (2015)
Tricholoma portentosum	X							Melgar et al. (2014)
Tricholoma terreum					X			Turfan et al. (2018)
Xerocomus badius	X, ●		X, ▲				▲	Dimitrijevic et al. (2016), Gąsecka et al. (2017), Mleczek, Siwulski, Mikołajczak, Gąsecka, Sobieralski, et al. (2015), Mleczek, Siwulski, Mikołajczak, Goliński, et al. (2015), Mleczek, Magdziak, et al. (2016)
Xerocomus chrysenteron	X							Dimitrijevic et al. (2016)

(*Continued*)

TABLE 4.13 Data on the mean content (mg kg^{-1} dry matter) of total *arsenic* in fruiting bodies of wild-growing mushrooms collected from unpolluted (X), geologically specific (●), and anthropogenically contaminated (▲) sites and in cultivated species published since 2010. (Continued)

Species	<0.5	0.5–1	1–2	2–5	5–10	10–50	50–100	References
Xerocomus rubellus	X							Zhang, Liu, et al. (2015)
Cultivated								
Agaricus bisporus (cremini, portobello, white)	X	X						Huang et al. (2015), Li et al. (2019), Mleczek, Rzymski, et al. (2018), Seyfferth, McClatchy, and Paukett (2016)
Agrocybe chaxinggu	X							Huang et al. (2015)
Agrocybe cylindracea	X							Niedzielski et al. (2017)
A. mellea	X							Huang et al. (2015)
A. auricula-judae	X			X				Huang et al. (2015), Mleczek, Rzymski, et al. (2018)
Auricularia polytricha	X							Niedzielski et al. (2017)
Auricularia thailandica	X							Bandara et al. (2017)
Clitocybe maxima		X						Niedzielski et al. (2017)
Flammulina velutipes	X		X					Huang et al. (2015), Li et al. (2019), Niedzielski et al. (2017)
Grifola frondosa	X							Niedzielski et al. (2017)
Hericium erinaceus	ND			X				Niedzielski et al. (2017), Turfan et al. (2018)
Hypsizygus marmoreus	X							Li et al. (2019)

L. sulphureus	X							Niedzielski et al. (2017)
L. edodes	X	X	X		X			Gonçalves et al. (2014), Huang et al. (2015), Li et al. (2019), Melgar et al. (2014), Mleczek, Siwulski, Rzymski, Niedzielski, et al. (2017), Mleczek, Rzymski, et al. (2018), Turfan et al. (2018)
Pholiota nameko	X	X						Huang et al. (2015), Niedzielski et al. (2017)
Pleurotus eryngii	X	X						Gonçalves et al. (2014), Li et al. (2019), Rashid et al. (2018)
Pleurotus floridanus	X							Khani et al. (2017)
P. ostreatus	X	X		X				Gonçalves et al. (2014), Huang et al. (2015), Li et al. (2019), Mleczek, Rzymski, et al. (2018), Rashid et al. (2018), Turfan et al. (2018)
Trametes versicolor	ND							Niedzielski et al. (2017)
Tremella fuciformis	X		X					Huang et al. (2015), Mleczek, Rzymski, et al. (2018), Niedzielski et al. (2017)
Volvariella volvacea	X							Mleczek, Rzymski, et al. (2018)

C, Caps; *ND*, below limit of detection; *S*, stipes; X^m, median value.

reported. Stijve and Bourqui (1991) observed the highest mean levels of 82 and 8.4 mg kg^{-1} DM in *Laccaria amethystina* and *Laccaria laccata*, respectively, among 5 cultivated and 74 wild-growing species. The respective maximum contents were 250 and 81 mg kg^{-1} DM. Within 83 species, Slekovec and Irgolic (1996) determined the highest levels (mg kg^{-1} DM) in *L. amethystina* (26–125), *L. laccata* (11–33), *Boletus cavipes* (11.6), and *Ramaria botrytis* (10.0). The caps contained approximately double arsenic content compared to the stipes. Vetter (2004) observed eight saprobic genera (*Agaricus*, *Calvatia*, *Collybia*, *Laccaria*, *Langermannia*, *Lepista*, *Lycoperdon*, and *Macrolepiota*) as bioaccumulators.

The main research interest has focused on the genus *Laccaria*. Vetter (2004) reported for *L. amethystina* a mean content of 59.3 and a maximum level of 147 mg kg^{-1} DM. An even higher mean level of 145 mg kg^{-1} DM was determined by Ayaz et al. (2011). Similar contents, namely 135 and 71 mg kg^{-1} DM, were quantified by Zhang, Li, Yang, Liu, and Wang (2015) in caps and stipes, respectively. Larsen, Hansen, and Gössler (1998) found extreme arsenic content of 1420 mg kg^{-1} DM in *L. amethystina* growing in a heavily polluted site formerly used for wood impregnation with a mixture containing $arsenic^{V}$ oxide As_2O_5. The water-extractable (bioavailable) arsenic in the contaminated topsoil was present as arsenate ($As^{V}O_4^{(3-)}$). The values reported by Zhang et al. (2015) for *Laccaria vinaceoavellanea* were 163 and 60.7 mg kg^{-1} DM in caps and stipes, respectively. The mean levels for *L. laccata* from three sampling sites varied between 14 and 143 mg kg^{-1} DM in caps and between 6.1 and 22 mg kg^{-1} DM in stipes.

4.2.1.2 Bioconcentration in fruiting bodies

Hyperaccumulation of arsenic in *Cyanoboletus pulverulentus* (syn. *Boletus* or *Xerocomus pulverulentus*) was reported by Braeuer et al. (2018). The mean total arsenic content was 250 ± 260, median 160, and range 2.4–1300 mg kg^{-1} DM. The majority of arsenic was accumulated in the spore-forming part of fruiting bodies. However, they did not find any significant correlation between arsenic content in fruiting bodies and in the underlying soils. The BCF for total arsenic varied very widely between 3 and 102 in 36 samples. Arsenic is present in mushrooms in both organic and inorganic compounds (Fig. 4.2). Inorganic arsenites (As^{III}) and arsenates (As^{V}) are toxic for humans. Organoarsenic compounds are of low toxicity, for example, arsenobetaine is nontoxic (Popowich, Zhang, & Le, 2016). Information on the bioaccumulation rate of arsenic in fruiting bodies has been limited. Mleczek, Niedzielski, Siwulski, et al. (2016) carried out experiments with four cultivated species aiming to detect the effects growing substrates supplementation with various doses of $NaAs^{III}O_2$, $Na_2HAs^{V}O_4$, or dimethylarsinic acid on fruiting body biomass and arsenic bioaccumulation

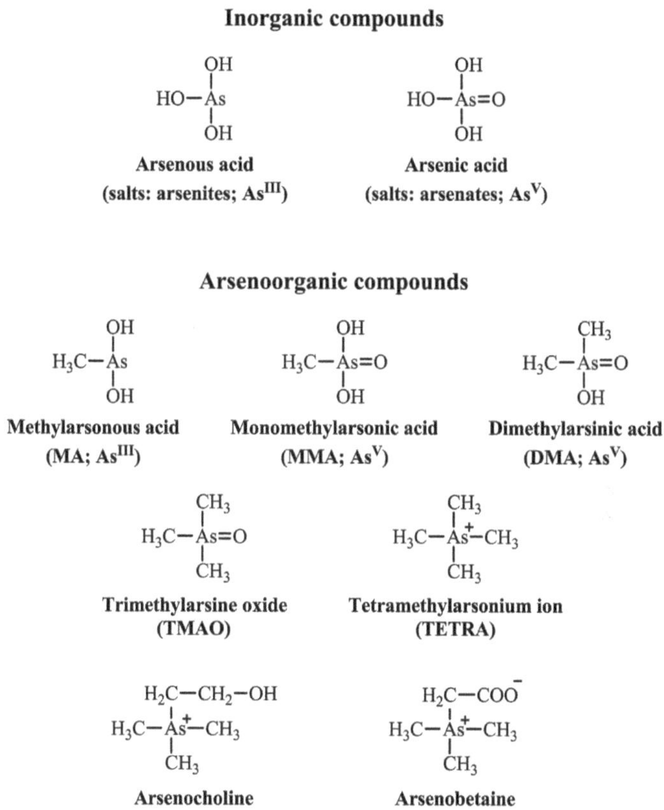

FIGURE 4.2 Arsenic compounds identified in mushrooms.

in the fruiting bodies. *A. bisporus* showed high resistance with low levels of arsenic accumulation compared with *P. ostreatus*, *P. eryngii*, and *H. erinaceus*. Thus it is necessary to check the level of substrates contamination with arsenic.

Arsenic probably is not distributed uniformly throughout the fruiting body. Li et al. (2019) localized most of arsenic in the surface coat of cap in *L. edodes*, while in the junction of stipe and cap in *P. ostreatus*. The respective total arsenic contents were 2.58 and 0.35 mg kg^{-1} DM, mostly in inorganic forms. The results differ from a report by Seyfferth et al. (2016) who localized arsenic mainly in spore-baring part of *L. edodes*.

4.2.1.3 Speciation of arsenic compounds

Larsen et al. (1998) accounted in *L. amethystina* 68%–74% dimethylarsinic acid (DMA), 0.3%–2.9% monomethylarsonic acid (MMA), 0.6%–2.0% trimethylarsine oxide (TMAO), and 0.1%–6.1% arsenic acid of total arsenic.

The unextractable fraction of arsenic ranged between 15% and 32%. TMAO was reported in mushrooms for the first time. Šlejkovec, Byrne, Stijve, Goessler, and Irgolic (1997) identified arsenobetaine (AB) as the main arsenocompound in various puffballs, *Agaricus* spp., and *M. procera*, DMA in *L. laccata* and *V. volvacea*, arsenocholine, and tetramethylarsonium ions in *Sparassis crispa*. Braeuer, Borovička, and Goessler (2018) found MMA, TMAO, and methylarsonous acid as the main arsenic compounds in three inedible species of the genus *Elaphomyces*.

Niedzielski, Mleczek, Magdziak, Siwulski, and Kozak (2013) determined contents of inorganic As^{III} and As^{V} and dimethylarsinic acid in widely consumed *X. badius* collected from 15 unpolluted and 4 polluted sites in Poland. In the former fruiting bodies the level was below 0.5 mg kg^{-1} DM for each of the arsenic forms, whereas in the latter mushrooms it was up to 27.1, 40.5 and 88.3 mg kg^{-1} DM for As^{III}, As^{V}, and dimethylarsinic acid, respectively. In their following work (Mleczek, Niedzielski, Rzymski, et al., 2016), the contents of total arsenic and proportions of inorganic As^{III} and As^{V} and organic arsenocompounds were compared in fruiting bodies of *X. badius* collected from seven unpolluted and three contaminated sites over 4 consecutive years. The latter sites were in the vicinity of an ironwork site (A), a coal mine (B), and a floating tailing deposit (C). The mean content of total arsenic in fruiting bodies from the unpolluted sites was 0.14 ± 0.07 mg kg^{-1} DM, whereas mean levels were around 50, 300, and 430 mg kg^{-1} DM in mushrooms collected from A, B and C, respectively. The fruiting bodies from site A contained at least 70% of As^{V} from total arsenic. The inorganic forms, As^{III} and As^{V}, prevailed in mushrooms from B and C sites. BCFs of 0.02–2.63, 2.05–3.3, 6.8–14.3, and 0.18 were determined for the unpolluted (background) sites, and site A, B and C, respectively. Thus *X. badius* was found to accumulate health-threatening levels of arsenic when growing in arsenic-polluted sites.

Different proportions of arsenic compounds in cultivated *A. bisporus* were reported by Seyfferth et al. (2016). In the white type they found 39%–94%, 12%–25%, and 7%–20% of inorganic arsenic, DMA, and arsenobetaine, respectively. The respective values for crimini were 65%–70%, 20%–28%, and 6%–11% and those for portobello 42%–47%, 12%–24%, and 2%–12%.

Arsenobetaine was the main arsenocompound in *L. edodes*, accounting 92.7% total arsenic (Chen, Guo, & Liu, 2017). This is in contrast with data reported by Llorente-Mirandes, Barbero, Rubio, and López-Sánchez (2014) who observed a mean proportion of 84% inorganic arsenic of the total content of the element. Similarly, Chen et al. (2018) reported the proportion of inorganic arsenic as about 33% from total arsenic content, with highly prevailing As^{III}, in both fresh and dried *L. edodes*, whereas arsenobetaine, MMA, and DMA formed minor shares and arsenocholine was mostly undetectable.

Some research works tried to elucidate biochemical pathways of arsenic compounds uptake and transformation in mushrooms. A series of papers has dealt with arsenobetaine (AB), which probably acts as an osmolyte in certain species to help maintain fruiting body structure. Generally, it is unknown whether mushrooms produce or accumulate AB from the surrounding environment. Nearing, Koch, and Reimer (2014) found AB as the major arsenocompound in the families *Agaricaceae* and *Lycoperdaceae*. However, AB was absent in log-growing species, suggesting that the microbial community may influence arsenic speciation in mushrooms. Mycelia of *A. bisporus*, *S. crispa*, and *Suillus luteus* were, therefore, cultured axenically and exposed to AB, arsenate, or dimethylarsenoyl acetic acid. The mycelia accumulated all arsenic compounds. Few biotransformations were observed. It is, thus, unlikely that mycelium is responsible for biosynthesizing AB (Nearing, Koch, & Reimer, 2015). In a following work (Nearing, Koch, & Reimer, 2016) the researchers studied the uptake and transformation of arsenic from a substrate with high level of arsenate. Arsenobetaine was found to be the major arsenocompound in *A. bisporus* at the earliest growth stage of fruiting (the primordium). Arsenobetaine was found exclusively in the fruiting body tissues of *A. bisporus* and *Agaricus campestris*. Thus AB formation seems to take place during the reproductive life stage, that is, the fruiting body formation, of the tested species.

Recently, Braeuer, Borovička, Glasnov, et al. (2018) detected in three species of the genus *Ramaria* minor levels of homoarsenocholine, a novel arsenic compound, together with dimethylarsinoyl acetate and trimethylarsonio propionate, the compounds known so far only from marine samples. The latter compounds were firstly identified within gilled fungi in *Cystoderma carcharias* (Borovička et al., 2019).

4.2.1.4 Effects of mushroom cooking

Blanching of *A. fulva* fresh caps for 15 min decreased the total arsenic content by 86% of the initial value. However, pickling somewhat increased the released proportion (Drewnowska, Falandysz, et al., 2017). Naturally, the leachate should be discarded. The high leachability is given by good solubility of main arsenic compounds in water.

Llorente-Mirandes, Llorens-Muñoz, Funes-Collado, and Sahuquillo (2016) determined arsenic in gastric and gastrointestinal bioaccessible fractions obtained after simulating human digestion by means of an in vitro physiologically based extraction test. Total arsenic contents in *L. edodes*, *A. bisporus*, and *P. ostreatus* decreased by 53%–71% and about by 11% in boiled and griddled mushrooms, respectively. High bioaccessibility of arsenic was observed in raw, boiled, and griddled mushrooms, ranging from 80% to 100% for gastrointestinal extracts.

4.2.1.5 Conclusion

According to the available data, the contents of total arsenic in most tested species were low. However, *Laccaria* spp. and *C. pulverulentus* were proven to be highly efficient bioaccumulators. Possibly other species, as shown in *X. badius*, may accumulate high levels of arsenocompounds if grown on substrates contaminated with inorganic arsenic. Reports on proportions of toxic inorganic fractions and less toxic organoarsenic compounds vary widely. Moreover, high bioaccessibility of arsenic was observed in both raw and cooked mushrooms. Thus elevated content of arsenic in fruiting bodies must be prevented.

4.2.2 Barium (Ba)

Data on barium contents in mushrooms published since 2010 are given in Table 4.14. The most frequent levels both in cultivated and wild-growing species are below 2 mg kg^{-1} DM. The contents above 10 mg kg^{-1} DM refer to fruiting bodies originated from geologically specific regions, namely quartzite acidic soils (Campos & Tejera, 2011) and soils from the Circum-Pacific Mercuriferous Belt (Falandysz, Zhang, Wiejak, et al., 2017). These data fit well with those published until 2010.

As results from very limited information show, barium is distributed evenly in caps and stipes. Reported BCFs are below 0.5 (e.g., Campos and Tejera, 2011 for 15 species and Mleczek, Siwulski, Stuper-Szablewska, Sobieralski, et al., 2013 for 6 species). Probably no accumulating species has yet been proved.

Blanching of *A. fulva* fresh caps for 15 min decreased barium content by 24% of the initial value (Drewnowska, Falandysz, et al., 2017). This is a relatively low proportion compared with numerous other metals.

4.2.3 Beryllium (Be)

Beryllium does not belong among elements often determined in fruiting bodies. In a comprehensive study, Seeger, Schleicher, and Schweinshaut (1984) determined the metal in 489 wild-growing species, edible, inedible, and toxic. Mean content was only 0.08 ± 0.002 mg kg^{-1} DM, ranging from <0.05 (limit of detection) to 0.57 mg kg^{-1} DM. No beryllium was detected in 27% of the samples. Old fruiting bodies contained more beryllium than young ones. The contents were usually somewhat higher in the flesh of caps than in stipes and spore-forming parts. The level of 0.041 ± 0.041 mg kg^{-1} DM was observed in *Auricularia auricula-judae*, with a maximum level of 0.155 mg kg^{-1} DM (Gabriel, Rychlovský, & Krenželok, 1995). Falandysz, Sapkota, Dryżalowska, et al. (2017) recently reported the value of 0.014 mg kg^{-1} DM in caps of *M. procera* and Alaimo et al. (2018) determined 0.01 and 0.02 mg kg^{-1} DM in *Clitopilus prunulus* and *Boletus appendiculatus*, respectively.

TABLE 4.14 Data on the mean content (mg kg^{-1} dry matter) of *barium* in fruiting bodies of wild-growing mushrooms collected from unpolluted (X), geologically specific (●), and anthropogenically contaminated (▲) sites and in cultivated species published since 2010.

Species	<2	2–5	5–10	10–25	25–50	References
Wild growing						
Agaricus arvensis	X					Ayaz et al. (2011)
Agaricus campestris		$▲^{C,S}$		●		Campos and Tejera (2011), Zsigmond et al. (2018)
Agaricus sylvicola				●		Campos and Tejera (2011)
Amanita caesarea				●		Campos and Tejera (2011)
Amanita fulva	$X^{C,S}$					Campos and Tejera (2011), Falandysz, Drewnowska, et al. (2017)
Amanita ponderosa	X					Salvador et al. (2018)
Amanita rubescens				●		Campos and Tejera (2011)
Boletus appendiculatus	$X^{S,Cm}$					Alaimo et al. (2018)
Boletus edulis	X, $X^{C,S}$	X	X, $X^{S,C}$			Ayaz et al. (2011), Cvetkovic et al. (2015), Falandysz et al. (2011), Frankowska et al. (2010), Giannaccini et al. (2012), Mleczek, Siwulski, Stuper-Szablewska, Sobieralski, et al. (2013), Wang et al. (2015b), Zhang et al. (2010)
Boletus luridus			$●^{S}$	$●^{C}$		Falandysz, Zhang, Wiejak, et al. (2017)

(*Continued*)

TABLE 4.14 Data on the mean content (mg kg^{-1} dry matter) of *barium* in fruiting bodies of wild-growing mushrooms collected from unpolluted (X), geologically specific (●), and anthropogenically contaminated (▲) sites and in cultivated species published since 2010. (Continued)

Species	<2	2–5	5–10	10–25	25–50	References
Boletus magnificus		●[S,C]				Falandysz, Zhang, Wiejak, et al. (2017)
Boletus tomentipes		●[C]			●[S]	Falandysz, Zhang, Wiejak, et al. (2017)
Cantharellus cibarius	X, ▲	X		●		Ayaz et al. (2011), Cvetkovic et al. (2015), Drewnowska and Falandysz (2015), Falandysz and Drewnowska (2015a), Falandysz, Chudzińska, et al. (2017), Mleczek, Siwulski, Stuper-Szablewska, Sobieralski, et al. (2013), Mleczek, Niedzielski, Kalač, Budka, et al. (2016)
Cantharellus tubaeformis	X					Ayaz et al. (2011), Falandysz, Chudzińska, et al. (2017)
Clitocybe geotropa				●		Campos and Tejera (2011)
Clitocybe gibba				●		Campos and Tejera (2011)
Clitopilus prunulus		X[m]				Alaimo et al. (2018)
Ganoderma lucidum				●		Campos and Tejera (2011)
Hydnum imbricatum	X[C,S]					Mędyk, Chudzińska, et al. (2017)
Hydnum repandum	X					Ayaz et al. (2011)
Hygrophorus russula				●		Campos and Tejera (2011)

Laccaria laccata		X				Ayaz et al. (2011)
Lactarius deliciosus		X		●		Campos and Tejera (2011), Mleczek, Siwulski, Stuper-Szablewska, Sobieralski, et al. (2013)
Lactarius piperatus	X					Cvetkovic et al. (2015)
Lactarius sanguifluus				●		Campos and Tejera (2011)
Leccinum aurantiacum	X					Mleczek, Siwulski, Stuper-Szablewska, Sobieralski, et al. (2013)
Leccinum duriusculum	$X^{C,S}$					Jarzyńska and Falandysz (2012a)
Leccinum griseum	$X^{C,S}$					Jarzyńska and Falandysz (2012b)
Leccinum scabrum	●, $X^{C,S}$					Falandysz (2018), Mleczek, Niedzielski, Kalač, Budka, et al. (2016)
Lepista nuda	X				●	Ayaz et al. (2011), Campos and Tejera (2011)
Macrolepiota procera	$X^{C,S}$	X^{C}	X	●		Campos and Tejera (2011), Falandysz, Sapkota, Dryżalowska et al. (2017), Giannaccini et al. (2012), Gucia et al. (2012), Jarzyńska et al. (2011), Kojta et al. (2011), Kułdo et al. (2014)
Marasmius oreades			X	●		Campos and Tejera (2011), Cvetkovic et al. (2015)
Pleurotus ostreatus	▲					Mleczek, Niedzielski, Kalač, Budka, et al. (2016)
Suillus bovinus	▲					Mleczek, Niedzielski, Kalač, Budka, et al. (2016)

(Continued)

TABLE 4.14 Data on the mean content (mg kg^{-1} dry matter) of *barium* in fruiting bodies of wild-growing mushrooms collected from unpolluted (X), geologically specific (●), and anthropogenically contaminated (▲) sites and in cultivated species published since 2010. (Continued)

Species	<2	2–5	5–10	10–25	25–50	References
Suillus luteus	X					Mleczek, Siwulski, Stuper-Szablewska, Sobieralski, et al. (2013)
Suillus variegatus	$X^{S,C}$					Szubstarska et al. (2012)
Tricholoma equestre				●		Campos and Tejera (2011)
Xerocomus badius	X, ▲, $▲^{C,S}$		X			Kojta et al. (2012), Mleczek, Siwulski, Stuper-Szablewska, Sobieralski, et al. (2013), Mleczek, Siwulski, Kaczmarek, et al. (2013), Mleczek, Siwulski, Mikołajczak, Gąsecka, Sobieralski, et al. (2015), Mleczek, Magdziak, et al. (2016)
Xerocomus subtomentosus	$X^{C,S}$					Jarzyńska et al. (2012)
Cultivated						
Agaricus bisporus (white)		X				Mleczek, Rzymski, et al. (2018)
Agrocybe cylindracea	X					Niedzielski et al. (2017)
Auricularia auricula-judae			X			Mleczek, Rzymski, et al. (2018)
Auricularia polytricha	X					Niedzielski et al. (2017)
Clitocybe maxima	X					Niedzielski et al. (2017)
Flammulina velutipes	X					Niedzielski et al. (2017)

Grifola frondosa		X				Niedzielski et al. (2017)
Hericium erinaceus	X					Niedzielski et al. (2017)
Laetiporus sulphureus		X				Niedzielski et al. (2017)
Lentinula edodes	X	X				Gonçalves et al. (2014), Mleczek, Siwulski, Rzymski, Niedzielski, et al. (2017), Mleczek, Rzymski, et al. (2018)
Pholiota nameko	X					Niedzielski et al. (2017)
Pleurotus eryngii	X					Gonçalves et al. (2014)
P. ostreatus	X	X				Gonçalves et al. (2014), Mleczek, Rzymski, et al. (2018)
Trametes versicolor		X				Niedzielski et al. (2017)
Tremella fuciformis	X	X				Mleczek, Rzymski, et al. (2018), Niedzielski et al. (2017)
Volvariella volvacea		X				Mleczek, Rzymski, et al. (2018)

C, Caps; *S*, stipes; X^m, median value.

According to the limited data, beryllium contents in mushrooms are comparable with those in vegetables and have no toxicological significance.

4.2.4 Cadmium (Cd)

Cadmium belongs among the most frequently determined elements in mushrooms due to its deleterious effects on human health. Data published since 2010 are collated in Table 4.15. Moreover, several papers reported mean contents >15 (all data in mg kg^{-1} DM): Sarikurkcu et al. (2011) reported 54.2 in *A. arvensis*, Petkovšek and Pokorny (2013) 23.5 in *B. edulis* from the vicinity of an abandoned lead smelter, Sun et al. (2017) 15.1 ± 5.4 in *Leccinum griseum*, and Mleczek, Siwulski, Mikołajczak, Gąsecka, Sobieralski, et al. (2015) 16 ± 2 in *X. badius* from a heavily polluted site. Extremely high levels up to 600 mg kg^{-1} DM were determined in saprobic inedible *C. carcharias*, which can be considered as a cadmium hyperaccumulator (Borovička et al., 2019).

As results from Table 4.15 show, usual levels range between <1 and 5 mg kg^{-1} DM in wild-growing species, whereas contents >1 mg kg^{-1} DM are sparse within cultivated mushrooms. Wide ranges within a species in fruiting bodies collected from unpolluted sites can be seen, for example, in *A. fulva, B. edulis, M. procera*, and *X. badius*. Commonly, cadmium contents are higher in caps than in stipes. Melgar, Alonso, and García (2016) found significantly higher content of cadmium in spore-forming parts (H) of many tested species than in the rest of the fruiting body (RFB). Among 28 species, the most highly accumulating was *A. macrosporus* with 52.9 and 28.3 mg kg^{-1} DM in the H and RFB, respectively. A very detailed study of cadmium distribution within fruiting bodies of accumulating *A. macrosporus* was carried out by Thomet, Vogel, and Krähenbühl (1999).

Data in Table 4.15 fit well with results published prior to 2010 (for references see reviews Kalač, 2010; Kalač & Svoboda, 2000). Two papers should be mentioned here. Seeger (1978) reported data for 402 edible, inedible, and toxic species. Low cadmium contents predominated as 68% of the samples contained <2 mg kg^{-1} DM, 86.5% had <5 mg kg^{-1} DM. A paper by Cocchi, Vescovi, Petrini, and Petrini (2006) gives data for 60 species and 1194 samples, unfortunately expressed only in FM. Some species of the genus *Agaricus* show to be highly accumulating, for example, *A. arvensis, A. augustus, A. macrosporus, A. sylvaticus*, and *A. sylvicola*, mainly those yellowing after mechanical damage of tissues (group *flavescentes*).

It should be underlined that even medium-accumulating species can reach 10s and highly accumulating species hundreds mg kg^{-1} DM in polluted areas. For instance, Collin-Hansen et al. (2002) determined up to 126 mg kg^{-1} DM in *B. edulis* growing in the vicinity of a Norwegian zinc smelter, Svoboda, Havlíčková, and Kalač (2006) reported 149 ± 15.3 mg kg^{-1} DM in *A. sylvaticus* from a historical silver-mining area, and Kalač et al. (1991)

TABLE 4.15 Data on the mean content (mg kg^{-1} dry matter) of *cadmium* in fruiting bodies of wild-growing mushrooms collected from unpolluted (X), geologically specific (●), and anthropogenically contaminated (▲) sites and in cultivated species published since 2010.

Species	<1	1–2	2–5	5–10	10–15	References
Wild growing						
Agaricus arvensis			▲		X	Ayaz et al. (2011), Sarikurkcu et al. (2011), Schlecht and Säumel (2015)
Agaricus bisporus	X					Zhu et al. (2011)
Agaricus bitorquis			▲			Schlecht and Säumel (2015)
Agaricus campestris	X, $X^{S,C}$, $▲^{S,C}$	X	X, ▲			Kosanić et al. (2017), Muszyńska et al. (2018), Sarikurkcu et al. (2012), Schlecht and Säumel (2015), Severoglu et al. (2013), Širić, Humar, et al. (2016), Širić, Kasap, Bedeković, and Falandysz (2017), Zsigmond et al. (2018)
Agaricus subperonatus			▲			Schlecht and Säumel (2015)
Agrocybe aegerita	X					Zhu et al. (2011)
Agrocybe cylindracea			X			Sarikurkcu et al. (2012)
Albatrellus ovinus	X^S	X^C				Mędyk, Grembecka, et al. (2017)
Amanita caesarea		X				Sarikurkcu et al. (2010)
Amanita fulva	$X^{C,S}$	X^S	$X^{C,S}$		X^C	Falandysz, Drewnowska, et al. (2017)
Amanita ponderosa		X				Salvador et al. (2018)

(Continued)

TABLE 4.15 Data on the mean content (mg kg^{-1} dry matter) of *cadmium* in fruiting bodies of wild-growing mushrooms collected from unpolluted (X), geologically specific (●), and anthropogenically contaminated (▲) sites and in cultivated species published since 2010. (Continued)

Species	<1	1–2	2–5	5–10	10–15	References
Armillariella mellea		X, ▲	X			Radulescu et al. (2010), Širić, Humar, et al. (2016), Širić et al. (2017), Zavastin et al. (2018)
Armillariella solidipes			▲			Schlecht and Säumel (2015)
Boletus aestivalis		X, ▲		▲		Harangozo and Stanovič (2016), Schlecht and Säumel (2015), Širić et al. (2014), Širić, Humar, et al. (2016), Širić et al. (2017), Sun et al. (2017)
Boletus appendiculatus	X, $X^{S,Cm}$	X				Alaimo et al. (2018), Dimitrijevic et al. (2016)
Boletus bicolor	X					Sun et al. (2017)
Boletus edulis	X	X,X^{S}	X, $X^{S,C}$	X^{C}		Ayaz et al. (2011), Brzezicha-Cirocka et al. (2016), Cvetkovic et al. (2015), Dimitrijevic et al. (2016), Falandysz et al. (2011), Giannaccini et al. (2012), Kosanić et al. (2017), Frankowska et al. (2010), Mędyk, Grembecka, et al. (2017), Mleczek, Siwulski, Stuper-Szablewska, Rissmann, et al. (2013), Mleczek, Siwulski, Mikołajczak, Goliński, et al. (2015), Muszyńska et al. (2018), Širić, Humar, et al. (2016), Širić et al. (2017), Sun et al. (2017), Turfan et al. (2018), Vinichuk (2013), Wang et al. (2015b), Zavastin et al. (2018), Zhang et al. (2010)

Boletus flammans	X					Sun et al. (2017)
Boletus griseus						Sun et al. (2017)
Boletus impolitus	X					Dimitrijevic et al. (2016)
Boletus luridus	▲	●[S]	●[C]			Falandysz, Zhang, Wiejak, et al. (2017), Schlecht and Säumel (2015)
Boletus magnificus	●[S]	●[C]				Falandysz, Zhang, Wiejak, et al. (2017)
Boletus pinophilus	X					Dospatliev and Ivanova (2017)
Boletus pulverulentus			▲			Árvay et al. (2014)
Boletus regius	X					Dimitrijevic et al. (2016)
Boletus sinicus	X					Sun et al. (2017)
Boletus speciosus	X					Sun et al. (2017)
Boletus tomentipes	X[S,C], ●[C]	●[S]				Falandysz, Zhang, Wiejak, et al. (2017), Wang et al. (2015a)
Calocybe gambosa	X					Severoglu et al. (2013)
Calvatia gigantea	▲					Schlecht and Säumel (2015)
Cantharellus cibarius	X, ▲	X,▲	▲			Árvay et al. (2014), Ayaz et al. (2011), Brzezicha-Cirocka et al. (2016), Cvetkovic et al. (2015), Drewnowska and Falandysz (2015), Falandysz and Drewnowska (2015a), Falandysz, Chudzińska, et al. (2017), Harangozo and Stanovič (2016), Mleczek, Siwulski, Stuper-Szablewska, Rissmann, et al. (2013), Mleczek, Niedzielski, Kalač, Budka, et al. (2016), Muszyńska et al. (2018), Petkovšek and Pokorny (2013), Zavastin et al. (2018)

(*Continued*)

TABLE 4.15 Data on the mean content (mg kg^{-1} dry matter) of *cadmium* in fruiting bodies of wild-growing mushrooms collected from unpolluted (X), geologically specific (●), and anthropogenically contaminated (▲) sites and in cultivated species published since 2010. (Continued)

Species	<1	1–2	2–5	5–10	10–15	References
Cantharellus tubaeformis	X					Ayaz et al. (2011), Falandysz, Chudzińska, et al. (2017), Vinichuk (2013)
Clitocybe geotropa	X					Sarikurkcu et al. (2010)
Clitocybe inversa		X				Širić, Humar, et al. (2016), Širić et al. (2017)
Clitocybe nebularis		X				Širić, Humar, et al. (2016), Širić et al. (2017)
Clitopilus prunulus	X^{m}					Alaimo et al. (2018)
Collybia velutipes	X					Zhu et al. (2011)
Coprinus comatus	X		▲			Schlecht and Säumel (2015), Severoglu et al. (2013), Zhu et al. (2011)
Craterellus cornucopioides		X				Turfan et al. (2018)
Fistulina hepatica	▲					Radulescu et al. (2010)
Gomphidius glutinosus	$X^{S,C}$					Mędyk, Grembecka, et al. (2017)
Gomphus clavatus			X			Sarikurkcu et al. (2015)
Helvella leucopus			X	X		Gezer and Kaygusuz (2014), Sarikurkcu et al. (2012)
Hericium erinaceus	X					Zhu et al. (2011)
Hydnum imbricatum		X^{S}	X	X^{C}		Mędyk, Chudzińska, et al. (2017),Vinichuk (2013)
Hydnum repandum	ND,X					Ayaz et al. (2011), Severoglu et al. (2013)

Hypsizygus marmoreus	X					Zhu et al. (2011)
Laccaria laccata	X					Ayaz et al. (2011)
Lactarius deliciosus	X, ●		X			Aloupi et al. (2012), Çayir et al. (2010), Gezer and Kaygusuz (2014), Mleczek, Siwulski, Stuper-Szablewska, Rissmann, et al. (2013), Severoglu et al. (2013), Turfan et al. (2018)
Lactarius deterrimus	X					Vinichuk (2013), Širić, Humar, et al. (2016), Širić et al. (2017)
Lactarius piperatus			X			Cvetkovic et al. (2015)
Lactarius salmonicolor	X	X	$X^{S,C}$			Chowaniak et al. (2017), Sarikurkcu et al. (2011), Severoglu et al. (2013)
Lactarius sanguifluus	●					Aloupi et al. (2012)
Lactarius semisanguifluus	●					Aloupi et al. (2012)
Laetiporus sulphureus	X					Sarikurkcu et al. (2015), Turfan et al. (2018)
Leccinum aurantiacum	X	X				Brzezicha-Cirocka et al. (2016), Mleczek, Siwulski, Stuper-Szablewska, Rissmann, et al. (2013)
Leccinum crocipodium	X	X				Dimitrijevic et al. (2016), Sun et al. (2017)
Leccinum duriusculum	X^{S}	X^{C}				Jarzyńska and Falandysz (2012a)
Leccinum griseum		X^{S}	X^{C}			Jarzyńska and Falandysz (2012b)
Leccinum pseudoscabrum			X			Dimitrijevic et al. (2016)

(*Continued*)

TABLE 4.15 Data on the mean content (mg kg^{-1} dry matter) of *cadmium* in fruiting bodies of wild-growing mushrooms collected from unpolluted (X), geologically specific (●), and anthropogenically contaminated (▲) sites and in cultivated species published since 2010. (Continued)

Species	<1	1–2	2–5	5–10	10–15	References
Leccinum scabrum	X,▲	X, ▲				Harangozo and Stanovič (2016), Mędyk, Grembecka, et al. (2017), Mleczek, Siwulski, Mikołajczak, Goliński, et al. (2015), Mleczek, Niedzielski, Kalač, Budka, et al. (2016), Muszyńska et al. (2018), Schlecht and Säumel (2015)
Leccinum versipelle			X			Mędyk, Grembecka, et al. (2017)
Lentinula edodes	X					Zhu et al. (2011)
Lepista nuda	X					Ayaz et al. (2011)
Lepista sordida	X					Zhu et al. (2011)
Leucoagaricus leucothites			X			Sarikurkcu et al. (2010)
Lycoperdon perlatum	X	▲	X			Brzezicha-Cirocka et al. (2016), Mędyk, Grembecka, et al. (2017), Radulescu et al. (2010), Sarikurkcu et al. (2015)
Macrolepiota mastoidea			▲			Schlecht and Säumel (2015)
Macrolepiota procera	X,X^S	▲, X^S	▲, X^C, X	X^C	▲	Árvay et al. (2014), Falandysz, Sapkota, Dryżalowska et al. (2017), Giannaccini et al. (2012), Gucia et al. (2012), Harangozo and Stanovič (2016), Jarzyńska et al. (2011), Kojta et al. (2011), Kułdo et al. (2014), Petkovšek and Pokorny (2013), Sarikurkcu et al. (2015), Schlecht and Säumel (2015), Severoglu et al. (2013), Širić, Humar, et al. (2016), Širić et al. (2017)

Marasmius oreades	X					Cvetkovic et al. (2015), Turfan et al. (2018)
Morchella conica		X				Turfan et al. (2018)
Morchella esculenta	X		X			Gezer and Kaygusuz (2014), Rossbach et al. (2017), Sarikurkcu et al. (2012)
Pleurotus eryngii	X					Zhu et al. (2011)
Pleurotus nebrodensis	X					Zhu et al. (2011)
Pleurotus ostreatus	X, ▲	X				Gezer and Kaygusuz (2014), Mleczek, Niedzielski, Kalač, Budka, et al. (2016), Muszyńska et al. (2018), Radulescu et al. (2010), Severoglu et al. (2013), Zhu et al. (2011)
Polyporus squamosus	X					Sarikurkcu et al. (2011)
Ramaria aurea	X					Severoglu et al. (2013)
Ramaria botrytis		X				Turfan et al. (2018)
Ramaria stricta	X					Severoglu et al. (2013)
Russula delica	●					Aloupi et al. (2012)
Russula olivacea	▲					Harangozo and Stanovič (2016)
Russula vesca			▲			Schlecht and Säumel (2015)
Russula xerampelina	▲					Árvay et al. (2014), Harangozo and Stanovič (2016)
Sparassis crispa	X, ▲					Severoglu et al. (2013)

(Continued)

TABLE 4.15 Data on the mean content (mg kg^{-1} dry matter) of *cadmium* in fruiting bodies of wild-growing mushrooms collected from unpolluted (X), geologically specific (●), and anthropogenically contaminated (▲) sites and in cultivated species published since 2010. (Continued)

Species	<1	1–2	2–5	5–10	10–15	References
Suillus bellinii	●					Aloupi et al. (2012)
Suillus bovinus	X,X^S	X^C, ▲				Mędyk, Grembecka, et al. (2017), Mleczek, Niedzielski, Kalač, Budka, et al. (2016), Schlecht and Säumel (2015), Severoglu et al. (2013)
Suillus granulatus	X					Vinichuk (2013)
Suillus grevillei	▲	▲				Árvay et al. (2014), Harangozo and Stanovič (2016)
Suillus luteus	X,X^S	X^C,X	X			Gezer and Kaygusuz (2014), Mleczek, Siwulski, Stuper-Szablewska, Rissmann, et al. (2013), Mędyk, Grembecka, et al. (2017), Muszyńska et al. (2018)
Suillus variegatus	$X^{S,C}$					Szubstarska et al. (2012)
Terfezia claveryi	X					Kivrak (2015), Vahdani et al. (2017)
Terfezia olbiensis	X					Kivrak (2015)
Tirmania nivea		X				Vahdani et al. (2017)
Tirmania pinoyi	X					Bouatia et al. (2018)
Tricholoma equestre		X	X			Vinichuk (2013), Širić, Humar, et al. (2016), Širić et al. (2017)
Tricholoma imbricatum	X					Sarikurkcu et al. (2011)

Tricholoma terreum	X	X				Gezer and Kaygusuz (2014), Severoglu et al. (2013), Širić, Humar, et al. (2016), Širić et al. (2017), Turfan et al. (2018)
Volvariella volvacea	X					Zhu et al. (2011)
Xerocomus badius	X, ▲, ▲^{S,C}	X^C,X	X^S	▲		Dimitrijevic et al. (2016), Gąsecka et al. (2017), Harangozo and Stanovič (2016), Kojta et al. (2012), Mleczek, Siwulski, Stuper-Szablewska, Rissmann, et al. (2013), Mleczek, Siwulski, Kaczmarek, et al. (2013), Mleczek, Siwulski, Mikołajczak, Gąsecka, Sobieralski, et al. (2015), Mleczek, Siwulski, Mikołajczak, Goliński, et al. (2015), Mleczek, Magdziak, et al. (2016), Muszyńska et al. (2018), Petkovšek and Pokorny (2013), Proskura et al. (2017), Schlecht and Säumel (2015)
Xerocomus chrysenteron	X	X		▲		Dimitrijevic et al. (2016), Sarikurkcu et al. (2011), Schlecht and Säumel (2015)
Xerocomus subtomentosus	X^C		X^S	X^C		Jarzyńska et al. (2012), Mędyk, Grembecka, et al. (2017)
Cultivated						
A. bisporus (unspecified)	X					Huang et al. (2015)
A. bisporus (cremini, portobello, white)	X					Seyfferth et al. (2016)
Agrocybe chaxinggu	X					Huang et al. (2015)
Agrocybe cylindracea	X					Niedzielski et al. (2017)
A. mellea	X					Huang et al. (2015)
Auricularia auricula-judae	X					Huang et al. (2015)
Auricularia polytricha	X					Niedzielski et al. (2017)

(*Continued*)

TABLE 4.15 Data on the mean content (mg kg^{-1} dry matter) of *cadmium* in fruiting bodies of wild-growing mushrooms collected from unpolluted (X), geologically specific (●), and anthropogenically contaminated (▲) sites and in cultivated species published since 2010. (Continued)

Species	<1	1–2	2–5	5–10	10–15	References
Auricularia thailandica	X					Bandara et al. (2017)
Clitocybe maxima	X					Niedzielski et al. (2017)
Flammulina velutipes	X					Huang et al. (2015), Niedzielski et al. (2017)
Grifola frondosa		X				Niedzielski et al. (2017)
H. erinaceus	X					Niedzielski et al. (2017), Turfan et al. (2018)
L. sulphureus	X					Niedzielski et al. (2017)
L. edodes	X	X				Gonçalves et al. (2014), Huang et al. (2015), Mleczek, Siwulski, Rzymski, Niedzielski, et al. (2017), Seyfferth et al. (2016), Turfan et al. (2018)
Pholiota nameko	X					Huang et al. (2015), Niedzielski et al. (2017)
P. eryngii	X					Gonçalves et al. (2014), Rashid et al. (2018)
Pleurotus floridanus	X					Khani et al. (2017)
P. ostreatus	X	X				Gonçalves et al. (2014), Huang et al. (2015), Rashid et al. (2018), Turfan et al. (2018)
Trametes versicolor	X					Niedzielski et al. (2017)
Tremella fuciformis	X					Huang et al. (2015), Niedzielski et al. (2017)

C, Caps; *S*, stipes; X^m, median value.

found $12 \pm 8.1\ mg\ kg^{-1}$ DM in *Amanita rubescens* in the vicinity of a lead smelter.

All the papers giving BCFs concur that mushrooms bioaccumulate cadmium; however, the reported values of BCF differ. Most probably, various methods of underlying soil sampling participate in the observed differences (see Section 2.1.2). Great variability in BCF within a species exists among sampling sites. For instance, BCF varied between 1 and 38 within 24 sampling sites of *A. ponderosa* (Salvador et al., 2018). Similarly, values in the range of 3.2–22 for four sites were observed by Falandysz and Drewnowska (2015a) for *C. cibarius*. The reported BCF values for numerous tested species range from single digits (Širić, Humar, et al., 2016; Širić et al., 2017) to tens (Melgar et al., 2016). The latter article gives extreme BCF values of 1399 and 741 in *A. macrosporus*, 701 and 266 in *A. sylvicola* for spore-forming parts and the rest of fruiting bodies, respectively.

Increasing cadmium levels in cultivated *A. subrufescens* were observed with increasing cadmium and also phosphorus contents in the substrate and in overgrown fruit bodies, particularly during the first flush (Huang, Ben, Yu, Wu, & Liu, 2008).

The information on chemical forms of cadmium in mushrooms has been very limited. Meisch and Schmitt (1986) isolated from *A. macrosporus* cadmium-mycophosphatin, a phosphoglycoprotein of molecular weight 12 kDa lacking sulfur, with a high proportion of acidic amino acids, glucose, and galactose. Moreover, four low-molecular glycoproteins containing sulfur and binding cadmium were isolated. No metallothioneins were found in fruiting bodies of cultivated *A. bisporus* (Esser & Brunnert, 1986). Collin-Hansen et al. (2002) found metallothionein-like proteins in virtually all samples of seven species, both mycorrhizal and saprobic. In a further work (Collin-Hansen, Andersen, & Steinnes, 2003), a novel cadmium-binding protein, not belonging to the metallothionein family, was isolated from *B. edulis*.

Several papers reported leaching of cadmium from mushrooms during common culinary treatments. Svoboda, Kalač, Špička, and Janoušková (2002) investigated leaching from fresh, air-dried, freeze-dried, and deep-frozen slices of *X. badius*. Soaking the mushrooms in a 0.3% table-salt solution at ambient temperature for 5, 10, or 15 min or repeatedly for 3×5 min and boiling in the same solution for 15, 30, or 60 min were tested. Short-time boiling was observed as a more efficient operation than soaking. For instance, 58% of the initial content of the element in fresh mushrooms was released during boiling of frozen slices for 15 min, whereas only 38% was released during soaking for 15 min. Cadmium was leached to the greatest extent from the most destroyed tissues of frozen slices, but less so from fresh or freeze-dried tissues. The release to water was more extensive for cadmium than for lead and mercury. Further experiments were carried out by Drewnowska et al. (2017) with *C. cibarius*. Fruiting bodies were cut vertically into four or three parts. Blanching of fresh chanterelles for 5 or 15 min caused a decrease of cadmium by around 11% ± 7% to 36% ± 7% of the initial content, respectively, while blanching deep-frozen fruiting bodies caused a decrease by around 40% ± 6%. The rate of cadmium decrease was similar for both the tested times of blanching. Pickling blanched chanterelles with a diluted vinegar marinade had a pronounced effect on further cadmium leaching. The total leaching rate from fresh and deep-frozen fruiting bodies was between 77% ± 7% and 91% ± 4% in fresh mushrooms, respectively. Similarly, blanching of *A. fulva* caps for 15 min and followed by pickling caused cadmium leaching at rates of 77% and 95%, respectively (Drewnowska, Hanć, et al., 2017).

While the initial information on bioaccessibility of cadmium from mushrooms reported only a low proportion, up to 10%, further works observed comparable and higher absorption from mushrooms than from inorganic cadmium salts (Lind, Glynn, Engman, & Jorhem, 1995; Mitra, Purkayastha, Chatterjee, & Bhattacharyya, 1995; Seeger, Schiefelbein, Seuffert, & Zant, 1986). Muszyńska et al. (2018) observed a transfer of 23.6% of total cadmium to gastric juice from *X. badius* biomass enriched with cadmium and lead. Nevertheless, the topic needs further research.

4.2.5 Lead (Pb)

Lead also belongs among the widely determined elements. Data published since 2010 are given in Table 4.16. Contents of lead up to 5 mg kg^{-1} DM are common in both cultivated and wild-growing species. The higher levels occur mainly in mushrooms growing in polluted sites; however, some species have been repeatedly found to contain elevated contents, including *A. sylvaticus*, *L. nuda*, *L. perlatum*, and *M. rhacodes* (García, Alonso, & Melgar, 2009; Kalač, Wittingerová, Stašková, Šimák, & Bastl, 1989; Svoboda et al., 2006). Petkovšek and Pokorny (2013) observed higher lead levels in saprobic than in mycorrhizal species. Very high lead contents, even 100–300 mg kg^{-1}DM, were determined in several species in the vicinity of lead smelters (Kalač et al., 1991; Lepšová & Král, 1988; Liukkonen-Lilja, Kuusi, Laaksovirta, Lodenius, & Piepponen, 1986; Petkovšek & Pokorny, 2013). As results from Table 4.16 show, lead is distributed evenly in caps and stipes. No statistically significant differences in lead content in spore-forming parts and in the rest of fruiting bodies were observed (García et al., 2009).

Numerous papers (e.g., García et al., 2009; Mleczek, Siwulski, Stuper-Szablewska, Rissmann, et al., 2013; Širić, Humar, et al., 2016; Širić et al., 2017) concur that values of BCF for lead are very low, often ≤ 0.1.

Only partial information is available on the isotopic ratio of $^{206}Pb/^{207}Pb$ in fruiting bodies of several mushroom species. The ratio enables to separate possible lead sources, that is, background lead derived from underlying bedrock, lead originating from former use of leaded petrol, or from smelter-derived fly ash. Each source of lead has its own isotopic signature.

TABLE 4.16 Data on the mean content (mg kg^{-1} dry matter) of *lead* in fruiting bodies of wild-growing mushrooms collected from unpolluted (X), geologically specific (●), and anthropogenically contaminated (▲) sites and in cultivated species published since 2010.

Species	<1	1–2	2–5	5–10	10–20	References
Wild growing						
Agaricus arvensis		X		▲		Sarikurkcu et al. (2011), Schlecht and Säumel (2015)
Agaricus bisporus			X			Zhu et al. (2011)
Agaricus bitorquis					▲	Schlecht and Säumel (2015)
Agaricus campestris	X	X	X, ●, $▲^{S,C}$	X^{C},▲		Campos and Tejera (2011), Kosanić et al. (2017), Muszyńska et al. (2018), Sarikurkcu et al. (2012), Schlecht and Säumel (2015), Severoglu et al. (2013), Širić, Humar, et al. (2016), Širić et al. (2017), Zsigmond et al. (2018)
Agaricus sylvicola			●			Campos and Tejera (2011)
Agaricus subperonatus					▲	Schlecht and Säumel (2015)
Agrocybe aegerita			X			Zhu et al. (2011)
Agrocybe cylindracea			X			Sarikurkcu et al. (2012)
Albatrellus ovinus		$X^{C,S}$				Mędyk, Grembecka, et al. (2017)
Amanita caesarea			●, X			Campos and Tejera (2011), Sarikurkcu et al. (2010)

(*Continued*)

TABLE 4.16 Data on the mean content (mg kg^{-1} dry matter) of *lead* in fruiting bodies of wild-growing mushrooms collected from unpolluted (X), geologically specific (●), and anthropogenically contaminated (▲) sites and in cultivated species published since 2010. (Continued)

Species	<1	1–2	2–5	5–10	10–20	References
Amanita fulva		X	X^{S}	X^{C}		Falandysz, Drewnowska, et al. (2017)
Amanita ponderosa			X			Salvador et al. (2018)
Amanita rubescens		●				Campos and Tejera (2011)
Armillariella mellea	X			▲		Radulescu et al. (2010), Širić, Humar, et al. (2016), Širić et al. (2017), Zavastin et al. (2018)
Armillariella solidipes	▲					Schlecht and Säumel (2015)
Boletus aestivalis		X, ▲	X, ▲			Harangozo and Stanovič (2016), Schlecht and Säumel (2015), Širić et al. (2014), Širić, Humar, et al. (2016), Širić et al. (2017)
Boletus appendiculatus	X, $X^{S,Cm}$					Alaimo et al. (2018), Dimitrijevic et al. (2016), Sun et al. (2017)
Boletus bicolor	X					Sun et al. (2017)
Boletus edulis	X	X		X,▲	X	Dimitrijevic et al. (2016), Giannaccini et al. (2012), Mędyk, Grembecka, et al. (2017), Mleczek, Siwulski, Stuper-Szablewska, Rissmann, et al. (2013), Mleczek, Siwulski, Mikołajczak, Goliński, et al. (2015), Petkovšek and Pokorny (2013), Širić, Humar, et al. (2016), Širić et al. (2017), Sun et al. (2017), Zavastin et al. (2018)
Boletus flammans	X					Sun et al. (2017)
Boletus griseus	X					Sun et al. (2017)

Boletus impolitus	X					Dimitrijevic et al. (2016)
Boletus luridus		●[S,C]	▲			Falandysz, Zhang, Wiejak, et al. (2017), Schlecht and Säumel (2015)
Boletus magnificus	●[C,S]					Falandysz, Zhang, Wiejak, et al. (2017)
Boletus pinophilus	X					Dospatliev and Ivanova (2017)
Boletus regius	X					Dimitrijevic et al. (2016)
Boletus sinicus	X					Sun et al. (2017)
Boletus speciosus	X					Sun et al. (2017)
Boletus tomentipes	●[C]	●[S]				Falandysz, Zhang, Wiejak, et al. (2017)
Calocybe gambosa			X			Severoglu et al. (2013)
Calvatia gigantea			▲			Schlecht and Säumel (2015)
Cantharellus cibarius	▲, X	X, ▲	X, ●,▲	X		Árvay et al. (2014), Campos and Tejera (2011), Cvetkovic et al. (2015), Drewnowska and Falandysz (2015), Falandysz and Drewnowska (2015a), Falandysz, Chudzińska, et al. (2017), Harangozo and Stanovič (2016), Mleczek, Siwulski, Stuper-Szablewska, Rissmann, et al. (2013), Muszyńska et al. (2018), Petkovšek and Pokorny (2013), Zavastin et al. (2018)
Cantharellus tubaeformis	X					Falandysz, Chudzińska, et al. (2017)
Clitocybe geotropa			X,●			Campos and Tejera (2011), Sarikurkcu et al. (2010)
Clitocybe gibba				●		Campos and Tejera (2011)
Clitocybe inversa		X				Širić, Humar, et al. (2016), Širić et al. (2017)
Clitocybe nebularis		X				Širić, Humar, et al. (2016), Širić et al. (2017)

(*Continued*)

TABLE 4.16 Data on the mean content (mg kg^{-1} dry matter) of *lead* in fruiting bodies of wild-growing mushrooms collected from unpolluted (X), geologically specific (●), and anthropogenically contaminated (▲) sites and in cultivated species published since 2010. (Continued)

Species	<1	1–2	2–5	5–10	10–20	References
Clitopilus prunulus	X^{m}					Alaimo et al. (2018)
Collybia velutipes	X					Zhu et al. (2011)
Coprinus comatus		X	▲	X		Schlecht and Säumel (2015), Severoglu et al. (2013), Zhu et al. (2011)
Craterellus cornucopioides			X			Turfan et al. (2018)
Cyanoboletus pulverulentus		▲				Árvay et al. (2014)
Fistulina hepatica	▲					Radulescu et al. (2010)
Ganoderma lucidum			●			Campos and Tejera (2011)
Gomphidius glutinosus				$X^{S,C}$		Mędyk, Grembecka, et al. (2017)
Gomphus clavatus			X			Sarikurkcu et al. (2015)
Helvella leucopus	X		X			Gezer and Kaygusuz (2014)
Hericium erinaceus			X			Zhu et al. (2011), Sarikurkcu et al. (2012)
Hydnum imbricatum		$X^{C,S}$				Mędyk, Chudzińska, et al. (2017)
Hydnum repandum			X			Severoglu et al. (2013)
Hygrophorus russula			●			Campos and Tejera (2011)
Hypsizigus marmoreus			X			Zhu et al. (2011)

Lactarius deliciosus	●	X	●, X			Aloupi et al. (2012), Campos and Tejera (2011), Çayir et al. (2010), Gezer and Kaygusuz (2014), Mleczek, Siwulski, Stuper-Szablewska, Rissmann, et al. (2013), Severoglu et al. (2013), Turfan et al. (2018)
Lactarius deterrimus	X					Širić, Humar, et al. (2016), Širić et al. (2017)
Lactarius piperatus				X		Cvetkovic et al. (2015)
Lactarius salmonicolor		X, $X^{S,C}$	X			Chowaniak et al. (2017), Sarikurkcu et al. (2011), Severoglu et al. (2013)
Lactarius sanguifluus	●		●			Aloupi et al. (2012), Campos and Tejera (2011)
Lactarius semisanguifluus	●					Aloupi et al. (2012)
Laetiporus sulphureus		X				Sarikurkcu et al. (2015), Turfan et al. (2018)
Leccinum aurantiacum	X					Mleczek, Siwulski, Stuper-Szablewska, Rissmann, et al. (2013)
Leccinum crocipodium	X		X			Dimitrijevic et al. (2016), Sun et al. (2017)
Leccinum duriusculum	$X^{S,C}$					Jarzyńska and Falandysz (2012a)
Leccinum griseum	$X^{S,C}$					Jarzyńska and Falandysz (2012b)
Leccinum pseudoscabrum		X				Dimitrijevic et al. (2016)
Leccinum scabrum		X, ▲	X, ▲			Harangozo and Stanovič (2016), Mędyk, Grembecka, et al. (2017), Mleczek, Siwulski, Mikołajczak, Goliński, et al. (2015), Muszyńska et al. (2018), Schlecht and Säumel (2015)
Leccinum versipelle			X			Mędyk, Grembecka, et al. (2017)

(*Continued*)

TABLE 4.16 Data on the mean content (mg kg^{-1} dry matter) of *lead* in fruiting bodies of wild-growing mushrooms collected from unpolluted (X), geologically specific (●), and anthropogenically contaminated (▲) sites and in cultivated species published since 2010. (Continued)

Species	<1	1–2	2–5	5–10	10–20	References
Lentinula edodes	X					Zhu et al. (2011)
Lepista nuda				●		Campos and Tejera (2011)
Lepista sordida			X			Zhu et al. (2011)
Leucoagaricus leucothites			X			Sarikurkcu et al. (2010)
Lycoperdon perlatum			X, ▲		X	Mędyk, Grembecka, et al. (2017), Radulescu et al. (2010), Sarikurkcu et al. (2015)
Macrolepiota mastoidea			▲			Schlecht and Säumel (2015)
Macrolepiota procera	▲, X^{S}	X, $X^{C,S}$,●	$X^{S,C}$,X, ▲	X,	▲	Árvay et al. (2014), Campos and Tejera (2011), Falandysz, Sapkota, Dryżalowska et al. (2017), Giannaccini et al. (2012), Gucia et al. (2012), Harangozo and Stanovič (2016), Kojta et al. (2011), Kułdo et al. (2014), Sarikurkcu et al. (2015), Schlecht and Säumel (2015), Severoglu et al. (2013), Širić, Humar, et al. (2016), Širić et al. (2017)
Marasmius oreades			●	X		Campos and Tejera (2011), Cvetkovic et al. (2015)
Morchella conica	X					Turfan et al. (2018)
Morchella esculenta	X					Gezer and Kaygusuz (2014), Sarikurkcu et al. (2012)
Pleurotus eryngii					X	Zhu et al. (2011)
Pleurotus nebrodensis			X			Zhu et al. (2011)

Pleurotus ostreatus	X, ▲		X			Gezer and Kaygusuz (2014), Muszyńska et al. (2018), Severoglu et al. (2013), Tel-Çayan et al. (2017), Zhu et al. (2011)
Polyporus squamosus	X					Sarikurkcu et al. (2011)
Ramaria aurea			X			Severoglu et al. (2013)
Ramaria botrytis		X				Turfan et al. (2018)
Ramaria stricta			X			Severoglu et al. (2013)
Russula delica	●					Aloupi et al. (2012)
Russula olivacea		▲				Harangozo and Stanovič (2016)
Russula vesca			▲			Schlecht and Säumel (2015)
Russula xerampelina		▲				Árvay et al. (2014), Harangozo and Stanovič (2016)
Sparassis crispa		▲	X			Schlecht and Säumel (2015), Severoglu et al. (2013)
Suillus bellini	●					Aloupi et al. (2012)
Suillus bovinus			X, $X^{S,C}$			Mędyk, Grembecka, et al. (2017), Muszyńska et al. (2018), Severoglu et al. (2013)
Suillus grevillei	▲		▲			Árvay et al. (2014), Harangozo and Stanovič (2016)
Suillus luteus	X	X		$X^{C,S}$		Gezer and Kaygusuz (2014), Mędyk, Grembecka, et al. (2017), Mleczek, Siwulski, Stuper-Szablewska, Rissmann, et al. (2013)
Suillus variegatus	$X^{C,S}$					Szubstarska et al. (2012)

(*Continued*)

TABLE 4.16 Data on the mean content (mg kg^{-1} dry matter) of *lead* in fruiting bodies of wild-growing mushrooms collected from unpolluted (X), geologically specific (●), and anthropogenically contaminated (▲) sites and in cultivated species published since 2010. (Continued)

Species	<1	1–2	2–5	5–10	10–20	References
Terfezia claveryi	X					Vahdani et al. (2017)
Tirmania nivea	X					Vahdani et al. (2017)
Tirmania pinoyi	X					Bouatia et al. (2018)
Tricholoma equestre	X^S	X^C	●			Campos and Tejera (2011), Širić et al. (2017)
Tricholoma fracticum	X					Tel-Çayan et al.(2017)
Tricholoma imbricatum			X			Sarikurkcu et al. (2011)
Tricholoma portentosum	X					Širić, Humar, et al. (2016)
Tricholoma terreum	X		X			Gezer and Kaygusuz (2014), Severoglu et al. (2013), Širić, Humar, et al. (2016), Širić et al. (2017), Turfan et al. (2018)
Volvariella volvacea		X				Zhu et al. (2011)
Xerocomus badius	X, X^C,▲, ▲^{C,S}	X, X^S,▲	$X^{C,S}$, ▲	▲	▲	Dimitrijevic et al. (2016), Gąsecka et al. (2017), Harangozo and Stanovič (2016), Kojta et al. (2012), Mleczek, Siwulski, Stuper-Szablewska, Rissmann, et al. (2013), Mleczek, Siwulski, Kaczmarek, et al. (2013), Mleczek, Siwulski, Mikołajczak, Gąsecka, Sobieralski, et al. (2015), Mleczek, Siwulski, Mikołajczak, Goliński, et al. (2015), Mleczek, Magdziak, et al. (2016), Muszyńska et al. (2018), Petkovšek and Pokorny (2013), Podlasińska et al. (2015), Proskura et al. (2017), Schlecht and Säumel (2015)

Xerocomus chrysenteron		X, ▲	X			Dimitrijevic et al. (2016), Sarikurkcu et al. (2011), Schlecht and Säumel (2015)
Xerocomus subtomentosus	X[C]		X[C,S]			Jarzyńska et al. (2012), Mędyk, Grembecka, et al. (2017)
Cultivated						
A. arvensis	X					Rzymski, Mleczek, Siwulski, Jasińska, et al. (2017)
A. bisporus (unspecified)			X			Huang et al. (2015)
A. bisporus (brown—cremini, portobello)	X					Rzymski, Mleczek, Siwulski, Jasińska, et al. (2017), Seyfferth et al., 2016
A. bisporus (white)	X		X			Mleczek, Rzymski, et al. (2018), Rzymski, Mleczek, Siwulski, Jasińska, et al. (2017), Seyfferth et al. (2016)
Agaricus subrufescens	X					Rzymski, Mleczek, Siwulski, Jasińska, et al. (2017)
Agrocybe chaxinggu		X				Huang et al. (2015)
A. cylindracea		X				Niedzielski et al. (2017)
A. mellea			X			Huang et al. (2015)
Auricularia auricula-judae	X		X			Huang et al. (2015), Mleczek, Rzymski, et al. (2018)
Auricularia polytricha	X					Niedzielski et al. (2017)
Auricularia thailandica	X					Bandara et al. (2017)
Clitocybe maxima	X					Niedzielski et al. (2017)

(Continued)

TABLE 4.16 Data on the mean content (mg kg^{-1} dry matter) of *lead* in fruiting bodies of wild-growing mushrooms collected from unpolluted (X), geologically specific (●), and anthropogenically contaminated (▲) sites and in cultivated species published since 2010. (Continued)

Species	<1	1–2	2–5	5–10	10–20	References
Flammulina velutipes		X	X			Huang et al. (2015), Niedzielski et al. (2017)
Grifola frondosa	X					Niedzielski et al. (2017)
H. erinaceus	X	X				Niedzielski et al. (2017), Turfan et al. (2018)
L. sulphureus		X				Niedzielski et al. (2017)
L. edodes	X	X	X			Gonçalves et al. (2014), Huang et al. (2015), Mleczek, Siwulski, Rzymski, Niedzielski, et al. (2017), Mleczek, Rzymski, et al. (2018), Seyfferth et al., 2016, Turfan et al. (2018)
Pholiota nameko	X	X				Huang et al. (2015), Niedzielski et al. (2017)
P. eryngii	X					Gonçalves et al. (2014), Rashid et al. (2018)
Pleurotus floridanus		X				Khani et al. (2017)
P. ostreatus	X		X			Gonçalves et al. (2014), Huang et al. (2015), Mleczek, Rzymski, et al. (2018), Rashid et al. (2018)
Trametes versicolor	X					Niedzielski et al. (2017)
Tremella fuciformis	X	X				Huang et al. (2015), Mleczek, Rzymski, et al. (2018), Niedzielski et al. (2017)
V. volvacea			X			Mleczek, Rzymski, et al. (2018)

C, Caps; *S*, stipes; X^m, median value.

The isotopic composition of lead in soils, thus, reflects the mixture of all participating lead sources. Komárek et al. (2007) observed that lead originating from recent air pollution is present mainly in the exchangable/acid-extractable fraction of organic horizons and is taken up by fruiting bodies. This was proved in *B. edulis*, where faster lead accumulation had occurred compared with *X. badius* and *X. chrysenteron*. In a work by Borovička et al. (2014), the $^{206}Pb/^{207}Pb$ isotopic ratio in fruiting bodies of *Agaricus bernardii*, *A. campestris*, and *Agaricus xanthodermus* ranged widely and did not reflect the organomineral topsoil horizon at particular sites. A detailed study of lead uptake was conducted in 19 samples of *A. bernardii* collected from an urban area in Prague, Czech Republic. The isotopic ratio varied in a surprisingly wide range of 1.124–1.175. In five samples characterized by low $^{206}Pb/^{207}Pb$ isotopic ratio, lead was undoubtedly taken from the topsoil layer (0–5 cm), corresponding with the former use of leaded petrol. In most of the remaining samples lead had to be transported from lower depths.

Samples of *Trametes* spp. collected between 1852 and 2008 in central and southern Victoria (Wu, Taylor, Handley, & Gulson, 2016a) and in the Greater Sydney region (Wu, Taylor, Handley, & Wu, 2016), Australia, helped to evaluate long-term atmospheric lead contamination sources. Lead isotopic composition $^{206}Pb/^{207}Pb$ data indicate that the environmental impact from leaded-petrol use during 1932–2002 persisted until the final sampling period of 2002–08.

Similarly as cadmium (Section 4.2.4), lead was leached by soaking and boiling to a greater extent from frozen slices of *X. badius* than from the fresh, air-dried, or freeze-dried slices. For instance, 57% of the initial content of the element in fresh mushrooms was released during boiling of frozen slices for 15 min, whereas only 23% was released during soaking for 15 min (Svoboda et al., 2002). Blanching of *A. fulva* caps for 15 min and followed by pickling caused lead leaching at rates of 62% and 85%, respectively (Drewnowska, Falandysz, et al., 2017).

Information on lead bioavailability from mushrooms is insufficient. Muszyńska et al. (2018) observed a transfer of 21.5% of total lead to gastric juice from *X. badius* biomass enriched with cadmium and lead.

4.2.6 Mercury (Hg)

Mercury ranks among the most frequently determined elements in mushrooms. The data here deal with total mercury content, that is, both inorganic and organic species. As results from Table 4.17 show, usual contents range between <0.5 and 5 mg kg^{-1} DM. Very similar values, mostly <0.5 mg kg^{-1} DM, were observed until 2010 (for a review, see Kalač, 2010 and references therein). Some species of genera *Agaricus* and *Boletus*, *L. nuda* and *M. procera* have showed to be mercury bioaccumulators. The reported contents in cultivated species are low (Table 4.17).

TABLE 4.17 Data on the mean content (mg kg^{-1} dry matter) of total *mercury* in fruiting bodies of wild-growing mushrooms collected from unpolluted (X), geologically specific (●), and anthropogenically contaminated (▲) sites and in cultivated species published since 2010.

Species	<0.5	0.5–1	1–2	2–5	5–10	10–20	References
Wild growing							
Agaricus campestris			X				Širić, Humar, et al. (2016), Širić et al. (2017)
Agrocybe aegerita	$X^{S,C}$						Ostos, Pérez-Rodríguez, Arroyo, and Moreno-Rojas (2015)
Amanita caesarea		X^{S}		X^{C}			Ostos et al. (2015)
Amanita fulva	$X^{S,C}$, X						Falandysz and Drewnowska (2015b), Nasr, Malloch, and Arp (2012)
Amanita rubescens	X^{S}	X^{C}					Drewnowska, Jarzyńska, Kojta, and Falandysz (2012)
Amanita vaginata	$X^{S,C}$						Drewnowska, Nnorom, and Falandysz (2014)
Armillariella mellea	X						Širić, Humar, et al. (2016), Širić et al. (2017), Zavastin et al. (2018)
Armillariella solidipes	$X^{S,C}$						Falandysz et al. (2013)
Boletus aestivalis			X^{S}	X, X^{C}			Falandysz, Krasińska, Pankavec, and Nnorom (2014), Harangozo and Stanovič (2016), Širić et al. (2014), Širić, Humar, et al. (2016), Širić et al. (2017)
Boletus auripes			$●^{S,C}$				Falandysz, Zhang, Wang, Saba, et al. (2015)
Boletus appendiculatus			X		X^{S}	X^{C}	Dimitrijevic et al. (2016), Ostos et al. (2015)

Boletus edulis		X, ▲	X, X^{S}	X, X^{S,C}, ●^{S}	X, ●^{C}		Árvay et al. (2017), Dimitrijevic et al. (2016), Falandysz, Zhang, Wang, Saba, et al. (2015), Frankowska et al. (2010), Giannaccini et al. (2012), Mleczek, Siwulski, Stuper-Szablewska, Rissmann, et al. (2013), Mleczek, Siwulski, Mikołajczak, Goliński, et al. (2015), Nasr et al. (2012), Širić, Humar, et al. (2016), Širić et al. (2017), Turfan et al. (2018), Zavastin et al. (2018), Zhang et al. (2010)
Boletus ferrugineus			●^{S}	●^{C}			Falandysz, Zhang, Wang, Saba, et al. (2015)
Boletus griseus			●^{S}	●^{C}			Falandysz, Zhang, Wang, Saba, et al. (2015)
Boletus impolitus		X, X^{S}	X^{C}				Dimitrijevic et al. (2016), Falandysz et al. (2014)
Boletus luridus	X^{S}	X^{C}		●^{S}	●^{C}		Falandysz et al. (2014), Falandysz, Zhang, Wang, Saba, et al. (2015), Falandysz, Zhang, Wiejak, et al. (2017)
Boletus magnificus		●^{S}	●^{S}	●^{C}			Falandysz, Zhang, Wang, Saba, et al. (2015), Falandysz, Zhang, Wiejak, et al. (2017)
Boletus pinophilus			X^{S}	X^{C}			Falandysz et al. (2014)
Boletus pulverulentus						▲	Árvay et al. (2014)
Boletus purpureus				●^{S}	●^{C}		Falandysz, Zhang, Wang, Saba, et al. (2015)
Boletus regius				X			Dimitrijevic et al. (2016)
Boletus speciosus			●^{S}	●^{C}			Falandysz, Zhang, Wang, Saba, et al. (2015)
Boletus tomentipes			●^{S}	●^{S,C}			Falandysz, Zhang, Wang, Saba, et al. (2015), Falandysz, Zhang, Wiejak, et al. (2017)

(*Continued*)

TABLE 4.17 Data on the mean content (mg kg^{-1} dry matter) of total *mercury* in fruiting bodies of wild-growing mushrooms collected from unpolluted (X), geologically specific (●), and anthropogenically contaminated (▲) sites and in cultivated species published since 2010. (Continued)

Species	<0.5	0.5–1	1–2	2–5	5–10	10–20	References
Boletus umbriniporus		$●^{S}$	$●^{C}$				Falandysz, Zhang, Wang, Saba, et al. (2015)
Cantharellus cibarius	X, $X^{S,C}$		X, ▲			▲	Árvay et al. (2014), Drewnowska and Falandysz (2015), Falandysz and Drewnowska (2015a), Falandysz, Widzicka, et al. (2012), Harangozo and Stanovič (2016), Mleczek, Siwulski, Stuper-Szablewska, Rissmann, et al. (2013), Nasr et al. (2012), Ostos et al. (2015), Zavastin et al. (2018)
Cantharellus tubaeformis	X						Nasr et al. (2012)
Clitocybe inversa			X				Širić, Humar, et al. (2016), Širić et al. (2017)
Clitocybe nebularis			X				Širić, Humar, et al. (2016), Širić et al. (2017)
Coprinus comatus			X^{S}	X^{C}			Falandysz (2016)
Cortinarius caperatus		X^{S}	X^{C}				Falandysz (2014)
Craterellus cornucopioides			X				Turfan et al. (2018)
Hydnum repandum	X						Nasr et al. (2012)
Laccaria amethystina	$X^{S,C}$						Kojta and Falandysz (2016b)
Laccaria laccata	$●^{S,C}$, $X^{S,C}$						Falandysz et al. (2016), Kojta and Falandysz (2016b)
Lactarius camphoratus		X					Nasr et al. (2012)
Lactarius deliciosus	$X^{S,C}$	X					Falandysz (2017), Mleczek, Siwulski, Stuper-Szablewska, Rissmann, et al. (2013)

Lactarius deterrimus	X^{S,C}	X, X^{C}					Falandysz (2017), Ostos et al. (2015), Rieder, Brunner, Horvat, Jacobs, and Frey (2011), Širić et al. (2017)
Lactarius volemus			●^{S}	●^{C}			Falandysz (2017)
Leccinum atrostipiatum		●^{S}	●^{C}				Falandysz et al. (2015a)
Leccinum chromapes			●^{S}	●^{C}			Falandysz et al. (2015a)
Leccinum crocipodium				X			Dimitrijevic et al. (2016)
Leccinum duriusculum	X^{S,C}						Falandysz et al. (2015a)
Leccinum extremiorientale			●^{S}	●^{C}			Falandysz et al. (2015a)
Leccinum griseum	X^{S,C}	X^{C}					Jarzyńska and Falandysz (2012b), Krasińska and Falandysz (2015)
Leccinum pseudoscabrum		X					Dimitrijevic et al. (2016)
Leccinum quercinum		X^{S}	X^{C}				Falandysz, Zhang, Wang, Krasińska, et al. (2015)
Leccinum rufum		X^{S,C}	X, X^{C}				Falandysz, Kowalewska, Nnorom, Drewnowska, & Jarzyńska (2012), Falandysz, Zhang, Wang, Krasińska, et al. (2015), Mleczek, Siwulski, Stuper-Szablewska, Rissmann, et al. (2013)
Leccinum rugosiceps			●^{S}	●^{C}			Falandysz, Zhang, Wang, Krasińska, et al. (2015)
Leccinum scabrum	X, X^{S,C}, ●^{C,S}				▲		Falandysz, Zhang, Wang, Krasińska, et al. (2015), Falandysz et al. (2016), Harangozo and Stanovič (2016), Mleczek, Siwulski, Mikołajczak, Goliński, et al. (2015), Nasr et al. (2012)

(*Continued*)

TABLE 4.17 Data on the mean content (mg kg^{-1} dry matter) of total *mercury* in fruiting bodies of wild-growing mushrooms collected from unpolluted (X), geologically specific (●), and anthropogenically contaminated (▲) sites and in cultivated species published since 2010. (Continued)

Species	<0.5	0.5–1	1–2	2–5	5–10	10–20	References
Leccinum versipelle	$●^{S}$, X^{S}	$●^{C}$, $X^{S,C}$					Falandysz, Zhang, Wang, Krasińska, et al. (2015), Krasińska and Falandysz (2016)
Leccinum vulpinum	X^{S}	X^{C}					Falandysz, Zhang, Wang, Krasińska, et al. (2015)
Lycoperdon perlatum			X				Falandysz, Nnorom, Jarzyńska, Romińska, and Damps (2012)
Macrocybe gigantea			$X^{S,C}$				Wiejak, Wang, Zhang, and Falandysz (2014)
Macrolepiota procera			X, $X^{S,C}$	X, $X^{S,C}$	X^{C}	▲	Árvay et al. (2014), Árvay et al. (2017), Falandysz, Sapkota, Dryżalowska et al. (2017), Giannaccini et al. (2012), Harangozo and Stanovič (2016), Kojta et al. (2011), Kułdo et al. (2014), Ostos et al. (2015), Rieder et al. (2011), Širić, Humar, et al. (2016), Širić et al. (2017)
Marasmius oreades				X			Turfan et al. (2018)
Pleurotus eryngii	$X^{S,C}$						Ostos et al. (2015)
Ramaria botrytis					X		Turfan et al. (2018)
Russula cyanoxantha					X		Rieder et al. (2011)
Russula nigricans				X			Rieder et al. (2011)
Russula olivacea					▲		Harangozo and Stanovič (2016)
Russula xerampelina					▲	▲	Árvay et al. (2014), Harangozo and Stanovič (2016)
Suillus bovinus	$X^{S,C}$						Saba, Falandysz, and Nnorom (2016b)

Suillus granulatus	$X^{S,C}$						Saba, Falandysz, and Nnorom (2016c)
Suillus grevillei		X				▲	Árvay et al. (2014), Harangozo and Stanovič (2016), Nasr et al. (2012)
Suillus luteus	$X^{S,C}$		X				Chudzyński, Jarzyńska, Stefańska, and Falandysz (2011), Mleczek, Siwulski, Stuper-Szablewska, Rissmann, et al. (2013), Saba, Falandysz, and Nnorom (2016a)
Suillus variegatus	$X^{S,C}$						Saba et al. (2016c)
Terfezia arenaria	X						Ostos et al. (2015)
Terfezia claveryi	X						Vahdani et al. (2017)
Tirmania nivea		X					Vahdani et al. (2017)
Tricholoma equestre		X, $X^{S,C}$					Maćkiewicz and Falandysz (2012), Širić, Humar, et al. (2016), Širić et al. (2017)
Tricholoma terreum	X						Širić, Humar, et al. (2016), Širić et al. (2017), Turfan et al. (2018)
Xerocomus badius	X, $X^{S,C}$, ▲^{S}	X, ▲, ▲^{C}	X, ▲	▲		▲	Dimitrijevic et al. (2016), Falandysz, Kojta, et al. (2012), Gąsecka et al. (2017), Harangozo and Stanovič (2016), Kojta et al. (2012), Mleczek, Siwulski, Stuper-Szablewska, Rissmann, et al. (2013), Mleczek, Siwulski, Kaczmarek, et al. (2013), Mleczek, Siwulski, Mikołajczak, Gąsecka, Sobieralski, et al. (2015), Mleczek, Siwulski, Mikołajczak, Goliński, et al. (2015), Mleczek, Magdziak, et al. (2016), Podlasińska et al. (2015), Rieder et al. (2011)
Xerocomus chrysenteron	X, $X^{S,C}$						Dimitrijevic et al. (2016), Dryżałowska and Falandysz (2014), Kojta et al. (2015)
Xerocomus ferrugineus	$X^{S,C}$						Kojta et al. (2015)

(*Continued*)

TABLE 4.17 Data on the mean content (mg kg^{-1} dry matter) of total *mercury* in fruiting bodies of wild-growing mushrooms collected from unpolluted (X), geologically specific (●), and anthropogenically contaminated (▲) sites and in cultivated species published since 2010. (Continued)

Species	<0.5	0.5–1	1–2	2–5	5–10	10–20	References
Xerocomus spadiceus		●^{S}	●^{C}				Kojta et al. (2015)
Xerocomus subtomentosus	X^{S,C}						Chojnacka, Drewnowska, Jarzyńska, Nnorom, and Falandysz (2012), Jarzyńska et al. (2012)
Xerocomus versicolor	X^{S,C}	●^{S}	●^{C}				Kojta et al. (2015)
Cultivated							
Agaricus bisporus	X						Huang et al. (2015)
Agrocybe chaxinggu	X						Huang et al. (2015)
A. mellea	X						Huang et al. (2015)
Auricularia auricula-judae	X						Huang et al. (2015)
Auricularia nigricans	X						Falandysz et al. (2016)
Auricularia thailandica	X						Bandara et al. (2017)
Flammulina velutipes	X						Huang et al. (2015)
Hericium erinaceus				X			Turfan et al. (2018)
Lentinula edodes	X			X			Huang et al. (2015), Turfan et al. (2018)
M. gigantea	X^{S,C}						Wiejak et al. (2014)
Pholiota nameko	X						Huang et al. (2015)
P. eryngii	X						Rashid et al. (2018)
Pleurotus ostreatus	X						Huang et al. (2015), Rashid et al. (2018)
Tremella fuciformis	X						Huang et al. (2015)

C, Caps; *S*, stipes.

Obviously considerably higher levels were observed in fruiting bodies growing in soils highly contaminated with mercury. For instance, extreme contents were repeatedly determined in several mushroom species collected from the vicinity of an abandoned mercury smelter in Slovakia. Árvay et al. (2014) reported mean contents of 20, 23, and 52 mg kg^{-1} DM in *C. cibarius*, *M. procera*, and *S. grevillei*, respectively. The respective maximum contents were 146, 144, and 177 mg kg^{-1} DM. Similarly, Harangozo and Stanovič (2016) in the same area determined median levels of 11.1, 17.4, 31.4, and 74.2 mg kg^{-1} DM in *X. badius*, *S. grevillei*, *M. procera*, and *B. aestivalis*, respectively. An extreme content of 182 mg kg^{-1} DM was observed in an individual sample of *B. aestivalis*. The results prove previous data reported by Kalač et al. (1996), who observed the highest mean values of 29.3, 32.4, and 84.7 mg kg^{-1} DM in *M. procera*, *B. edulis*, and *L. nuda*, respectively.

Falandysz, Zhang, Wang, Saba, et al. (2015) reported elevated mercury levels in 21 species of the genus *Boletus* growing in the Yunnan province of China within the Circum-Pacific Mercuriferous Belt.

4.2.6.1 Distribution within fruiting bodies

Mercury is distributed unevenly within fruiting bodies. As results from Table 4.17 show, the contents in caps are generally higher than in stipes. The values of mercury ratios in caps to stipes are collated in Table 4.18. The data originate from numerous papers from the laboratory of Professor Jerzy Falandysz, University of Gdańsk, Poland between 2007 and 2015 (Falandysz, Zhang, Wang, Krasińska, et al., 2015).

Another researchers separated fruiting body to spore-forming part (H) and the rest of fruiting body (RFB). Alonso, Salgado, García, and Melgar (2000) observed in eight wild-growing species a mean H/RFB ratio of 2.13, with a maximum value of 5.14 in *M. procera*. Surprisingly, no statistically significant differences between mercury contents in the Hs and in the RFBs of 28 wild-growing species were found in a further report from the same laboratory (Melgar, Alonso, & García, 2009). The mean H/RFB value of 1.74 was determined by Árvay et al. (2015) in 12 species growing in an area polluted from historical mining and smelting of polymetallic ores including mercury.

4.2.6.2 Bioconcentration in fruiting bodies

According to Nasr and Arp (2011), the total mercury level in fruiting bodies of wild-growing species is strongly affected by species and further by developmental stage, cap versus stipe, total organic sulfur both in fruiting bodies and in underlying soil, and also by total mercury and total carbon in the soil. Several papers reported lower bioconcentration potential of mushrooms at sites with elevated mercury content in the underlying substrates and higher bioconcentration at sites with lower contents in the substrates. Such relations were observed for *X. badius* (Falandysz, Kojta, et al., 2012) and *X. chrysenteron*

TABLE 4.18 Ratio of mercury contents in caps and stipes ($R_{C/S}$) (Falandysz, Zhang, Wang, Krasińska, et al., 2015).

Species	Number of samples	$R_{C/S}$
Amanita rubescens	272	1.1 ± 0.4–1.7 ± 0.8
Amanita fulva	831	1.3 ± 0.4–2.5 ± 1.1
Amanita vaginata	92	1.2 ± 0.4–2.1 ± 0.5
Armillariella solidipes	955	1.1 ± 0.4–1.7–0.3
Boletus edulis	173	1.0 ± 0.7–3.2 ± 2.1
Cortinarius caperatus	715	1.8 ± 0.4–3.2 ± 0.9
Leccinum griseum	110	1.3 ± 0.7–2.3 ± 0.9
Leccinum rufum	126	1.4 ± 0.1–2.3 ± 0.7
Leccinum scabrum	240	1.7 ± 0.4–2.9 ± 1.0
Macrolepiota procera	348	1.1 ± 0.2–4.9 ± 5.1
Suillus grevillei	121	3.1 ± 1.1
Suillus luteus	383	1.8 ± 0.4–3.3 ± 0.8
Tricholoma equestre	149	1.1 ± 0.1–1.9 ± 1.8
Xerocomus badius	221	1.8 ± 0.8
Xerocomu chrysenteron	640	0.86 ± 0.55–2.8 ± 2.5
Xerocomus subtomentosus	247	1.0 ± 0.4–2.9 ± 1.8

(Dryżałowska & Falandysz, 2014). For instance, in *A. fulva*, classified as a weak mercury bioaccumulator, were determined BCF values of 1.2–3.6 for caps and 0.66–1.7 for stipes with elevated mercury level in underlying soils, while BCF of 11–25 for caps and 7–12 for stipes in fruiting bodies growing in less contaminated soils (Falandysz & Drewnowska, 2015b). Statistical analysis of data sets available worldwide on mercury in *C. comatus* rendered an interesting information (Falandysz, 2016). Wide ranges of BCF values, 8–10 for caps and 4–74 for stipes, were observed. In spite of this, the analysis showed a positive correlation between the degree of soils' and fruiting bodies' contamination. *C. comatus* could be, thus, considered as a sensitive species with a bioindication potency for soils polluted with mercury. A similar course, decreasing BCF with increasing mercury concentration in the substrate, appeared during experimental cultivation of *Stropharia rugosoannulata* (Gabriel, Švec, Kolihová, Tlustoš, & Száková, 2016).

In contrarst, Rzymski, Mleczek, Siwulski, Gąsecka, and Niedzielski (2016) found mercury uptake increasing in a content-dependent manner in

A. bisporus, *H. erinaceus*, and *P. ostreatus* cultivated on substrates supplemented with mercury at levels of 0.1–0.5 mM (20.1–100.3 mg Hg kg^{-1} DM of the substrate) as $mercury^{II}$ nitrate. Maximum mercury contents of 116, 53, and 44 mg kg^{-1} DM in *A. bisporus*, *H. erinaceus*, and *P. ostreatus*, respectively, were determined in caps of fruiting bodies cultivated at substrates with 0.5 mM of added mercury.

According to the available data, mushroom species can be classified into groups of weak, medium, and extensive bioaccumulators of mercury. *C. cibarius* is a representative of the first group. The determined BCF from various sites varied between 0.1 and 5.9 (Falandysz & Drewnowska, 2015a; Falandysz, Widzicka, et al., 2012). *Armillariella solidipes* with BCF 1.8–15 for caps and 0.9–4.5 for stipes can be characterized also as a moderate mercury accumulator (Falandysz et al., 2013). *Lactarius deliciosus* and *Lactarius volemus* can be classified as medium accumulators (Falandysz, 2017). Naturally, the greatest interest has been focused on the extensive bioaccumulators. Data for several species are collated in Table 4.19.

4.2.6.3 Mercury speciation

Mercury is released into the atmosphere by natural and anthropogenic processes at annual global levels above 6000 tons and can be distributed over long distances and then deposited. Mercury and its compounds, in particular monomethylmercury (commonly methylmercury, CH_3Hg, or, more accurately, $CH_3Hg^{(+)}$) are highly toxic for microorganisms, animals, and humans. Methylation of mercury proceeds mainly under anoxic conditions by bacterial activity. Methylmercury is lipophillic in nature and is thus accumulated in living organisms more efficiently than inorganic species. Methylmercury is more toxic than the inorganic counterparts; recent values of tolerable weekly intake are 4 and 1.3 μg kg^{-1} bodyweight for inorganic mercury and CH_3Hg, respectively.

High toxicity of CH_3Hg raised the interest of researchers since the early period of trace elements investigation in mushrooms in the 1970's. Stijve and Besson (1976) determined the methylmercury proportion from total mercury as 1.2%–16.4% in 14 species of the genus *Agaricus*; however, this was mostly up to 10%. Minagawa, Sasaki, Takizawa, Tamura, and Oshina (1980) reported a proportion of 2.9%–9.1% in *Collybia* spp. growing in the vicinity of an acetaldehyde-producing plant, using mercury salts as catalysts. Low CH_3Hg contents ranging between 0.01 and 3.7 mg kg^{-1} DM were observed by Bargagli and Baldi (1984) in mushrooms in an Italian mercury-ore mining area. Kojo and Lodenius (1989) reported CH_3Hg proportion up to 10% in only four fruiting bodies of three *Agaricus* species. A wider range of 0.4%–19% was reported by Fischer, Rapsomanikis, Andreae, and Baldi (1995) in mushrooms from a former mercury-mining area in Germany. Methylmercury in widely consumed *X. badius* and *L. scabrum* showed the proportion of only

TABLE 4.19 Bioconcentration factor (BCF) for *mercury* of several highly accumulative wild-growing mushroom species.

Species	BCF	Reference
Agaricus campestris	14	Širić, Humar, et al. (2016)
	28^{C}, 35^{S}	Širić et al. (2017)
Boletus aestivalis	24	Širić, Humar, et al. (2016)
	42^{C}, 35^{S}	Širić et al. (2017)
Boletus edulis	11 − 132	Mleczek, Siwulski, Stuper-Szablewska, Rissmann, et al. (2013)
	27	Širić, Humar, et al. (2016)
	42^{C}, 39^{S}	Širić et al. (2017)
Cortinarius caperatus	$18–120^{C}$, $7.3. – 42^{S}$	Falandysz (2014)
Lactarius deliciosus	8–98	Mleczek, Siwulski, Stuper-Szablewska, Rissmann, et al. (2013)
Leccinum rufum	12 − 150	Mleczek, Siwulski, Stuper-Szablewska, Rissmann, et al. (2013)
Lycoperdon perlatum	9.6–280	Falandysz, Nnorom, et al. (2012)
Macrolepiota procera	140^{C}, 51^{S}	Kułdo et al. (2014)
	14	Širić, Humar, et al. (2016)
	25^{C}, 19^{S}	Širić et al. (2017)
Suillus luteus	11–141	Mleczek, Siwulski, Stuper-Szablewska, Rissmann, et al. (2013)
Xerocomus badius	13–170	Mleczek, Siwulski, Stuper-Szablewska, Rissmann, et al. (2013)

C, Caps; *S*, stipes.

0.7%–1.3%. The authors also showed, for the first time, the ability to methylate mercury in *C. comatus* and *Coprinus radians*.

Further data on CH_3Hg were published after a gap. Rieder et al. (2011) observed a highly significant correlation between total and methylmercury contents in fruiting bodies. The proportion of CH_3Hg from total mercury varied from 0.3% in *Lactarius deterrimus* and *S. luteus* to 11.3% in *Lycoperdon pyriforme*. The mean proportion was 4.5%. A higher mean proportion of 14.3% was found by Ruiz-de-Cenzano, López-Salazar, Cervera, and de la Guardia (2016) in *L. deliciosus*.

Overall, the most reported percentages of methylmercury from total mercury in mushrooms are up to 10%.

4.2.6.4 Mercury shrinkage during mushroom storage and cooking

Nasr et al. (2012) observed a mean decrease of mercury content by 21% from various freeze-dried mushroom species after air-dry storage for 1 year; the reduction during the following two years was low.

About 10% of the initial content of mercury was released from *X. badius* slices to a table-salt solution during soaking at ambient temperature for 5−15 min. Boiling was a more efficient treatment resulting in 15%−25% shrinkage of mercury during the initial 15 min. Prolonged boiling had only a limited effect to further decrease the mercury level. Higher shrinkage was observed from frozen and air-dried slices than from fresh or freeze-dried counterparts due to the different disruption of tissues and cells. The decrease of mercury content was lower than those of cadmium and lead (Svoboda et al., 2002). Comparable decreases by 10% and 19% after boiling of *B. edulis* for 15 and 30 min, respectively, and 40% after frying, were observed by Melgar et al. (2009). Reduction of the mercury level in *A. fulva* by 10% followed boiling for 10 min (Falandysz & Drewnowska, 2015b).

Blanching, that is, boiling for 5 or 15 min, of fresh sliced *C. cibarius* resulted in mercury decrease by about 15% of the initial content, while shrinkage up to 35% was observed in deep-frozen slices. Following pickling of blanched slices in a diluted vinegar marinade for 30 days had only a low, if any, effect on additional removal of mercury. The element was more effectively released in boiling water from fresh caps of *A. fulva* than from *C. cibarius*. Following pickling of blanched *A. fulva* had no additional effect on mercury leaching (Falandysz & Drewnowska, 2017).

Simulated pan-frying for 20 min decreased mercury content in *X. badius* and *X. chrysenteron* by about 33% of the initial level in frozen and then thawed mushrooms (Cibulka, Čurdová, Miholová, & Stěhulová, 1999).

Testing the strategy to reduce mercury absorption (bioaccessibility) from foods after gastrointestinal digestion, Jadán-Piedra, Alcántara, et al. (2017) and Jadán-Piedra, Baquedano, Puig, Vélez, and Devesa (2017) reported good results after the addition of various strains of lactic acid bacteria or *Sacharomyces cerevisiae* to consumed mushrooms. The respective reduction levels were up to 68% and 19%−77%, respectively. In seafood, another source of dietary inorganic mercury and methylmercury, the application of the microorganisms did not reduce the bioaccessibility.

4.2.7 Silver (Ag)

Data of Table 4.20 show that the most frequent silver contents are up to 2 and <0.5 mg kg^{-1} DM in wild-growing and cultivated species, respectively. Levels over 5 mg kg^{-1} DM were observed only in *X. badius* growing in polluted sites (Kojta et al., 2012; Mleczek, Siwulski, Mikołajczak, Gąsecka,

TABLE 4.20 Data on the mean content (mg kg^{-1} dry matter) of *silver* in fruiting bodies of wild-growing mushrooms collected from unpolluted (X), geologically specific (●), and anthropogenically contaminated (▲) sites and in cultivated species published since 2010.

Species	<0.5	0.5–1	1–2	2–5	5–10	>10	References
Wild growing							
Agaricus arvensis					X		Ayaz et al. (2011)
Agaricus campestris					▲^{S}	▲^{C}, X^{S,C}	Zsigmond et al. (2018)
Amanita fulva		X^{C,S}					Falandysz, Drewnowska, et al. (2017)
Amanita ponderosa			X				Salvador et al. (2018)
Armillariella mellea		X					Zavastin et al. (2018)
Boletus appendiculatus			X^{Sm}	X	X^{Cm}		Alaimo et al. (2018), Dimitrijevic et al. (2016)
Boletus edulis			X	X	X		Ayaz et al. (2011), Brzezicha-Cirocka et al. (2016), Dimitrijevic et al. (2016), Mędyk, Grembecka, et al. (2017), Mleczek, Siwulski, Mikołajczak, Goliński, et al. (2015), Zavastin et al. (2018)
Boletus impolitus			X				Dimitrijevic et al. (2016)
Boletus luridus		●^{S}		●^{C}			Falandysz, Zhang, Wiejak, et al. (2017)
Boletus magnificus	●^{S}		●^{C}				Falandysz, Zhang, Wiejak, et al. (2017)
Boletus regius				X			Dimitrijevic et al. (2016)
Boletus tomentipes				●^{S,C}			Falandysz, Zhang, Wiejak, et al. (2017)

Cantharellus cibarius	X, ▲, ND	X					Ayaz et al. (2011), Brzezicha-Cirocka et al. (2016), Drewnowska and Falandysz (2015), Falandysz and Drewnowska (2015a), Falandysz, Chudzińska, et al. (2017), Mleczek, Niedzielski, Kalač, Budka, et al. (2016), Zavastin et al. (2018)
Cantharellus tubaeformis	ND,X						Ayaz et al. (2011), Falandysz, Chudzińska, et al. (2017)
Clitopilus prunulus				X^{m}			Alaimo et al. (2018)
Hydnum imbricatum	$X^{S,C}$						Mędyk, Chudzińska, et al. (2017)
Hydnum repandum	ND						Ayaz et al. (2011)
Laccaria laccata	ND						Ayaz et al. (2011)
Leccinum aurantiacum		X					Brzezicha-Cirocka et al. (2016)
Leccinum crocipodium	X						Dimitrijevic et al. (2016)
Leccinum duriusculum	X^{S}	X^{C}					Jarzyńska and Falandysz (2012a)
Leccinum griseum	X^{S}	X^{C}					Jarzyńska and Falandysz (2012b)
Leccinum pseudoscabrum				X			Dimitrijevic et al. (2016)
Leccinum scabrum	X, ▲			X			Mędyk, Grembecka, et al. (2017), Mleczek, Siwulski, Mikołajczak, Goliński, et al. (2015), Mleczek, Niedzielski, Kalač, Budka, et al. (2016)
Leccinum versipelle		X					Mędyk, Grembecka, et al. (2017)

(Continued)

TABLE 4.20 Data on the mean content (mg kg^{-1} dry matter) of *silver* in fruiting bodies of wild-growing mushrooms collected from unpolluted (X), geologically specific (●), and anthropogenically contaminated (▲) sites and in cultivated species published since 2010. (Continued)

Species	<0.5	0.5–1	1–2	2–5	5–10	>10	References
Lepista nuda		X					Ayaz et al. (2011)
Lycoperdon perlatum		X	X				Brzezicha-Cirocka et al. (2016), Mędyk, Grembecka, et al. (2017)
Macrolepiota procera			X^{C}	$X^{C,S}$	X^{S}		Falandysz, Sapkota, Dryżalowska et al. (2017), Gucia et al. (2012), Kojta et al. (2011), Kułdo et al. (2014), Stefanović et al. (2016)
Pleurotus ostreatus	▲						Mleczek, Niedzielski, Kalač, Budka, et al. (2016)
Suillus bovinus	$X^{C,S}$, ▲						Mędyk, Grembecka, et al. (2017), Mleczek, Niedzielski, Kalač, Budka, et al. (2016)
Suillus variegatus	$X^{S,C}$						Szubstarska et al. (2012)
Xerocomus badius		X	$▲^{S}$	X	$▲^{C}$	▲	Dimitrijevic et al. (2016), Kojta et al. (2012), Mleczek, Siwulski, Mikołajczak, Gąsecka, Sobieralski, et al. (2015), Mleczek, Siwulski, Mikołajczak, Goliński, et al. (2015)
Xerocomus chrysenteron	X						Dimitrijevic et al. (2016)
Xerocomus subtomentosus	X^{C}			$X^{S,C}$			Jarzyńska et al. (2012), Mędyk, Grembecka, et al. (2017)

Cultivated							
Agrocybe cylindracea	X						Niedzielski et al. (2017)
Auricularia polytricha	X						Niedzielski et al. (2017)
Clitocybe maxima	X						Niedzielski et al. (2017)
Flammulina velutipes	X						Niedzielski et al. (2017)
Grifola frondosa	X						Niedzielski et al. (2017)
Hericium erinaceus	X						Niedzielski et al. (2017)
Laetiporus sulphureus	X						Niedzielski et al. (2017)
Lentinula edodes			X				Mleczek, Siwulski, Rzymski, Niedzielski, et al. (2017)
Pholiota nameko	X						Niedzielski et al. (2017)
Trametes versicolor	X						Niedzielski et al. (2017)
Tremella fuciformis	X						Niedzielski et al. (2017)

C, Caps; *ND*, below limit of detection; *S*, stipes.

Sobieralski, et al., 2015; Mleczek, Siwulski, Mikołajczak, Goliński, et al., 2015). Values similar to the data in Table 4.20 were reported during the period 2000–09 (for references, see Kalač, 2010). Several species were observed as silver bioaccumulators, for example, *Amanita strobiliformis*, *A. arvensis*, *A. campestris*, *A. augustus*, or *M. procera*. For instance, *A. campestris* from 38 ± 25 (range 1.7–150) mg kg^{-1} DM, while fruiting bodies 24 ± 13 (range 3.4–43) mg kg^{-1} DM (Falandysz, Bona, & Danisiewicz, 1994a).

Borovička et al. (2010) determined median silver contents of 0.79 and 2.94 mg kg^{-1} DM in mycorrhizal and saprobic mushrooms, respectively, from pristine areas, whereas a median of 24.7 mg kg^{-1} DM was observed for both groups in fruiting bodies collected from the vicinity of a long-operating lead smelter. The highest level of 304–692 mg kg^{-1} DM was found in *Amanita* spp. of the section *Vaginatae*. Elevated silver levels compared with data in Table 4.20 were reported by Kubrová et al. (2014) in mushrooms from a former uranium and historical silver-mining area. Mean contents were 1.07 and 9.83 mg kg^{-1} DM in mycorrhizal and saprobic species, respectively. The highest level of 53.9 mg kg^{-1} DM in individual species was determined in *A. arvensis*.

Mycorrhizal species *A. strobiliformis*, edible but consumed only to a limited extent, was identified as a silver hyperaccumulator with commonly hundreds mg kg^{-1} DM (Borovička, Řanda, Jelínek, & Dunn, 2007). Beneš, Hložková, Matěnová, Borovička, and Kotrba (2016) determined in *A. strobiliformis* growing in two parks in Prague 67 ± 15 and 284 ± 64 mg kg^{-1} DM. The element was sequestered by 3.4 kDa metallothionein. More information on intracellular silver sequestration in *A. strobiliformis* with metallothioneins was reported by Osobová et al. (2011). Virtually all silver in inedible *Amanita submembranacea* was found to be intercellular and sequestered in the major 7 kDa and the minor 3.3 kDa complexes (Borovička et al., 2007).

Generally, silver belongs among the elements bioaccumulated in fruiting bodies. The reported BCF values vary very widely, not only among species, but also in dependence on presence of other metals in growing substrate. For instance, BCF up to 10 was observed in *X. badius*, but was <0.5 in *B. edulis* and *X. chrysenteron* growing in a site polluted from a long-operated lead smelter (Komárek et al., 2007). In contrast, Falandysz and Danisiewicz (1995) determined BCF of 10–670 and 7.5–400 for caps and stipes, respectively, of wild-growing *A. campestris*. The BCF values showed a significantly decreasing trend with an increase of silver content in the substrates. This observation was proved in *A. bisporus* cultivated on compost enriched with silver nitrate at levels of silver 0.01–10.3 mg kg^{-1} DM. The highest BCF values of 120 and 230 were observed in caps and stipes, respectively, of fruiting bodies produced on the compost with the lowest level of supplemented silver (Falandysz, Bona, & Danisiewicz, 1994b). On the contrary, Kubrová et al. (2014), using sequential extraction, inferred that the accumulation of silver in fruiting bodies apparently does not depend on its total content and chemical fractionation in substrates.

An interesting comparison was reported by Andersson, Reimann, Flem, Englmaier, and Fabian (2018). The median content of silver in inedible *Lactarius rufus* of 0.72 mg kg^{-1} DM was 195 times higher than the median of 15 plant materials growing at the same sampling sites.

According to the data in Table 4.20, silver is distributed evenly in caps and stipes.

Silver was leached from fresh caps of *A. fulva* by 70% and 90% of the initial content in blanching water for 15 min and then to a pickling vinegar solution during 30 days, respectively (Drewnowska, Falandysz, et al., 2017).

4.2.8 Thallium (Tl)

The most comprehensive study on thallium content in mushrooms, entailing 421 edible, inedible, and toxic species was carried out by Seeger and Gross (1981). Over 85% of the samples had a thallium level below the limit of detection of 0.25 mg kg^{-1} DM, while only 4.3% of the samples had over 2 mg kg^{-1} DM. The maximum observed contents were 5.5 mg kg^{-1} DM in several samples. Similar values are apparent from data published since 2010 (Table 4.21). Most contents are below 0.3 mg kg^{-1} DM. The same levels were published in several papers prior to 2010 (for references, see Kalač, 2010). Fruiting bodies of a white strain of *Hypsizygus marmoreus* had significantly higher thallium contents than a gray strain cultivated under the same experimental conditions (Mleczek, Siwulski, Rzymski, Budka, et al., 2018).

No bioconcentration of thallium in fruiting bodies was observed in five wild, edible species (Seeger & Gross, 1981). Information on the element distribution between caps and stipes is limited; however, it seems from data in Table 4.21 that the levels in stipes are usually higher than those in caps.

Thallium was leached from fresh caps of *A. fulva* to blanching water during 15 min and then to a pickling vinegar solution during 30 days by 80% and 95%, respectively, of the initial content in fresh caps (Drewnowska, Falandysz, et al., 2017).

Overall, the limited data report low levels of thallium in fruiting bodies.

4.2.9 Estimation of intake of the main deleterious elements

Information on tolerable intake of main detrimental elements was given in Section 2.4.

As results from previous information show, the contents of the deleterious elements in mushrooms, particularly in wild-growing species, vary widely. The consideration of a possible health hazard is, therefore, rather speculative. Data from Table 4.22 thus have to be taken as general information. Within the variables, the usual content of an element in mushrooms is

TABLE 4.21 Data on the mean content (mg kg^{-1} dry matter) of *thallium* in fruiting bodies of wild-growing mushrooms collected from unpolluted (X), geologically specific (●), and anthropogenically contaminated (▲) sites and in cultivated species published since 2010.

Species	<0.1	0.1–0.3	0.3–0.5	0.5–1.0	1–2	References
Wild growing						
Amanita fulva	$X^{C,S}$	X^{S}				Drewnowska, Falandysz, et al. (2017), Falandysz, Drewnowska, et al. (2017)
Armillariella mellea	X					Zavastin et al. (2018)
Boletus appendiculatus		$X^{C,Sm}$				Alaimo et al. (2018)
Boletus edulis	X					Zavastin et al. (2018)
Boletus luridus	$●^{C}$	$●^{S}$				Falandysz, Zhang, Wiejak, et al. (2017)
Boletus magnificus	$●^{C,S}$					Falandysz, Zhang, Wiejak, et al. (2017)
Boletus tomentipes	$●^{C}$	$●^{S}$				Falandysz, Zhang, Wiejak, et al. (2017)
Cantharellus cibarius	X		X			Falandysz, Chudzińska, et al. (2017), Zavastin et al. (2018)
Cantharellus tubaeformis	X					Falandysz, Chudzińska, et al. (2017)
Clitopilus prunulus	X^{m}					Alaimo et al. (2018)
Hydnum imbricatum	X^{C}	X^{S}				Mędyk, Chudzińska, et al. (2017)
Macrolepiota procera	X^{C}					Falandysz, Sapkota, Dryżalowska et al. (2017)
Pleurotus ostreatus	X					Tel-Çayan et al.(2017)
Tricholoma fracticum		X				Tel-Çayan et al.(2017)
Xerocomus badius					▲	Mleczek, Siwulski, Mikołajczak, Gąsecka, Sobieralski, et al. (2015)
Cultivated						
Lentinula edodes				X		Mleczek, Siwulski, Rzymski, Niedzielski, et al. (2017)

C, Caps; *S*, stipes; X^{m}, median value.

TABLE 4.22 Estimation of the daily intake (mg day^{-1}) and the contribution (%) to the Provisional Tolerable Weekly Intake (PTWI) of main detrimental elements from wild-growing mushrooms.

Element	Usual content (mg kg^{-1} DM)	Content in a single serving (mg)	PTWI (mg kg^{-1} bodyweight)	PTWI for a 60 kg adult (mg)	Proportion of PTWI from a single serving (%)
Arsenic	1.0	0.025	0.015	0.9	2.8
Cadmium	2.5	0.0625	0.058	0.348	18.0
Mercury (total)	2.0	0.050	0.004	0.24	20.8
Lead	2.5	0.0625	0.025	1.5	4.2

Specifications: nonaccumulating species; usual level of an element from Tables 4.13 and 4.15–4.17; a single serving of 250 g FM (approximately 25 g DM); a 60 kg adult.

the weakest guess. The estimation can change markedly in species accumulating an element. Only one mushroom serving of 25 g DM (i.e., about 250 g fresh matter) would fulfill the provisional tolerable weekly intake (PTWI) values of arsenic, cadmium, total mercury, and lead at contents of 36, 13.9, 9.6, and 60 mg kg^{-1} DM, respectively, calculated for an adult weighing 60 kg. Such a scenario seems to be of low probability; however, consumption frequency is often high during wild mushroom harvest season and mushrooms are not the only source of deleterious elements.

Generally, cultivated mushrooms are of low risk.

4.3 Nutritionally nonessential elements

This section deals with a number of mineral elements considered recently as nutritionally unimportant. Nevertheless, the classification can change with increasing knowledge on their roles in human nutrition and health. The contents of most of these elements in mushrooms are low and very low, even at the very limit of quantification of the recent sophisticated analytical methods and instruments.

4.3.1 Aluminum (Al)

Aluminum belongs among medium-determined elements in mushrooms. Data in Table 4.23 show a wide range of the contents from <25 mg kg^{-1} DM in most of the cultivated and a proportion of wild-growing species to >500 mg kg^{-1} DM in several reports. The highest contents of 3310, 2080, and 1850 mg kg^{-1} DM were reported by Durkan et al. (2011) in *P. ostreatus*,

TABLE 4.23 Data on the mean content (mg kg^{-1} dry matter) of *aluminum* in fruiting bodies of wild-growing mushrooms collected from unpolluted (X), geologically specific (●), and anthropogenically contaminated (▲) sites and in cultivated species published since 2010.

Species	<25	25–50	50–75	75–100	100–150	150–200	200–500	>500	References
Wild growing									
Agaricus arvensis							X		Ayaz et al. (2011)
Agaricus bisporus							X		Durkan et al. (2011)
Agaricus bitorquis								X	Durkan et al. (2011)
Agaricus campestris		$X^{C,S}$, ●			X	$▲^{C,S}$	X		Campos and Tejera (2011), Durkan et al. (2011), Sarikurkcu et al. (2012), Zsigmond et al. (2018)
Agaricus sylvicola		●							Campos and Tejera (2011)
Agrocybe aegerita							X		Durkan et al. (2011)
Agrocybe cylindracea		X							Sarikurkcu et al. (2012)
Amanita caesarea		●							Campos and Tejera (2011)
Amanita fulva				$X^{C,S}$					Falandysz, Drewnowska, et al. (2017)
Amanita ponderosa							X		Salvador et al. (2018)
Amanita rubescens			●						Campos and Tejera (2011)
Armillariella mellea						X			Durkan et al. (2011)
Boletus appendiculatus				X, X^{Sm}	X^{Cm}				Alaimo et al. (2018), Dimitrijevic et al. (2016)

Boletus edulis	X^{C}	X, X^{S}	X, X^{C}	$X, X^{C,S}$					Ayaz et al. (2011), Cvetkovic et al. (2015), Dimitrijevic et al. (2016), Falandysz et al. (2011), Frankowska et al. (2010), Mleczek, Siwulski, Stuper-Szablewska, Sobieralski, et al. (2013), Turfan et al. (2018), Zhang et al. (2010)
Boletus impolitus			X						Dimitrijevic et al. (2016)
Boletus regius			X						Dimitrijevic et al. (2016)
Cantharellus cibarius		X, ▲		●		X	X		Ayaz et al. (2011), Campos and Tejera (2011), Cvetkovic et al. (2015), Drewnowska and Falandysz (2015), Falandysz and Drewnowska (2015a), Mleczek, Siwulski, Stuper-Szablewska, Sobieralski, et al. (2013), Mleczek, Niedzielski, Kalač, Budka, et al. (2016)
Cantharellus tubaeformis						X			Ayaz et al. (2011)
Clitocybe geotropa				●					Campos and Tejera (2011)
Clitocybe gibba					●				Campos and Tejera (2011)
Clitopilus prunulus							X^{m}		Alaimo et al. (2018)
Craterellus cornucopioides						X			Turfan et al. (2018)
Ganoderma lucidum				●					Campos and Tejera (2011)
Helvella leucopus							X		Sarikurkcu et al. (2012)
Hydnum repandum						X			Ayaz et al. (2011)

(Continued)

TABLE 4.23 Data on the mean content (mg kg^{-1} dry matter) of *aluminum* in fruiting bodies of wild-growing mushrooms collected from unpolluted (X), geologically specific (●), and anthropogenically contaminated (▲) sites and in cultivated species published since 2010. (Continued)

Species	<25	25–50	50–75	75–100	100–150	150–200	200–500	>500	References
Hygrophorus russula				●					Campos and Tejera (2011)
Laccaria amethystina							X		Durkan et al. (2011)
Laccaria laccata								X	Ayaz et al. (2011), Durkan et al. (2011)
Lactarius deliciosus		X	●						Campos and Tejera (2011), Mleczek, Siwulski, Stuper-Szablewska, Sobieralski, et al. (2013), Turfan et al. (2018)
Lactarius piperatus				X					Cvetkovic et al. (2015)
Lactarius sanguifluus			●						Campos and Tejera (2011)
Laetiporus sulphureus		X	X						Durkan et al. (2011), Turfan et al. (2018)
Leccinum aurantiacum		X							Mleczek, Siwulski, Stuper-Szablewska, Sobieralski, et al. (2013)
Leccinum crocipodium		X							Dimitrijevic et al. (2016)
Leccinum duriusculum		$X^{C,S}$							Jarzyńska and Falandysz (2012a)
Leccinum griseum	X^{S}	X^{C}							Jarzyńska and Falandysz (2012b)
Leccinum pseudoscabrum								X	Dimitrijevic et al. (2016)
Leccinum scabrum	▲		X^{S}	X^{C}					Falandysz (2018), Mleczek, Niedzielski, Kalač, Budka, et al. (2016)

Lepista nuda				●	X				Ayaz et al. (2011), Campos and Tejera (2011), Durkan et al. (2011)
Lycoperdon perlatum					X				Durkan et al. (2011)
Macrolepiota procera			●	$X^{S,C}$		X^{S}	$X^{S,C}$		Campos and Tejera (2011), Gucia et al. (2012), Kojta et al. (2011), Kułdo et al. (2014)
Marasmius oreades			X	●			X		Campos and Tejera (2011), Cvetkovic et al. (2015), Gucia et al. (2012), Turfan et al. (2018)
Morchella conica			X						Turfan et al. (2018)
Morchella esculenta	X		X						Rossbach et al. (2017), Sarikurkcu et al. (2012)
Pleurotus ostreatus	▲							X	Durkan et al. (2011), Mleczek, Niedzielski, Kalač, Budka, et al. (2016), Tel-Çayan et al.(2017)
Ramaria botrytis		X							Turfan et al. (2018)
Suillus bovinus	▲						X		Durkan et al. (2011), Mleczek, Niedzielski, Kalač, Budka, et al. (2016)
Suillus luteus			X						Mleczek, Siwulski, Stuper-Szablewska, Sobieralski, et al. (2013)
Suillus variegatus		X^{S}	X^{C}						Szubstarska et al. (2012)
Terfezia claveryi	X								Kivrak (2015)
Terfezia olbiensis	X								Kivrak (2015)
Tricholoma equestre					●				Campos and Tejera (2011)

(Continued)

TABLE 4.23 Data on the mean content (mg kg^{-1} dry matter) of *aluminum* in fruiting bodies of wild-growing mushrooms collected from unpolluted (X), geologically specific (●), and anthropogenically contaminated (▲) sites and in cultivated species published since 2010. (Continued)

Species	<25	25–50	50–75	75–100	100–150	150–200	200–500	>500	References
Tricholoma fracticum		X							Tel-Çayan et al.(2017)
Tricholoma terreum				X					Turfan et al. (2018)
Xerocomus badius	X, ▲^{C}	X, ▲, ▲^{S}		X			▲		Dimitrijevic et al. (2016), Kojta et al. (2012), Mleczek, Siwulski, Stuper-Szablewska, Sobieralski, et al. (2013), Mleczek, Siwulski, Mikołajczak, Gąsecka, Sobieralski, et al. (2015), Mleczek, Magdziak, et al. (2016)
Xerocomus chrysenteron				X				X	Dimitrijevic et al. (2016), Durkan et al. (2011)
Xerocomus subtomentosus		X^{S,C}							Jarzyńska et al. (2012)
Cultivated									
A. arvensis	X								Rzymski, Mleczek, Siwulski, Jasińska, et al. (2017)
A. bisporus (brown)	X								Rzymski, Mleczek, Siwulski, Jasińska, et al. (2017)
A. bisporus (white)	X								Mleczek, Rzymski, et al. (2018), Rzymski, Mleczek, Siwulski, Jasińska, et al. (2017)
Agaricus subrufescens	X								Rzymski, Mleczek, Siwulski, Jasińska, et al. (2017)
A. cylindracea	X								Niedzielski et al. (2017)

Auricularia auricula-judae					X				Mleczek, Rzymski, et al. (2018)
Auricularia polytricha	X								Niedzielski et al. (2017)
Clitocybe maxima	X								Niedzielski et al. (2017)
Flammulina velutipes	X								Niedzielski et al. (2017)
Grifola frondosa	X								Niedzielski et al. (2017)
Hericium erinaceus	X								Niedzielski et al. (2017), Turfan et al. (2018)
L. sulphureus	X								Niedzielski et al. (2017)
Lentinula edodes	X	X		X					Gonçalves et al. (2014), Mleczek, Siwulski, Rzymski, Niedzielski, et al. (2017), Mleczek, Rzymski, et al. (2018), Turfan et al. (2018)
Pholiota nameko	X								Niedzielski et al. (2017)
Pleurotus eryngii				X					Gonçalves et al. (2014)
P. ostreatus	X	X		X					Gonçalves et al. (2014), Mleczek, Rzymski, et al. (2018), Turfan et al. (2018)
Trametes versicolor	X								Niedzielski et al. (2017)
Tremella fuciformis	X								Niedzielski et al. (2017)
Volvariella volvacea		X							Mleczek, Rzymski, et al. (2018)

C, Caps; *S*, stipes; X^m, median value.

A. bitorquis, and *X. chrysenteron*, respectively. Data in papers published until 2009 were similar to those in Table 4.23. Wide variations within individual species were recorded in all the articles. *A. rubescens*, *M. rhacodes*, *L. scabrum*, and *S. variegatus* seem to be the species accumulating aluminum. Higher levels of aluminum have been observed in caps as compared to stipes in some species; however, with no generalizing relationship.

Information on aluminum bioconcentration in fruiting bodies has been insufficient. Rudawska and Leski (2005) reported BCF values in the range of 0.07–3.13 and 0.26–1.12 for *S. luteus* and *X. badius*, respectively. A comparable range of 0.1–2.5 was observed for *A. ponderosa* collected from 24 sites (Salvador et al., 2018).

Aluminum contents in fruiting bodies can be overestimated due to the risk of contamination with soil particles in many wild-growing species. Such contamination is virtually unavoidable in difficult-to-clean fruiting bodies such as cup mushrooms, truffles, false truffles, and gilled mushrooms developing underground (Stijve, Goessler, & Dupuy, 2004). Moreover, contamination of sample with aluminum during the analytical procedure could arise during combustion of DM in a muffle furnace used formerly for sample mineralization.

4.3.2 Antimony (Sb)

A survey by Parisis and van den Heede (1992) determined up to 0.15, 0.15, and 0.32 mg kg^{-1} DM of antimony in *A. rubescens*, *L. nuda*, and *L. amethystina*, respectively. Borovička, Řanda, and Jelínek (2006) compared antimony levels in fruiting bodies from unpolluted sites and from areas contaminated from historical mining and smelting of silver ores. The contents were generally below 0.1 mg kg^{-1} DM from the unpolluted sites, whereas considerably higher levels, up to hundreds mg kg^{-1} DM, were observed in the contaminated areas. A unique ability to accumulate antimony in fruiting bodies was found in genera *Suillus* and inedible *Chalciporus*. Very low contents of 0.01–0.31 mg kg^{-1} DM were determined in *X. badius* (Mleczek, Magdziak et al., 2016), caps of *M. procera* (Falandysz, Sapkota, Dryżałowska, et al., 2017), in three *Boletus* species growing in polymetallic soils (Falandysz, Zhang, Wiejak, et al., 2017), and in *B. appendiculatus* and *Clitopilus prunulus* (Alaimo et al., 2018). Surprisingly high levels of 15.6, 15.6, and 26.1 mg kg^{-1} DM were observed by Cvetkovic et al. (2015) in *B. edulis*, *C. cibarius*, and *M. oreades*, respectively. High contents ranging between 2.2 and 4.7 mg kg^{-1} DM were reported by Turfan et al. (2018) in eight wild and three cultivated species.

Within cultivated mushrooms, Gonçalves et al. (2014) reported 0.03, 0.03, and 0.04 mg kg^{-1} DM in *L. edodes*, *P. eryngii*, and *P. ostreatus*, respectively, and Mleczek, Siwulski, Rzymski, Niedzielski, et al. (2017) determined 0.26 mg kg^{-1} DM in *L. edodes*.

In a survey by Sousa Ferreira, Costa Ferreira, Cervera, and de la Guardia (2009), approximately two thirds of antimony occurred in the inorganic compounds of Sb^{V} and the rest as inorganic Sb^{III} in five commercial mushroom samples.

4.3.3 Bismuth (Bi)

Bismuth is another element with very limited available data. Trace contents of $<0.1\ mg\ kg^{-1}$ DM were determined in both wild-growing species (Alaimo et al., 2018; Falandysz, Sapkota, Dryżałowska, et al., 2017; Mleczek, Niedzielski, Kalač, Budka, et al., 2016; Zavastin et al., 2018) and cultivated mushrooms (Gonçalves et al., 2014). Higher levels of 0.44, 0.45, and $1.40\ mg\ kg^{-1}$ DM were reported by Dimitrijevic et al. (2016) in *B. edulis*, *B. regius*, and *B. rhodoxanthus*, respectively. Mleczek, Siwulski, Rzymski, Niedzielski, et al. (2017) found $0.18\ mg\ kg^{-1}$ DM in cultivated *L. edodes*.

4.3.4 Bromine (Br)

In a pioneering survey, Stijve, Diserens, Oberson, and de Meijer (1998) determined elevated levels of natural inorganic bromide ($mg\ kg^{-1}$ DM) in following species (with at least five fruiting bodies per species): 20.7 (2.6–92), 54 (15–91), 79 (27–232), and 124 (20–192) in *L. laccata*, *A. rubescens*, *Lepista inversa*, and *Lepista gilva*, respectively. Moreover, further species, namely of the genus *Agaricus*, seem to be bromide accumulators; however, only one to three fruiting bodies were analyzed. Usual bromide contents in numerous edible species were $<5\ mg\ kg^{-1}$ DM. Twenty years later, Turfan et al. (2018) reported contents mostly up to $10\ mg\ kg^{-1}$ DM; however, they found contents of 41.5, 115, and $220\ mg\ kg^{-1}$ DM in *M. oreades*, *R. botrytis*, and *B. edulis*, respectively.

4.3.5 Cesium (Cs)

Data on nonradioactive cesium published since 2010 are given in Table 4.24. Unfortunately, only three papers reported cesium content in wild-growing species and information for cultivated mushrooms is lacking from this period. The most frequent contents are $2–10\ mg\ kg^{-1}$ DM. These results fit well with the comprehensive data reported by Seeger and Schweinshaut (1981) who determined cesium in 433 wild-growing edible, inedible, and toxic mushroom species. Mean content was $7\ mg\ kg^{-1}$ DM, about half of the samples contained $3–12\ mg\ kg^{-1}$ DM. No differences were observed between cesium content of young and old fruiting bodies. In seven tested species, the highest cesium content was determined in the flesh of caps, whereas the lowest level in gills and stipes. A record content of $308\ mg\ kg^{-1}$ DM was noticed in a single sample of *Cortinarius alboviolaceus*. Klán,

TABLE 4.24 Data on the mean content (mg kg^{-1} dry matter) of *cesium* in fruiting bodies of wild-growing mushrooms collected from unpolluted (X) or geologically specific (●) sites published since 2010.

Species	<2	2–5	5–10	10–25	25–50	50–100	References
Wild growing							
Agaricus campestris		●					Campos and Tejera (2011)
Agaricus sylvicola			●				Campos and Tejera (2011)
Amanita caesarea		●					Campos and Tejera (2011)
Amanita rubescens			●				Campos and Tejera (2011)
Boletus luridus				●[S]		●[C]	Falandysz, Zhang, Wiejak, et al. (2017)
Boletus magnificus	●[S,C]						Falandysz, Zhang, Wiejak, et al. (2017)
Boletus tomentipes	●[C,S]						Falandysz, Zhang, Wiejak, et al. (2017)
Cantharellus cibarius		X			●		Campos and Tejera (2011), Falandysz, Chudzińska, et al. (2017)
Cantharellus tubaeformis		X					Falandysz, Chudzińska, et al. (2017)
Clitocybe geotropa			●				Campos and Tejera (2011)
Clitocybe gibba		●					Campos and Tejera (2011)
Ganoderma lucidum			●				Campos and Tejera (2011)

Hydnum imbricatum				X^S	X^C		Mędyk, Chudzińska, et al. (2017)
Hygrophorus russula		●					Campos and Tejera (2011)
Lactarius deliciosus			●				Campos and Tejera (2011)
Lactarius sanguifluus				●			Campos and Tejera (2011)
Lepista nuda		●					Campos and Tejera (2011)
Macrolepiota procera	X^C					●	Campos and Tejera (2011), Falandysz, Sapkota, Dryżalowska et al. (2017)
Marasmius oreades		●					Campos and Tejera (2011)
Tricholoma equestre					●		Campos and Tejera (2011)

C, Caps; *S*, stipes.

Řanda, Benada, and Horyna (1988) found lower levels, commonly $<1.0 \text{ mg kg}^{-1}$ DM, in wild species. Wide ranges of cesium content within the individual species were observed in both articles.

Klán et al. (1988) reported very low BCFs, mostly <0.05.

Occurrence of radioactive isotopes of cesium are provided in Chapter 5, Radioactivity.

4.3.6 Gallium (Ga)

Very limited data on gallium match trace levels up to 1 mg kg^{-1} DM in cultivated (Gonçalves et al., 2014; Niedzielski et al., 2017) and wild-growing species (Falandysz, Sapkota, Dryżałowska, et al., 2017; Mleczek, Niedzielski, Kalač, Budka, et al., 2016). Higher contents of $0.24\text{–}3.36 \text{ mg kg}^{-1}$ DM were determined by Tel-Çayan et al. (2017) in wild, but mostly inedible, species. They found the highest value in *Gyromitra esculenta*, the species with doubtful edibility due to the occurrence of carcinogenic gyromitrin. Similar contents of $1.0\text{–}2.4 \text{ mg kg}^{-1}$ DM were reported by Campos and Tejera (2011) in mushrooms growing in quartzite acidic soils.

4.3.7 Germanium (Ge)

Very scarce information on germanium in mushrooms indicates contents at the same limit of detection. Contents of only up to 0.03 mg kg^{-1} DM were determined by Mleczek, Niedzielski, Kalač, Budka, et al. (2016) and Falandysz, Sapkota, Dryżałowska, et al. (2017) in several wild-growing species.

4.3.8 Gold (Au)

Gold content in mushrooms also ranks among trace elements with only a few reports. Borovička, Řanda, and Jelínek (2005) determined gold in 154 samples of 89 species growing in nonauriferous and unpolluted areas. The contents were mostly $<0.02 \text{ mg kg}^{-1}$ DM. Within the mycorrhizal species, the highest levels of 0.14, 0.15, and 0.24 mg kg^{-1} DM were found in *A. strobiliformis*, *Russula claroflava*, and *B. edulis*, respectively. Among the saprobic species, the highest contents of 0.16 and 0.19 mg kg^{-1} DM were observed in *Langermannia gigantea* and *M. esculenta*, respectively. Comparable gold content, mostly below 0.05 mg kg^{-1} DM, were also determined by Mleczek, Niedzielski, Kalač, Budka, et al. (2016). The detected gold levels in mushrooms are considerably higher than in vascular plants.

Noticeably higher contents were reported from a site of a gold deposit (Borovička, Dunn, et al., 2010). Median values of gold content were elevated in this site, with 1.4-times in mycorrhizal and 4.4-times in saprobic species, compared with mushrooms from nonauriferous areas. The maximum contents (mg kg^{-1} DM) in the individual samples were 0.61 in *B. edulis* among the mycorrhizal species and 4.23, 5.54, and 7.74 in *A. sylvaticus*, *A. arvensis*, and *L. perlatum*, respectively, within saprobic species. Generally, saprobic species are more efficient at accumulating gold than mycorrhizal mushrooms.

4.3.9 Indium (In)

Pioneering data on indium levels in mushrooms were published recently by a Polish laboratory using inductively coupled plasma optical emission spectrometry. Contents up to 0.25 mg kg^{-1} DM were determined in wild-growing species (Mleczek, Niedzielski, Kalač, Budka, et al., 2016). Comparable levels were observed in three cultivated *Agaricus* spp. (Rzymski, Mleczek, Siwulski, Jasińska, et al., 2017), cultivated *L. edodes* (Mleczek, Siwulski, Rzymski, Niedzielski, et al., 2017), and six cultivated *Pleurotus* spp. (Siwulski et al., 2017). Elevated contents up to several mg kg^{-1} DM were found in various cultivated species (Mleczek, Rzymski et al., 2018; Niedzielski et al., 2017).

4.3.10 Lithium (Li)

As results from Table 4.25 show, usual lithium contents in wild-growing species vary between nondetectable levels and 0.3 mg kg^{-1} DM; however, contents up to 1.5 mg kg^{-1} DM have been recorded since 2010. Surprisingly, elevated levels were observed also in cultivated species. These data fit well with the contents observed by Vetter (2005) in 38 wild-growing species in Hungary. About 25% of the samples contained <0.03 mg kg^{-1} DM and the mean content of all fruiting bodies was 0.19 mg kg^{-1} DM. Somewhat elevated levels were observed in *A. strobiliformis* and *C. cornucopioides*; nevertheless, these species cannot be included among bioaccumulators. Wang et al. (2015b) reported mean lithium contents of 1.06 and 1.14 mg kg^{-1} DM in caps and stipes, respectively, of *B. edulis* from five sites.

Lithium as a drug shows mood-stabilizing effects, antiviolent behavior, and can restore normal brain function in some people. Enrichment of mushrooms with the element can provide its promising dietary source, since foods naturally rich in lithium are limited.

Assunção et al. (2012) cultivated *P. ostreatus* in a substrate based on coffee husks enriched with 0−500 mg lithium chloride per kilogram. Lithium content in the fruiting bodies increased linearly in all three harvest flushes. Mean lithium solubility determined by in vitro gastrointestinal digestion was 27.5%, 70.5%, and 0% in nonenriched (control), enriched fruiting bodies,

TABLE 4.25 Data on the mean content (mg kg^{-1} dry matter) of *lithium* in fruiting bodies of wild-growing mushrooms collected from unpolluted (X), geologically specific (●), and anthropogenically contaminated (▲) sites and in cultivated species published since 2010.

Species	<0.05	0.05–0.1	0.1–0.3	0.3–0.5	0.5–0.75	0.75–1.0	1.0–1.5	References
Wild growing								
Agaricus arvensis		X						Ayaz et al. (2011)
Armillariella mellea		X						Zavastin et al. (2018)
Boletus appendiculatus		$X^{S,Cm}$						Alaimo et al. (2018)
Boletus edulis	X	X	X				$X^{C,S}$	Ayaz et al. (2011), Cvetkovic et al. (2015), Giannaccini et al. (2012), Wang et al. (2015b), Zavastin et al. (2018)
Boletus luridus					●			Falandysz, Zhang, Wiejak, et al. (2017)
Boletus magnificus			●					Falandysz, Zhang, Wiejak, et al. (2017)
Boletus tomentipes			●					Falandysz, Zhang, Wiejak, et al. (2017)
Cantharellus cibarius	▲	X			X			Ayaz et al. (2011), Cvetkovic et al. (2015), Falandysz, Chudzińska, et al. (2017), Mleczek, Niedzielski, Kalač, Budka, et al. (2016)
Cantharellus tubaeformis	X	X						Ayaz et al. (2011), Falandysz, Chudzińska, et al. (2017), Zavastin et al. (2018)
Clitopilus prunulus			X^{m}					Alaimo et al. (2018)

Hydnum imbricatum	X^C	X^S						Mędyk, Chudzińska, et al. (2017)
Hydnum repandum		X						Ayaz et al. (2011)
Laccaria laccata			X					Ayaz et al. (2011)
Leccinum scabrum	▲							Mleczek, Niedzielski, Kalač, Budka, et al. (2016)
Lepista nuda	X							Ayaz et al. (2011)
Macrolepiota procera			X		X^C			Falandysz, Sapkota, Dryżalowska et al. (2017), Giannaccini et al. (2012)
Marasmius oreades							X	Cvetkovic et al. (2015)
Pleurotus ostreatus		▲						Mleczek, Niedzielski, Kalač, Budka, et al. (2016)
Xerocomus badius	▲	X						Mleczek, Magdziak, et al. (2016)
Cultivated								
Lentinula edodes				X		X		Gonçalves et al. (2014), Mleczek, Siwulski, Rzymski, Niedzielski, et al. (2017)
Pleurotus eryngii							X	Gonçalves et al. (2014)
P. ostreatus							X	Gonçalves et al. (2014)

C, Caps; *S*, stipes; X^m, median value.

and lithium carbonate (drug used in psychiatry), respectively. In a further work from the same Brazilian laboratory (Vieira et al., 2013), *P. ostreatus* cultivated in the previous substrate, fortified with 500 mg LiCl per kg, contained 37.5 mg kg^{-1} DM of lithium, while the element was undetectable in the nonfortified variant.

Mleczek, Siwulski, Rzymski, Budzyńska, et al. (2017) fortified substrates of cultivated *Ganoderma lucidum*, *P. eryngii*, and *P. ostreatus* with 1.7–6.9 mg lithium kg^{-1} in the forms of lithium acetate (CH_3COOLi) or lithium carbonate (Li_2CO_3). The latter compound was a more available source of lithium; however, it had a greater adverse effect on the growth of fruiting bodies. Substrate supplementation with lithium acetate resulted in limited or no growth retardation, but decreased the uptake of lithium. The most promising results were obtained for *G. lucidum*, which accumulated lithium up to 73.6 ± 10.9 mg kg^{-1} DM using lithium carbonate. The lithium levels accumulated in the fruiting bodies were not high enough for application in psychiatric treatments, but they could potentially support calming down behavior. In a further study from the same Polish laboratory (Rzymski, Niedzielski, Siwulski, Mleczek, et al., 2017), analogous tests were carried out with cultivation of *Agrocybe cylindracea* and *H. erinaceus*. The same levels of lithium as in the previous work were applied to substrates in the forms of lithium acetate or lithium chloride. Supplementation with the latter compound yielded more satisfactory results. Lithium contents were around 2 and 6 mg kg^{-1} DM in fruiting bodies of *A. cylindracea* and *H. erinaceus*, respectively, produced in the substrates supplemented with the element at levels of 5.2 and 6.9 mg kg^{-1}.

4.3.11 Platinum group elements

This group consists of six elements, namely ruthenium (Ru), rhodium (Rh), palladium (Pd), osmium (Os), iridium (Ir), and platinum (Pt); four of these, namely, Pt, Pd, Rh, and later also Ir have been used since the 1970s and 1980s in the United States and Europe, respectively, as vehicular converters. Environmental pollution with these traffic-related elements has steadily increased since that time. The elements are spread into the environment as a part of airborne, fine-particulate matter. The exposure to these metals may pose a health risk, especially at a chronic and subclinical levels. Platinum is a well-known allergen and palladium shows a strong sensitization potential.

Initial limited data on PGEs level in mushrooms determined in a Polish laboratory published since 2010, are included in Table 4.26. Although the contents are low, elevated platinum contents were surprisingly observed in several cultivated species. No information is available until now on the bioaccumulation or bioexclusion of the PGEs in mushrooms. Overall, investigation of these elements in mushrooms is in the pioneering stage.

TABLE 4.26 Data on the content (mg kg^{-1} dry matter) of *platinum group elements* (PGEs) in mushroom fruiting bodies published since 2010.

Species	Ru	Rh	Pd	Os	Ir	Pt	References
Wild growing							
Boletus edulis	–	–	–	–	–	<0.01	Mleczek, Siwulski, Mikołajczak, Goliński, et al. (2015)
Leccinum scabrum	–	–	–	–	–	<0.01	
Xerocomus badius	–	–	–	–	–	<0.01	
5 Species	0.02	0.03	0.02–0.04	0.01–0.02	0.06–0.27	0.01–0.02	Mleczek, Niedzielski, Kalač, Siwulski, et al. (2016)
Cultivated							
Lentinula edodes	0.06	0.08	0.10	0.09	0.38	0.90	Mleczek, Siwulski, Rzymski, Niedzielski, et al. (2017)
12 Species	ND	ND-0.30	ND	ND-0.20	ND	1.6–6.0	Niedzielski et al. (2017)
3 *Agaricus* spp.	ND	ND	ND	ND	ND	0.08–2.2	Rzymski, Mleczek, Siwulski, Jasińska, et al. (2017)
6 *Pleurotus* spp.	ND	0.01–0.60	ND	ND	ND	0.10-8.87	Siwulski et al. (2017)
14 Species	ND	ND	ND	0.01–0.29	0.01–0.94	0.7–7.2	Mleczek, Rzymski, et al. (2018)

ND, Nondetectable.

4.3.12 Rare-earth elements

Rare-earth elements (REEs) are often separated into two groups. Light REEs, which include lanthanum (La), cerium (Ce), praseodymium (Pr), neodymium (Nd), promethium (Pm), samarium (Sm), europium (Eu), and gadolinium (Gd). The group of heavy REEs consists of terbium (Tb), dysprosium (Dy), holmium (Ho), erbium (Er), thulium (Tm), ytterbium (Yb), and lutetium (Lu). These elements have been traditionally termed lanthanoids. Another system classifies REEs into three subgroups: light (La–Pm), middle (Sm–Dy), and heavy (Ho–Lu). Moreover, actinides scandium (Sc) and yttrium (Y) are also inserted among REEs. The significance of the REEs is related to their wide and increasing usage in new technologies and materials. Transport of these elements from the industry into the environment can occur. The REEs can be harmful for human health. Nevertheless, limits for foods have not been established until now. Biological materials contain REEs at the ultratrace levels of 0.1–10 $\mu g\ kg^{-1}$ fresh weight.

Data from the latest papers are given in Table 4.27. The level of the individual REEs is commonly <0.1 mg kg^{-1} DM and seldom exceed 1 mg kg^{-1} DM. The results fit well with previous reports, although these have been rare. Cerium, lanthanum, and neodymium were reported to occur at the highest contents. Stijve, Andrey, Lucchini, and Goessler (2002) observed significant differences of the sum of Ce, La, and Nd between tested cultivated and wild-growing species. The former group of 12 species contained mostly <0.1 mg kg^{-1} DM, whereas 19 from 35 species of the latter group showed >1 mg kg^{-1} DM. Similar results were observed by Aruguete, Aldstadt, and Mueller (1998) in *A. rubescens* and *A. flavorubescens*, Falandysz et al. (2001) in 6 wild-growing species, Borovička, Kubrová, Rohovec, Řanda, and Dunn (2011) who determined in 36 wild-growing species a sum of the REEs up to 0.36 mg kg^{-1} DM and Zocher, Kraemer, Merschel, and Bau (2018) in fruiting bodies in *S. luteus* containing total REEs up to 0.074 mg kg^{-1} DM. Very low level of biococentration factors of lanthanoids in wild-growing mushrooms were found by Yoshida and Muramatsu (1997).

Changes in the REEs content during the life cycle of fruiting bodies of inedible *Lactarius pubescens* were described recently by Grawunder and Gube (2018). They supposed REEs accumulation during growth stage and a way of their redistribution during degradation of fruiting bodies following release of spores.

Overall, the contents of the REEs in mushrooms are low. The dietary intake from mushrooms, thus, seems to be of no health risk.

4.3.13 Rhenium (Re)

The initial data on rhenium content also come from the Polish laboratory. The determined contents in numerous cultivated species varied between 0.02

TABLE 4.27 Data (mean or range) on the content (mg kg^{-1} dry matter) of rare-earth elements (REEs) in mushroom fruiting bodies published since 2010.

Species	Sc	Y	La	Ce	Pr	Nd	Sm	Eu	Gd	Tb	Dy	Ho	Er	Tm	Yb	Lu	References
Wild growing																	
15 Species[a]			–	4.2–27.8	–	0.6–10.4	–	–	–	–	–	–	–	–	–	–	Campos and Tejera (2011)
Xerocomus badius[b]	0.03/ 0.07	–	0.09/ 0.08	0.11/ 1.95	–	0.05/ 9.38	–	0.01/ 0.02	0.05/ 0.05	–	0.03/ 0.07	–	0.03/ 0.49	–	–	0.01/ 0.02	Mleczek, Magdziak, et al. (2016)
5 Species	–	0.02–0.03	0.01–0.06	0.02–0.15	0.02–0.07	0.07–0.23	0.02–0.11	-	0.02–0.03	0.01–0.02	-	0.03–0.11	0.18–0.75	0.01–0.12	0.01–0.02	0.01–0.03	Mleczek, Niedzielski, Kalač, Siwulski, et al. (2016)
Caps of *Macrolepiota procera*[c]	0.03	0.07	0.08	0.18	0.02	0.06	0.01	Tr	0.01	Tr	0.01	Tr	Tr	Tr	Tr	Tr	Falandysz, Sapkota, Mędyk, and Feng (2017)
6 Samples[d]	–	0.21–0.79	0.39–1.58	0.82–4.74	0.09–0.60	0.36–2.40	0.06–0.50	0.03–0.11	0.07–0.31	0.01–0.06	0.05–0.30	0.01–0.07	0.02–0.17	0.01–0.03	0.02–0.16	0.01–0.03	Fiket, Medunić, Turk, Ivanić, and Kniewald (2017)
Boletus edulis	–	0.02	0.02	0.02	Tr	0.01	Tr	Tr	Tr	Tr	Tr	Tr	Tr	Tr	Tr	Tr	Bau, Schmidt, Pack, Bendel, and Kraemer (2018)

(Continued)

TABLE 4.27 Data (mean or range) on the content (mg kg^{-1} dry matter) of rare-earth elements (REEs) in mushroom fruiting bodies published since 2010. (Continued)

Species	Sc	Y	La	Ce	Pr	Nd	Sm	Eu	Gd	Tb	Dy	Ho	Er	Tm	Yb	Lu	References
Cultivated																	
Cyclocybe cylindracea[e]	Tr	Tr	0.04	0.08	Tr	0.03	Tr	Tr	Tr	Tr	Tr	Tr	Tr	Tr	Tr	Tr	Koutrotsios, Danezis, Georgiou, and Zervakis (2018)
Lentinula edodes	0.02	0.02	0.10	0.80	0.39	1.70	0.04	0.04	0.03	0.01	Tr	0.07	0.50	0.04	Tr	Tr	Mleczek, Siwulski, Rzymski, Niedzielski, et al. (2017)
12 Species	–	–	Tr-0.08	–	0.02–1.8	0.11–0.45	–	–	Tr-0.05	–	–	0.04–0.30	–	–	–	–	Siwulski et al. (2017)
3 *Agaricus* spp.	0.01–0.03	Tr	–	–	–	1.1–2.2	–	–	–	–	–	–	0.31–0.39	–	–	–	Rzymski, Mleczek, Siwulski, Jasińska, et al. (2017)
Pleurotus ostreatus[e]	0.03	Tr	0.02	0.03	Tr	Tr	Tr	Tr	Tr	Tr	Tr	Tr	Tr	Tr	Tr	Tr	Koutrotsios et al. (2018)
6 *Pleurotus* spp.	0.03	–	–	–	–	0.41	–	–	–	–	–	–	0.38	–	–	0.02	Siwulski et al. (2017)
14 Species	0.01–0.05	0.01–0.14	0.06–0.37	0.05–0.68	–	0.27–4.29	–	0.01–0.09	–	–	–	–	0.02–3.59	0.01–0.10	–	0.01–0.03	Mleczek, Rzymski, et al. (2018)

Tr, Traces (<0.01 mg kg^{-1} DM).
Promethium is generally undetectable via recent analytical methods.
[a]*Geologically specific substrate.*
[b]*From unpolluted / polluted sites.*
[c]*Mean of 13 samples.*
[d]*Unspecified species.*
[e]*Cultivated on corn cobs.*

and 0.62 mg kg^{-1} DM with the most frequent level about 0.2 mg kg^{-1} DM (Mleczek, Siwulski, Rzymski, Niedzielski, et al., 2017; Mleczek, Rzymski, et al., 2018; Rzymski, Mleczek, Siwulski, Jasińska, et al., 2017; Siwulski et al., 2017).

The data are insufficient for an assessment of rhenium occurrence in mushrooms.

4.3.14 Rubidium (Rb)

Rubidium belongs to the relatively frequently determined elements in mushrooms. Data published since 2010 are collated in Table 4.28. The contents vary widely from <25 to 500 mg kg^{-1} DM. The *Boletaceae* family seems to be rich in this element. Generally low levels were observed in mushrooms growing in quartzite acidic soils (Campos & Tejera, 2011). The data of Table 4.28 fit well with the reports until 2009 (for references see the review by Kalač, 2010). Very high levels, 360–1700 mg kg^{-1} DM were determined in *C. cibarius* from four Polish sites (Drewnowska & Falandysz, 2015). An extreme content of 9750 mg kg^{-1} DM was reported by Turfan et al. (2018) in *R. botrytis*.

As results from Table 4.28 show, caps usually have higher rubidium contents than stipes. For instance, a mean cap to stem ratio of 3.1 was observed in *M. procera* by Kułdo et al. (2014). Limited information on values of BCF vary extremely. Drewnowska and Falandysz (2015) found a range of 710–6100 for *C. cibarius*, while Campos and Tejera (2011) found only 0.17–2.59. Furthermore, 9 of 15 wild-growing species were bioexcluders. Low levels of BCF, mostly <1.0, were also reported by Klán et al. (1988) for many wild-growing species.

Losses of rubidium by 85% and 98% of the initial content in fresh caps of *A. fulva* were observed during blanching in boiling water for 15 min and following pickling in a vinegar solution for 30 days, respectively (Drewnowska, Falandysz, et al., 2017).

4.3.15 Strontium

As results from Table 4.29 show, strontium contents of <2 mg kg^{-1} DM prevail in wild-growing and cultivated mushroom species, but levels of 2–5 mg kg^{-1} DM were also frequent. Higher contents of up to 30 mg kg^{-1} DM were determined primarily in mushrooms growing in quartzite acidic soils (Campos & Tejera, 2011). Seeger, Orth, and Schweinshaut (1982), in a comprehensive study of 433 edible, inedible, and toxic species, reported a mean level of 7.0 ± 0.43 mg kg^{-1} DM. Strontium content correlated with calcium content.

According to data in Table 4.29, distribution of strontium within fruiting bodies seems to be virtually even. Seeger et al. (1982) observed in eight

TABLE 4.28 Data on the mean content (mg kg − 1 dry matter) of *rubidium* in fruiting bodies of wild-growing mushrooms collected from unpolluted (X), geologically specific (●), and anthropogenically contaminated (▲) sites and in cultivated species published since 2010.

Species	<25	25–50	50–100	100–200	200–500	>500	References
Wild growing							
Agaricus campestris	●						Campos and Tejera (2011)
Agaricus sylvicola	●						Campos and Tejera (2011)
Amanita caesarea	●						Campos and Tejera (2011)
Amanita fulva				X^{S}	X^{C}		Falandysz, Drewnowska, et al. (2017)
Amanita rubescens			●				Campos and Tejera (2011)
Boletus appendiculatus	X		X^{Sm}	X^{Cm}			Alaimo et al. (2018), Dimitrijevic et al. (2016)
Boletus edulis			X	X		X	Dimitrijevic et al. (2016), Giannaccini et al. (2012), Turfan et al. (2018)
Boletus impolitus			X				Dimitrijevic et al. (2016)
Boletus luridus				$●^{S}$	$●^{C}$		Falandysz, Zhang, Wiejak, et al. (2017)
Boletus magnificus			$●^{S,C}$				Falandysz, Zhang, Wiejak, et al. (2017)
Boletus regius					X		Dimitrijevic et al. (2016)
Boletus tomentipes				$●^{S,C}$			Falandysz, Zhang, Wiejak, et al. (2017)
Cantharellus cibarius			●		X	X	Campos and Tejera (2011), Drewnowska and Falandysz (2015), Falandysz and Drewnowska (2015a), Falandysz, Chudzińska, et al. (2017)

Cantharellus tubaeformis					X		Falandysz, Chudzińska, et al. (2017)
Clitocybe geotropa	●						Campos and Tejera (2011)
Clitocybe gibba	●						Campos and Tejera (2011)
Clitopilus prunulus				X^{m}			Alaimo et al. (2018)
Craterellus cornucopioides						X	Turfan et al. (2018)
Hydnum imbricatum					X^{S}	X^{C}	Mędyk, Chudzińska, et al. (2017)
Hygrophorus russula		●					Campos and Tejera (2011)
Lactarius deliciosus			●		X		Campos and Tejera (2011), Turfan et al. (2018)
Lactarius sanguifluus		●					Campos and Tejera (2011)
Laetiporus sulphureus		X					Turfan et al. (2018)
Leccinum crocipodium			X				Dimitrijevic et al. (2016)
Leccinum duriusculum			X^{S}		X^{C}		Jarzyńska and Falandysz (2012a)
Leccinum griseum				X^{S}	X^{C}		Jarzyńska and Falandysz (2012b)
Leccinum pseudoscabrum				X			Dimitrijevic et al. (2016)
Leccinum scabrum			X^{S}		X^{C}		Falandysz (2018)
Lepista nuda	●						Campos and Tejera (2011)
Macrolepiota procera		$X^{C,S}$, ●, X	X^{S}	X^{C}			Campos and Tejera (2011), Falandysz, Sapkota, Dryżalowska et al. (2017), Giannaccini et al. (2012), Gucia et al. (2012), Kojta et al. (2011), Kułdo et al. (2014)

(*Continued*)

TABLE 4.28 Data on the mean content (mg kg − 1 dry matter) of *rubidium* in fruiting bodies of wild-growing mushrooms collected from unpolluted (X), geologically specific (●), and anthropogenically contaminated (▲) sites and in cultivated species published since 2010. (Continued)

Species	<25	25–50	50–100	100–200	200–500	>500	References
Marasmius oreades	●	X					Campos and Tejera (2011), Turfan et al. (2018)
Morchella conica				X			Turfan et al. (2018)
Ramaria botrytis						X	Turfan et al. (2018)
Suillus variegatus				X^S	X^C		Szubstarska et al. (2012)
Tricholoma terreum						X	Turfan et al. (2018)
Xerocomus badius			$▲^S$	X, $▲^C$			Dimitrijevic et al. (2016), Kojta et al. (2012)
Xerocomus chrysenteron			X				Dimitrijevic et al. (2016)
Xerocomus subtomentosus					$X^{S,C}$		Jarzyńska et al. (2012)
Cultivated							
Hericium erinaceus				X			Turfan et al. (2018)
Lentinula edodes	X	X			X		Gonçalves et al. (2014), Mleczek, Siwulski, Rzymski, Niedzielski, et al. (2017), Turfan et al. (2018)
Pleurotus eryngii			X				Gonçalves et al. (2014)
Pleurotus ostreatus			X		X		Gonçalves et al. (2014), Turfan et al. (2018)

C, Caps; *S*, stipes; X^m, median value.

TABLE 4.29 Data on the mean content (mg kg^{-1} dry matter) of *strontium* in fruiting bodies of wild-growing mushrooms collected from unpolluted (X), geologically specific (●), and anthropogenically contaminated (▲) sites and in cultivated species published since 2010.

Species	<2	2–5	5–10	10–20	20–30	References
Wild growing						
Agaricus arvensis	X					Ayaz et al. (2011)
Agaricus campestris	$X^{C,S}$	$▲^{C}$	$▲^{S}$	●		Campos and Tejera (2011), Zsigmond et al. (2018)
Agaricus sylvicola				●		Campos and Tejera (2011)
Amanita caesarea				●		Campos and Tejera (2011)
Amanita fulva	$X^{C,S}$					Falandysz, Drewnowska, et al. (2017)
Amanita rubescens				●		Campos and Tejera (2011)
Armillariella mellea	X					Zavastin et al. (2018)
Boletus appendiculatus	X, $X^{C,Sm}$					Alaimo et al. (2018), Dimitrijevic et al. (2016)
Boletus edulis	X, $X^{C,S}$	X, $X^{C,S}$				Ayaz et al. (2011), Cvetkovic et al. (2015), Dimitrijevic et al. (2016), Frankowska et al. (2010), Giannaccini et al. (2012), Mleczek, Siwulski, Stuper-Szablewska, Rissmann, et al. (2013), Wang et al. (2015b), Zavastin et al. (2018), Zhang et al. (2010)
Boletus impolitus	X					Dimitrijevic et al. (2016)
Boletus luridus	$●^{C,S}$					Falandysz, Zhang, Wiejak, et al. (2017)
Boletus magnificus	$●^{C,S}$					Falandysz, Zhang, Wiejak, et al. (2017)

(*Continued*)

TABLE 4.29 Data on the mean content (mg kg^{-1} dry matter) of *strontium* in fruiting bodies of wild-growing mushrooms collected from unpolluted (X), geologically specific (●), and anthropogenically contaminated (▲) sites and in cultivated species published since 2010. (Continued)

Species	<2	2–5	5–10	10–20	20–30	References
Boletus regius	X					Dimitrijevic et al. (2016)
Boletus tomentipes	●^{C}		●^{S}			Falandysz, Zhang, Wiejak, et al. (2017)
Cantharellus cibarius	X, X^{C,S}	X		●		Ayaz et al. (2011), Campos and Tejera (2011), Cvetkovic et al. (2015), Drewnowska and Falandysz (2015), Falandysz and Drewnowska (2015a), Falandysz et al. (2011), Falandysz, Chudzińska, et al. (2017), Mleczek, Siwulski, Stuper-Szablewska, Rissmann, et al. (2013), Zavastin et al. (2018)
Cantharellus tubaeformic	X	X				Ayaz et al. (2011), Falandysz, Chudzińska, et al. (2017)
Clitocybe geotropa				●		Campos and Tejera (2011)
Clitocybe gibba				●		Campos and Tejera (2011)
Clitopilus prunulus		X^{m}				Alaimo et al. (2018)
Ganoderma lucidum				●		Campos and Tejera (2011)
Helvella crispa		▲				Golubkina and Mironov (2018)
Hydnum imbricatum	X^{C,S}					Mędyk, Chudzińska, et al. (2017)
Hydnum repandum	X					Ayaz et al. (2011)
Hygrophorus russula				●		Campos and Tejera (2011)
Laccaria laccata		X				Ayaz et al. (2011)
Lactarius deliciosus	X				●	Campos and Tejera (2011), Mleczek, Siwulski, Stuper-Szablewska, Rissmann, et al. (2013)

Lactarius piperatus		X				Cvetkovic et al. (2015)
Lactarius sanguifluus				●		Campos and Tejera (2011)
Leccinum aurantiacum	X		▲			Golubkina and Mironov (2018), Mleczek, Siwulski, Stuper-Szablewska, Rissmann, et al. (2013)
Leccinum crocipodium	X					Dimitrijevic et al. (2016)
Leccinum duriusculum	$X^{C,S}$					Jarzyńska and Falandysz (2012a)
Leccinum griseum	$X^{C,S}$					Jarzyńska and Falandysz (2012b)
Leccinum pseudoscabrum		X				Dimitrijevic et al. (2016)
Leccinum scabrum	$X^{C,S}$	▲				Falandysz (2018), Golubkina and Mironov (2018)
Lepista nuda		X			●	Ayaz et al. (2011), Campos and Tejera (2011)
Macrolepiota procera	$X^{C,S}$		X	●		Campos and Tejera (2011), Falandysz, Sapkota, Dryżałowska et al. (2017), Giannaccini et al. (2012), Gucia et al. (2012), Jarzyńska et al. (2011), Kojta et al. (2011), Kułdo et al. (2014)
Marasmius oreades		X		●		Campos and Tejera (2011), Cvetkovic et al. (2015)
Morchella esculenta		▲				Golubkina and Mironov (2018)
Pleurotus ostreatus				X		Tel-Çayan et al. (2017)
Suillus granulatus	▲					Golubkina and Mironov (2018)
Suillus luteus	X		▲			Golubkina and Mironov (2018), Mleczek, Siwulski, Stuper-Szablewska, Rissmann, et al. (2013)
Suillus variegatus	$X^{C,S}$					Szubstarska et al. (2012)

(*Continued*)

TABLE 4.29 Data on the mean content (mg kg^{-1} dry matter) of *strontium* in fruiting bodies of wild-growing mushrooms collected from unpolluted (X), geologically specific (●), and anthropogenically contaminated (▲) sites and in cultivated species published since 2010. (Continued)

Species	<2	2–5	5–10	10–20	20–30	References
Tricholoma equestre				●		Campos and Tejera (2011)
Tricholoma fracticum				●		Tel-Çayan et al. (2017)
Xerocomus badius	X, ▲, ▲[C,S]	▲				Dimitrijevic et al. (2016), Kojta et al. (2012), Mleczek, Siwulski, Stuper-Szablewska, Rissmann, et al. (2013), Mleczek, Siwulski, Kaczmarek, et al. (2013), Mleczek, Siwulski, Mikołajczak, Gąsecka, Sobieralski, et al. (2015), Mleczek, Magdziak, et al. (2016)
Xerocomus chrysenteron		X				Dimitrijevic et al. (2016)
Xerocomus subtomentosus	X[S,C]					Jarzyńska et al. (2012)
Cultivated						
A. arvensis	X					Rzymski, Mleczek, Siwulski, Jasińska, et al. (2017)
Agaricus bisporus (brown)	X					Rzymski, Mleczek, Siwulski, Jasińska, et al. (2017)
A. bisporus (white)	X					Mleczek, Rzymski, et al. (2018), Rzymski, Mleczek, Siwulski, Jasińska, et al. (2017)
Agaricus subrufescens	X					Rzymski, Mleczek, Siwulski, Jasińska, et al. (2017)
Agrocybe cylindracea	X					Niedzielski et al. (2017)
Auricularia auricula-judae				X		Mleczek, Rzymski, et al. (2018)
Auricularia polytricha	X					Niedzielski et al. (2017)

Clitocybe maxima	X					Niedzielski et al. (2017)
Flammulina velutipes	X					Niedzielski et al. (2017)
Grifola frondosa			X			Niedzielski et al. (2017)
Hericium erinaceus	X					Niedzielski et al. (2017)
Laetiporus sulphureus	X					Niedzielski et al. (2017)
Lentinula edodes	X	X				Gonçalves et al. (2014), Mleczek, Siwulski, Rzymski, Niedzielski, et al. (2017), Mleczek, Rzymski, et al. (2018)
Pholiota nameko	X					Niedzielski et al. (2017)
Pleurotus eryngii	X					Gonçalves et al. (2014)
P. ostreatus	X					Gonçalves et al. (2014), Mleczek, Rzymski, et al. (2018)
Trametes versicolor			X			Niedzielski et al. (2017)
Tremella fuciformis	X	X				Mleczek, Rzymski, et al. (2018), Niedzielski et al. (2017)
Volvariella volvacea				X		Mleczek, Rzymski, et al. (2018)

C, Caps; *S*, stipes; X^m, median value.

tested species significantly decreasing levels of the element in the flesh of caps > stipe > gills; however, the differences were small. Kułdo et al. (2014) found a wider range of cap to stipe ratio of 4.4 ± 3.5 in *M. procera*, Wang et al. (2015b) reported the ratio of 0.09–3.14 in *B. edulis*, but a narrow range of 1.11–1.67 in four of the six tested sites.

M. procera was termed as a strontium bioexcluder with BCF values 0.96 and 0.16 for caps and stipes, respectively (Kułdo et al., 2014). On the contrary, Mleczek, Siwulski, Stuper-Szablewska, Rissmann, et al. (2013) reported BCF values of >1 for all six tested popular wild-growing species.

4.3.16 Tellurium (Te)

Data on tellurium content in mushroom arose in the past few years. Contents of <0.3 mg kg^{-1} DM were determined in 16 edible species growing along a heavily trafficked road (Mleczek, Niedzielski, Kalač, Budka, et al., 2016). The levels of 0.02 and 0.33 mg kg^{-1} DM were observed in *X. badius* from unpolluted and polluted sites, respectively (Mleczek, Magdziak, et al., 2016). Further data deal with cultivated species. The reported contents (mg kg^{-1} DM) were 2.9 in *L. edodes* (Mleczek, Siwulski, Rzymski, Niedzielski, et al., 2017), 1.3–3.1 in 3 *Agaricus* spp. (Rzymski, Mleczek, Siwulski, Jasińska, et al., 2017), 0.33–6.41 in 6 *Pleurotus* spp. (Siwulski et al., 2017), and 0.5–3.0 in 14 commercial species (Mleczek, Rzymski, et al., 2018).

4.3.17 Thorium (Th)

The range of 1.1–2.6 mg kg^{-1} DM was observed in 15 species growing in quartzite acidic soils (Campos & Tejera, 2011). Considerably lower levels, only up to tenths mg kg^{-1} DM were reported by Stijve et al. (2002), Borovička et al. (2011) yet hundredths mg kg^{-1} DM in 36 mycorrhizal and saprobic species from unpolluted sites. Similar values were determined by Kubrová et al. (2014) in mushrooms collected in an area of former uranium ore mining. Also Falandysz, Sapkota, Dryżałowska, et al. (2017) observed 0.029 mg kg^{-1} DM in the caps of *M. procera*. Thorium apparently is not accumulated in fruiting bodies.

Within cultivated species (all contents in mg kg^{-1} DM), Mleczek, Siwulski, Rzymski, Niedzielski, et al. (2018) determined 0.12 in *L. edodes*, Rzymski, Mleczek, Siwulski, Jasińska, et al. (2017) found 0.05–0.34 in 3 *Agaricus* spp., Siwulski et al. (2017) reported 0.01–0.38 in 6 *Pleurotus* spp., and Mleczek et al. (2018) up to 0.18 in 14 commercial species.

4.3.18 Tin (Sn)

Tin belongs among elements with very limited data. Wuilloud, Kannamkumarath, and Caruso (2004) determined 4.0, 5.0, and 5.1 mg kg^{-1}

DM in *A. bisporus*, *B. edulis*, and *L. edodes*, respectively, Durkan et al. (2011) found 3.0–4.5 mg kg^{-1} DM in numerous wild-growing species from Turkey. Similar data between 4.7 and 8.3 mg kg^{-1} DM reported Turfan et al. (2018) in eight wild and three cultivated species, also from Turkey. Other reports give lower levels (mg kg^{-1} DM), namely 0.21 and 0.29 in *T. olbiensis* and *T. claveryi*, respectively (Kivrak, 2015), 0.19 in caps of *M. procera* (Falandysz, Sapkota, Dryżałowska, et al., 2017), and 0.05–0.1 in cultivated *L. edodes*, *P. ostreatus*, and *P. eryngii* (Gonçalves et al., 2014).

4.3.19 Titanium (Ti)

Data on titanium are collected in Table 4.30. Usual contents are in ones of mg kg^{-1} DM in wild-growing species with elevated levels in caps of *M. procera* and in *L. laccata*. In the cultivated species the reported values are lower, commonly in the tenths mg kg^{-1} DM.

TABLE 4.30 Data on the mean content or range (mg kg^{-1} dry matter) of *titanium* in fruiting bodies of wild-growing species from unpolluted sites and in cultivated mushrooms published since 2010.

Species	Mean or range	References
Wild growing		
Agaricus arvensis	6.38	Ayaz et al. (2011)
Boletus edulis	2.68;1.56	Ayaz et al. (2011), Mleczek, Siwulski, Mikołajczak, Goliński, et al. (2015)
Cantharellus cibarius	5.58	Ayaz et al. (2011)
Cantharellus tubaeformis	4.25	Ayaz et al. (2011)
Hydnum repandum	6.79	Ayaz et al. (2011)
Laccaria laccata	13.5	Ayaz et al. (2011)
Leccinum scabrum	1.12	Mleczek, Siwulski, Mikołajczak, Goliński, et al. (2015)
Lepista nuda	2.18	Ayaz et al. (2011)
Macrolepiota procera (caps)	29	Falandysz, Sapkota, Dryżalowska et al. (2017)
Xerocomus badius	1.16	Mleczek, Siwulski, Mikołajczak, Goliński, et al. (2015)

(*Continued*)

TABLE 4.30 Data on the mean content or range (mg kg^{-1} dry matter) of *titanium* in fruiting bodies of wild-growing species from unpolluted sites and in cultivated mushrooms published since 2010. (Continued)

Species	Mean or range	References
Cultivated		
A. arvensis	0.12	Rzymski, Mleczek, Siwulski, Jasińska, et al. (2017)
Agaricus bisporus (brown)	0.12	Rzymski, Mleczek, Siwulski, Jasińska, et al. (2017)
A. bisporus (white)	0.15	Rzymski, Mleczek, Siwulski, Jasińska, et al. (2017)
Agaricus subrufescens	0.14	Rzymski, Mleczek, Siwulski, Jasińska, et al. (2017)
Lentinula edodes	0.19	Mleczek, Siwulski, Rzymski, Niedzielski, et al. (2017)
6 *Pleurotus* spp.	0.03–0.57	Siwulski et al. (2017)
14 Commercial species	0.08–2.14	Mleczek, Rzymski, et al. (2018)

4.3.20 Uranium (U)

As results from Table 4.31 show, usual uranium contents in wild-growing mushrooms are up to 2 mg kg^{-1} DM, in the cultivated species <1 mg kg^{-1} DM. However, the data originate from limited reports.

Very low uranium levels of <0.03 mg kg^{-1} DM were determined by Borovička et al. (2011). No significant differences were observed between contents in mycorrhizal and saprobic mushrooms collected from unpolluted sites. Somewhat higher median values, 0.063 and 0.082 mg kg^{-1} DM for mycorrhizal and saprobic species, respectively, were reported by Kubrová et al. (2014) in mushrooms growing in the area of a former uranium mining.

Apparently, uranium is not accumulated in fruiting bodies.

4.3.21 Vanadium (V)

Usual vanadium contents in wild-growing species are 0.1–0.5 mg kg^{-1} DM, whereas levels in the range of 0.5–2.0 mg kg^{-1} DM are less common (Table 4.32). Elevated contents were reported by Campos and Tejera (2011) in mushrooms growing in quartzite acidic soils. Wang et al. (2015b) determined ranges of 1.2–27.3 and 0.5–15.8 mg kg^{-1} DM in caps and stipes, respectively, of *B. edulis* collected from six sites in Yunnan Province, China.

TABLE 4.31 Data on the mean content (mg kg^{-1} dry matter) of *uranium* in fruiting bodies of wild-growing mushrooms collected from unpolluted (X), geologically specific (●), and anthropogenically contaminated (▲) sites and in cultivated species published since 2010.

Species	<1	1–2	2–5	5–10	>10	References
Wild growing						
Agaricus campestris		●				Campos and Tejera (2011)
Agaricus sylvicola		●				Campos and Tejera (2011)
Amanita caesarea		●				Campos and Tejera (2011)
Amanita rubescens		●				Campos and Tejera (2011)
Boletus appendiculatus	$X^{S,Cm}$					Alaimo et al. (2018)
Boletus edulis					X	Turfan et al. (2018)
Boletus luridus	●^{C,S}					Falandysz, Zhang, Wiejak, et al. (2017)
Boletus magnificus	●^{S,C}					Falandysz, Zhang, Wiejak, et al. (2017)
Boletus tomentipes	●^{C,S}					Falandysz, Zhang, Wiejak, et al. (2017)
Cantharellus cibarius	X	●				Campos and Tejera (2011), Falandysz, Chudzińska, et al. (2017)
Cantharellus tubaeformis	X					Falandysz, Chudzińska, et al. (2017)
Clitocybe geotropa	●					Campos and Tejera (2011)
Clitocybe gibba		●				Campos and Tejera (2011)

(*Continued*)

TABLE 4.31 Data on the mean content (mg kg^{-1} dry matter) of *uranium* in fruiting bodies of wild-growing mushrooms collected from unpolluted (X), geologically specific (●), and anthropogenically contaminated (▲) sites and in cultivated species published since 2010. (Continued)

Species	<1	1–2	2–5	5–10	>10	References
Clitopilus prunulus	X^{m}					Alaimo et al. (2018)
Craterellus cornucopioides				X		Turfan et al. (2018)
Hydnum imbricatum	$X^{S,C}$					Mędyk, Chudzińska, et al. (2017)
Hygrophorus russula		●				Campos and Tejera (2011)
Laccaria laccata	▲					Baumann et al. (2014)
Lactarius deliciosus		●		X		Campos and Tejera (2011), Turfan et al. (2018)
Lactarius sanguifluus		●				Campos and Tejera (2011)
Laetiporus sulphureus				X		Turfan et al. (2018)
Leccinum scabrum	▲					Baumann et al. (2014)
Leccinum versipelle	▲					Baumann et al. (2014)
Lepista nuda	●					Campos and Tejera (2011)
Macrolepiota procera	X^{C}	X	●			Campos and Tejera (2011), Falandysz, Chudzińska, et al. (2017), Falandysz, Sapkota, Dryżalowska et al. (2017)
Marasmius oreades	●		X			Campos and Tejera (2011), Turfan et al. (2018)
Morchella conica			X			Turfan et al. (2018)
Ramaria botrytis					X	Turfan et al. (2018)

Tricholoma equestre				●		Campos and Tejera (2011)
Tricholoma terreum				X		Turfan et al. (2018)
Cultivated						
Agrocybe cylindracea	X					Niedzielski et al. (2017)
Auricularia polytricha	X					Niedzielski et al. (2017)
Clitocybe maxima	X					Niedzielski et al. (2017)
Flammulina velutipes	X					Niedzielski et al. (2017)
Grifola frondosa	X					Niedzielski et al. (2017)
Hericium erinaceus	X		X			Niedzielski et al. (2017), Turfan et al. (2018)
L. sulphureus	X					Niedzielski et al. (2017)
Lentinula edodes		X		X		Mleczek, Siwulski, Rzymski, Niedzielski, et al. (2017), Turfan et al. (2018)
Pholiota nameko	X					Niedzielski et al. (2017)
Trametes versicolor	X					Niedzielski et al. (2017)
Tremella fuciformis	X					Niedzielski et al. (2017)

C, Caps; *S*, stipes; X^m, median value.

TABLE 4.32 Data on the mean content (mg kg^{-1} dry matter) of *vanadium* in fruiting bodies of wild-growing mushrooms collected from unpolluted (X) or geologically specific (●) sites and in cultivated species published since 2010.

Species	<0.1	0.1–0.5	0.5–1.0	1–2	2–5	5–10	>10	References
Wild growing								
Agaricus arvensis		X						Ayaz et al. (2011)
Agaricus campestris					●			Campos and Tejera (2011)
Agaricus sylvicola					●			Campos and Tejera (2011)
Amanita caesarea					●			Campos and Tejera (2011)
Amanita fulva		$X^{C,S}$						Falandysz, Drewnowska, et al. (2017)
Amanita rubescens					●			Campos and Tejera (2011)
Boletus appendiculatus		$X^{S,Cm}$						Alaimo et al. (2018)
Boletus edulis		X		X, X^{S}	X^{C}			Ayaz et al. (2011), Turfan et al. (2018), Wang et al. (2015b)
Boletus luridus					$●^{C,S}$			Falandysz, Zhang, Wiejak, et al. (2017)
Boletus magnificus			$●^{S}$	$●^{C}$				Falandysz, Zhang, Wiejak, et al. (2017)
Boletus tomentipes				$●^{C}$	$●^{S}$			Falandysz, Zhang, Wiejak, et al. (2017)
Cantharellus cibarius		X				●		Ayaz et al. (2011), Campos and Tejera (2011), Falandysz, Chudzińska, et al. (2017)
Cantharellus tubaeformis		X						Ayaz et al. (2011), Falandysz, Chudzińska, et al. (2017)
Clitocybe geotropa						●		Campos and Tejera (2011)

Clitocybe gibba						●		Campos and Tejera (2011)
Clitopilus prunulus				X^m				Alaimo et al. (2018)
Craterellus cornucopioides					X			Turfan et al. (2018)
Hydnum imbricatum			$X^{S,C}$					Mędyk, Chudzińska, et al. (2017)
Hydnum repandum		X						Ayaz et al. (2011)
Hygrophorus russula					●			Campos and Tejera (2011)
Laccaria laccata				X				Ayaz et al. (2011)
Lactarius deliciosus					X	●		Campos and Tejera (2011), Turfan et al. (2018)
Lactarius sanguifluus						●		Campos and Tejera (2011)
Laetiporus sulphureus			X					Turfan et al. (2018)
Lepista nuda			X				●	Ayaz et al. (2011), Campos and Tejera (2011)
Macrolepiota procera				X^C		●		Campos and Tejera (2011), Falandysz, Drewnowska, et al. (2017), Falandysz, Sapkota, Dryżalowska et al. (2017)
Marasmius oreades					X, ●			Campos and Tejera (2011), Turfan et al. (2018)
Morchella conica				X				Turfan et al. (2018)
Morchella esculenta		X						Rossbach et al. (2017)
Pleurotus ostreatus		X						Tel-Çayan et al.(2017)
Ramaria botrytis						X		Turfan et al. (2018)
Tricholoma equestre							●	Campos and Tejera (2011)

(Continued)

TABLE 4.32 Data on the mean content (mg kg^{-1} dry matter) of *vanadium* in fruiting bodies of wild-growing mushrooms collected from unpolluted (X) or geologically specific (●) sites and in cultivated species published since 2010. (Continued)

Species	<0.1	0.1–0.5	0.5–1.0	1–2	2–5	5–10	>10	References
Tricholoma fracticum			X					Tel-Çayan et al.(2017)
Tricholoma terreum					X			Turfan et al. (2018)
Cultivated								
Agrocybe cylindracea	X							Niedzielski et al. (2017)
Auricularia polytricha	X							Niedzielski et al. (2017)
Clitocybe maxima	X							Niedzielski et al. (2017)
Flammulina velutipes	X							Niedzielski et al. (2017)
Grifola frondosa	X							Niedzielski et al. (2017)
Hericium erinaceus	ND	X						Niedzielski et al. (2017), Turfan et al. (2018)
L. sulphureus	X							Niedzielski et al. (2017)
Lentinula edodes	X			X				Gonçalves et al. (2014), Turfan et al. (2018)
Pholiota nameko	X							Niedzielski et al. (2017)
Pleurotus eryngii		X						Gonçalves et al. (2014)
P. ostreatus		X		X				Gonçalves et al. (2014), Turfan et al. (2018)
Trametes versicolor	X							Niedzielski et al. (2017)
Tremella fuciformis	ND							Niedzielski et al. (2017)

C, Caps; *ND*, below limit of detection; *S*, stipes; X^m, median value.

Levels of <0.5 mg kg^{-1} DM were observed also in papers published until 2009 (for references, see Kalač, 2010).

No generalizing conclusion on vanadium distribution within fruiting bodies can be drawn from the available fractional information. Generally, it seems that the element is not accumulated in fruiting bodies. No edible species was so far identified as a discernible vanadium bioaccumulator, although some papers indicate that *C. comatus* may be. Natural scientists have been interested in the chemical structure and biological roles of amavadin, a natural complex vanadium compound, occurring particularly in potentially toxic *Amanita muscaria*.

There were reported hypoglycemic effects of *C. comatus* rich in vanadium on hyperglycemic mice (Han & Liu, 2009; Ma & Fu, 2009).

4.3.22 Zirconium (Zr)

Ayaz et al. (2011) determined in 7 wild-growing, edible species up to 0.72 mg kg^{-1} DM, Falandysz et al. (2017) found 1.1 mg kg^{-1} DM in caps of *M. procera*, while Campos and Tejera (2011) reported the range of 1.6–27.1 mg kg^{-1} DM in 15 species growing in quartzite acidic soils.

The contents (mg kg^{-1} DM) in cultivated species are low, namely 0.09 in *L. edodes* (Mleczek, Siwulski, Rzymski, Niedzielski, et al., 2017), 0.02–0.04 in 3 *Agaricus* spp. (Rzymski, Mleczek, Siwulski, Jasińska, et al., 2017), 0.01–0.54 in 6 *Pleurotus* spp. (Siwulski et al., 2017), and around 0.05 in 12 commercial species (Mleczek, Rzymski, et al., 2018).

According to the literature data, except for the report by Campos and Tejera (2011), zirconium belongs among the elements occurring in fruiting bodies at very low levels.

4.3.23 Elements with very limited data

Singular data on hafnium, niobium, tantalum, thulium, and tungsten contents are collated in Table 4.33. Except for the results by Campos and Tejera (2011) dealing with niobium in mushrooms growing in quartzite acidic soils, other papers report very low levels of the elements, generally near the limits of detection. However, the report by Turfan et al. (2018) gives considerably higher levels.

4.3.24 Conclusion

Tens of trace elements classified in this section are considered so far as nutritionally unimportant. Data for most of them are very limited, originate from a few reports, and only deal with several species. Only two elements, aluminum and rubidium, occur at usual contents of <25–500 mg kg^{-1} DM. Many further elements are present at very low levels, often <0.5 and even <0.1 mg kg^{-1} DM. Surprisingly, higher levels of several elements were reported in cultivated species than in those growing wildly. Such findings

TABLE 4.33 Contents (mg kg^{-1} dry matter) of elements with very limited data in mushroom fruiting bodies.

Element	Symbol	Reported content	Species with elevated content	References
Hafnium	Hf	0.02; 2.7–4.5		Falandysz, Sapkota, Dryżalowska et al. (2017), Turfan et al. (2018)
Niobium	Nb	0.05; 3.3–13.2	*Tricholoma equestre*	Falandysz, Sapkota, Dryżalowska et al. (2017), Campos and Tejera (2011)
Tantalum	Ta	0.016; 21–30		Falandysz, Sapkota, Dryżalowska et al. (2017), Turfan et al. (2018)
Thulium	Tm	0.01–0.19		Siwulski et al. (2017), Mleczek, Rzymski, et al. (2018)
Tungsten	W	0.02; ND-2.4		Falandysz, Sapkota, Dryżalowska et al. (2017); Turfan et al. (2018)

ND, Below limit of detection.

need to be elucidated by further research. Nutritional and health effects of this group of trace elements seem to be marginal due to their usually very low contents and limited consumption of mushrooms.

References

Alaimo, M. G., Dongarrà, G., La Rosa, A., Tamburo, E., Vasquez, G., & Varrica, D. (2018). Major and trace elements in *Boletus aereus* and *Clitopilus prunulus* growing on volcanic and sedimentary soils of Sicily (Italy). *Ecotoxicology and Environmental Safety*, *157*, 182–190.

Alonso, J., Salgado, J., García, M. A., & Melgar, M. J. (2000). Accumulation of mercury in edible macrofungi: Influence of some factors. *Archives of Environmental Contamination and Toxicology*, *38*, 158–162.

Alonso, J., Garcia, A., Pérez-López, M., & Melgar, M. J. (2003). The concentrations and bioconcentration factors of copper and zinc in edible mushrooms. *Archives of Environmental Contamination and Toxicology*, *44*, 180–188.

Aloupi, M., Koutrotsios, G., Koulousaris, M., & Kalogeropoulos, N. (2012). Trace metal contents in wild edible mushrooms growing on serpentine and volcanic soils on the island of Lesvos, Greece. *Ecotoxicology and Environmental Safety*, *78*, 184–194.

Andersson, M., Reimann, C., Flem, B., Englmaier, P., & Fabian, K. (2018). Element distribution in *Lactarius rufus* in comparison to the underlying substrate along a transect in southern Norway. *Applied Geochemistry*, *97*, 61–70.

Aruguete, D. M., Aldstadt, J. H., & Mueller, G. M. (1998). Accumulation of several heavy metals and lanthanides in mushrooms (Agaricales) from the Chicago region. *The Science of the Total Environment*, *224*, 43–56.

Árvay, J., Demková, L., Hauptvogel, M., Michalko, M., Bajčan, D., Stanovič, R., ... Trebichalský, P. (2017). Assessment of environmental and health risks in former polymetallic ore mining and smelting area, Slovakia: Spatial distribution and accumulation of mercury in four different ecosystems. *Ecotoxicology and Environmental Safety, 144*, 236–244.

Árvay, J., Tomáš, J., Hauptvogel, M., Kopernická, M., Kováčik, A., Bajčan, D., & Massányi, P. (2014). Contamination of wild-grown edible mushrooms by heavy metals in a former mercury-mining area. *Journal of Environmental Science and Health B, 49*, 815–827.

Árvay, J., Tomáš, J., Hauptvogel, M., Massányi, P., Harangozo, Ľ., Tóth, T., ... Bumbalová, M. (2015). Human exposure to heavy metals and possible public health risks via consumption of wild edible mushrooms from Slovak Paradise National Park, Slovakia. *Journal of Environmental Science and Health B, 50*, 833–843.

Assunção, L. S., da Luz, J. M. R., da Silva, M. C. S., Vieira, P. A. F., Bazzolli, D. M. S., Vanetti, M. C. D., & Kasuya, M. C. M. (2012). Enrichment of mushrooms: An interesting strategy for the acquisition of lithium. *Food Chemistry, 134*, 1123–1127.

Ayaz, F. A., Torun, H., Colak, A., Sesli, E., Millson, M., & Glew, R. H. (2011). Macro- and microlement contents of fruiting bodies of wild-edible mushrooms growing in the East Black Sea region of Turkey. *Food and Nutrition Sciences, 2*, 53–59.

Bach, F., Helm, C. V., Bellettini, M. B., Maciel, G. M., & Haminiuk, C. W. I. (2017). Edible mushrooms: A potential source of essential amino acids, glucans and minerals. *International Journal of Food Science and Technology, 52*, 2382–2392.

Bandara, A. R., Karunarathna, S. C., Mortimer, P. E., Hyde, K. D., Khan, S., Kakumyan, P., & Xu, J. (2017). First successful domestication and determination of nutritional and antioxidant properties of the red ear mushroom *Auricularia thailandica (Auriculariales, Basidiomycota). Mycological Progress, 16*, 1029–1039.

Bargagli, R., & Baldi, F. (1984). Mercury and methyl mercury in higher fungi and their relation with the substrata in a cinnabar mining area. *Chemosphere, 13*, 1059–1071.

Bau, M., Schmidt, K., Pack, A., Bendel, V., & Kraemer, D. (2018). The European Shale: An improved data set for normalisation of rare earth element and yttrium concentrations in environmental and biological samples from Europe. *Applied Geochemistry, 90*, 142–149.

Baumann, N., Arnold, T., & Haferburg, G. (2014). Uranium contents in plants and mushrooms grown on a uranium-contaminated site near Ronneburg in Eastern Thuringia/Germany. *Environmental Science and Pollution Research, 21*, 6921–6929.

Beneš, V., Hložková, K., Matěnová, M., Borovička, J., & Kotrba, P. (2016). Accumulation of Ag and Cu in *Amanita strobiliformis* and characteriziation of its Cu and Ag uptake transporter genes As*CTR2* and As*CTR3*. *Biometals, 29*, 249–264.

Borovička, J., Braeuer, S., Sácký, J., Kameník, J., Goessler, W., Trubač, J., ... Kotrba, P. (2019). Speciation analysis of elements accumulated in *Cystoderma carcharias* from clean and smelter-polluted sites. *Science of the Total Environment, 648*, 1570–1581.

Borovička, J., Dunn, C. E., Gryndler, M., Mihaljevič, M., Jelínek, E., Rohovec, J., ... Řanda, Z. (2010). Bioaccumulation of gold in macrofungi and ectomycorrhizae from the vivinity of the Mokrsko gold deposit, Czech Republic. *Soil Biology and Biochemistry, 42*, 83–91.

Borovička, J., Kotrba, M., Gryndler, M., Mihaljevič, M., Řanda, Z., Rohovec, J., ... Dunn, C. E. (2010). Bioaccumulation of silver in ectomycorrhizal and saprobic macrofungi from pristine and polluted areas. *Science of the Total Environment, 408*, 2733–2744.

Borovička, J., Kubrová, J., Rohovec, J., Řanda, Z., & Dunn, C. E. (2011). Uranium, thorium and rare earth elements in macrofungi: What are the genuine concentrations? *Biometals, 24*, 837–845.

Borovička, J., Mihaljevič, M., Gryndler, M., Kubrová, J., Žigová, A., Hršelová, H., & Řanda, Z. (2014). Lead isotopic signatures of saprotrophic macrofungi of various origins: Tracing for lead sources and possible applications in geomycology. *Applied Geochemistry*, *43*, 114–120.

Borovička, J., Řanda, Z., & Jelínek, E. (2005). Gold content of ectomycorrhizal and saprobic macrofungi from non-auriferous and unpolluted areas. *Mycological Research*, *109*, 951–955.

Borovička, J., Řanda, Z., & Jelínek, E. (2006). Antimony content of macrofungi from clean and polluted areas. *Chemosphere*, *64*, 1837–1844.

Borovička, J., Řanda, Z., Jelínek, E., & Dunn, C. E. (2007). Hyperaccumulation of silver by *Amanita strobiliformis* and related species of the section *Lepidella*. *Mycological Research*, *111*, 1339–1344.

Bouatia, M., Touré, H. A., Cheikh, A., Eljaoudi, R., Rahali, Y., Oulad Bouyahya Idrissi, M., . . . Draoui, M. (2018). Analysis of nutrient and antinutrient content of the truffle (*Tirmania pinoyi*) from Morocco. *International Food Research Journal*, *25*, 174–178.

Braeuer, S., Borovička, J., Glasnov, T., de la Cruz, G. G., Jensen, K. B., & Goessler, W. (2018). Homoarsenocholine – A novel arsenic compound detected for the first time in nature. *Talanta*, *188*, 107–110.

Braeuer, S., Borovička, J., & Goessler, W. (2018). A unique arsenic speciation profile in *Elaphomyces* spp. ("deer truffles") – trimethylarsine oxide and methylarsonous acid as a significant arsenic compounds. *Analytical and Bioanalytical Chemistry*, *410*, 2283–2290.

Braeuer, S., Goessler, W., Kameník, J., Konvalinková, T., Žigová, A., & Borovička, J. (2018). Arsenic hyperaccumulation and speciation in the edible ink stain bolete (*Cyanoboletus pulverulentus*). *Food Chemistry*, *242*, 225–231.

Brzezicha-Cirocka, J., Mędyk, M., Falandysz, J., & Szefer, P. (2016). Bio- and toxic elements in edible wild mushrooms from two regions of potentially different environmental conditions in eastern Poland. *Environmental Science and Pollution Research*, *23*, 21517–21522.

Campos, J. A., & Tejera, N. A. (2011). Bioconcentration factors and trace elements bioaccumulation in sporocarps of fungi collected from quartzite acidic soils. *Biological Trace Elements Research*, *143*, 540–554.

Çayir, A., Coşkun, M., & Coşkun, M. (2010). The heavy metal content of wild edible mushroom samples collected in Canakkale Province, Turkey. *Biological Trace Element Research*, *134*, 212–219.

Chansler, M. W., Mutanen, M., Morris, V. C., & Levander, O. A. (1986). Nutritional bioavailability to rats of selenium in Brazil nuts and mushrooms. *Nutrition Research*, *6*, 1419–1428.

Chen, S., Guo, Q., & Liu, L. (2017). Determination of arsenic species in edible mushrooms by high-performance liquid chromatography coupled to inductively coupled plasma mass spectrometry. *Food Analytical Methods*, *10*, 740–748.

Chen, S., Yuan, B., Xu, J., Chen, G., Hu, Q., & Zhao, L. (2018). Simultaneous separation and determination of six arsenic species in Shiitake (*Lentinus edodes*) mushrooms: Method development and applications. *Food Chemistry*, *262*, 134–141.

Chojnacka, A., Drewnowska, M., Jarzyńska, G., Nnorom, I. C., & Falandysz, J. (2012). Mercury in Yellow-cracking Boletes *Xerocomus subtomentosus* mushrooms and soils from spatially diverse sites: Assessment of bioconcentration potential by species and human intake. *Journal of Environmental Science and Health A*, *47*, 2094–2100.

Chowaniak, M., Niemiec, M., & Paluch, Ł. (2017). Bioconcentration of cadmium (Cd), copper (Cu), lead (Pb) and zinc (Zn) in *Lactarius salmonicolor* in the Western Carpathians. *Journal of Elementology*, *22*, 1537–1547.

Chudzyński, K., Jarzyńska, G., Stefańska, A., & Falandysz, J. (2011). Mercury content and bioconcentration potential of Slippery Jack, *Suillus luteus*, mushroom. *Food Chemistry, 125*, 986–990.

Cibulka, J., Čurdová, E., Miholová, D., & Stěhulová, I. (1999). Mercury loss from edible mushrooms after their model thermal treatment. *Czech Journal of Food Sciences, 17*, 238–240.

Cocchi, L., Vescovi, L., Petrini, L. E., & Petrini, O. (2006). Heavy metals in edible mushrooms in Italy. *Food Chemistry, 98*, 277–284.

Collin-Hansen, C., Andersen, R. A., & Steinnes, E. (2003). Isolation and N-terminal sequencing of a novel cadmium-binding protein from *Boletus edulis*. *Journal de Physique IV France, 107*, 311–314.

Collin-Hansen, C., Yttri, K. E., Andersen, R. A., Berthelsen, B. O., & Steinnes, E. (2002). Mushrooms from two metal-contaminated areas in Norway: Occurrence of metals and metallothionein-like proteins. *Geochemistry, Exploration, Environment, Analysis, 2*, 121–130.

Coşkuner, Y., & Özdemir, Y. (1997). Effects of canning processes on the elements content of cultivated mushrooms (*Agaricus bisporus*). *Food Chemistry, 60*, 559–562.

Cremades, O., Diaz-Herrero, M. M., Carbonero-Aguilar, P., Gutierrez-Gil, J. F., Fontiveros, E., Rodríguez-Morgado, B., & Bautista, J. (2012). Preparation and characterization of selenium-enriched mushroom aqueous extracts (MAEE) obtained from whit button mushroom (*Agaricus bisporus*). *Food Chemistry, 133*, 1538–1543.

Cvetkovic, J. S., Mitic, V. D., Stankov-Jovanovic, V. P., Dimitrijevic, M. V., & Nikolic-Mandic, S. D. (2015). Elemental composition of wild edible mushrooms from Serbia. *Analytical Letters, 48*, 2017–2121.

Dimitrijevic, M. V., Mitic, V. D., Cvetkovic, J. S., Stankov Jovanovic, V. P., Mutic, J. J., & Nikolic Mandic, S. D. (2016). Update on element content profiles in eleven wild edible mushrooms from family *Boletaceae*. *European Food Research and Technology, 242*, 1–10.

Dospatliev, L., & Ivanova, M. (2017). *Boletus pinophilus* growing in Bulgaria: Chemical profile and hazard index. *Comptes Rendus de l'Académie Bulgare des Sciences, 70*, 795–802.

Drewnowska, M., & Falandysz, J. (2015). Investigation on mineral composition and accumulation by popular edible mushroom common chantarelle (*Cantharellus cibarius*). *Ecotoxicology and Environmental Safety, 113*, 9–17.

Drewnowska, M., Falandysz, J., Chudzińska, M., Hanć, A., Saba, M., & Barałkiewicz, D. (2017). Leaching of arsenic and sixteen metallic elements from *Amanita fulva* mushrooms after food processing. *LWT – Food Science and Technology, 84*, 861–866.

Drewnowska, M., Hanć, A., Barałkiewicz, D., & Falandysz, J. (2017). Pickling of chantarelle *Cantharellus cibarius* mushrooms highly reduce cadmium contamination. *Environmental Science and Pollution Research, 24*, 21733–21738.

Drewnowska, M., Jarzyńska, G., Kojta, A. K., & Falandysz, J. (2012). Mercury in European Blushers, *Amanita rubescens*, mushrooms and topsoils: Bioconcentration potential and intake assessment. *Journal of Environmental Science and Health B, 47*, 466–474.

Drewnowska, M., Nnorom, I. C., & Falandysz, J. (2014). Mercury in the Grisette, *Amanita vaginata* Fr. and soil below the fruiting bodies. *Journal of Environmental Science and Health B, 49*, 521–526.

Dryżałowska, A., & Falandysz, J. (2014). Bioconcentration of mercury by mushroom *Xerocomus chrysenteron* from the spatially distant locations: Levels, possible intake and safety. *Ecotoxicology and Environmental Safety, 107*, 97–102.

Durkan, N., Ugulu, I., Unver, M. C., Dogan, Y., & Baslar, S. (2011). Concentrations of trace elements aluminum, boron, cobalt and tin in various edible mushroom species from Buyuk Menderes River Basin in Turkey by ICP-OES. *Trace Elements and Electrolytes, 28*, 242–248.

EFSA (European Food Safety Authority) (2017). *Dietary reference values for nutrients*. Summary report. 92 pp. https://doi.org/10.2903/sp.efsa.2017.e15121.

Egressy-Molnar, O., Ouerdane, L., Györfi, J., & Dernovics, M. (2016). Analogy of selenium enrichment and selenium speciation between selenized yeast *Saccharomyces cerevisiae* and *Hericium erinaceus* (lion's mane mushroom). *LWT – Food Science and Technology*, *68*, 306–312.

Elekes, C. C., & Busuioc, G. (2013). Influence of chemical composition of soil on metal accumulation in edible mushroom species of *Russula* genus. *Revue Roumaine de Chimie*, *58*, 629–637.

Esser, J., & Brunnert, H. (1986). Isolation and partial purification of cadmium-binding components from fruiting bodies of *Agaricus bisporus*. *Environmental Pollution*, *A41*, 263–275.

Falandysz, J. (2008). Selenium in edible mushrooms. *Journal of Environmental Science and Health C*, *26*, 256–299.

Falandysz, J. (2013). Review: On published data and methods for selenium in mushrooms. *Food Chemistry*, *138*, 242–250.

Falandysz, J. (2014). Distribution of mercury in Gypsy *Cortinarius caperatus* mushrooms from several populations: An efficient accumulator species and estimated intake of element. *Ecotoxicology and Environmental Safety*, *110*, 68–72.

Falandysz, J. (2016). Mercury bio-extraction by fungus *Coprinus comatus*: A possible bioindicator and mycoremediator of polluted soils?. *Environmental Science and Pollution Research*, *23*, 7444–7451.

Falandysz, J. (2017). Mercury accumulation of three *Lactarius* mushroom species. *Food Chemistry*, *214*, 96–101.

Falandysz, J. (2018). Mineral constituents in *Leccinum scabrum* from lowland locations in the central Europe and their relation to concentration in forest topsoil. *Journal of Environmental Science and Health B*, *53*, 546–560.

Falandysz, J., Bona, H., & Danisiewicz, D. (1994a). Silver content of wild-grown mushrooms from Northern Poland. *Zeitschrift für Lebensmittel Untersuchung und Forschung*, *199*, 222–224.

Falandysz, J., Bona, H., & Danisiewicz, D. (1994b). Silver uptake by *Agaricus bisporus* from an artificially enriched substrate. *Zeitschrift für Lebensmittel Untersuchung und Forschung*, *199*, 225–228.

Falandysz, J., & Borovička, J. (2013). Macro and trace mineral constituents and radionuclides in mushrooms: Health benefits ad risks. *Applied Microbiology and Biotechnology*, *97*, 477–501.

Falandysz, J., Chudzińska, M., Barałkiewicz, D., Drewnowska, M., & Hanć, D. (2017). Toxic elements and bio-metals in *Cantharellus* mushrooms from Poland and China. *Environmental Science and Pollution Research*, *24*, 11472–11482.

Falandysz, J., & Danisiewicz, D. (1995). Bioconcentration factors (BCF) of silver in wild *Agaricus campestris*. *Bulletin of Environmental Contamination and Toxicology*, *55*, 122–129.

Falandysz, J., & Drewnowska, M. (2015a). Macro and trace elements in Common Chanterelle (*Cantharellus cibarius*) mushroom from the European background areas in Poland: Composition, accumulation, dietary exposure and data review for species. *Journal of Environmental Science and Health B*, *50*, 374–387.

Falandysz, J., & Drewnowska, M. (2015b). Distribution of mercury in *Amanita fulva* (Schaeff.) Secr. mushrooms: Accumulation, loss in cooking and dietary intake. *Ecotoxicology and Environmental Safety*, *115*, 49–54.

Falandysz, J., & Drewnowska, M. (2017). Cooking can decrease mercury contamination of a mushroom meal: *Cantharellus cibarius* and *Amanita fulva*. *Environmental Science and Pollution Research*, *24*, 13352–13357.

Falandysz, J., Drewnowska, M., Chudzińska, M., & Barałkiewicz, D. (2017). Accumulation and distribution of metallic elements and metalloids in edible *Amanita fulva* mushrooms. *Ecotoxicology and Environmental Safety*, *137*, 265–271.

Falandysz, J., Drewnowska, M., Jarzyńska, G., Zhang, D., Zhang, Y., & Wang, J. (2012). Mineral constituents in Common Chanterelles and soils collected from a high mountain and lowland sites in Poland. *Journal of Mountain Science*, *9*, 697–705.

Falandysz, J., Frankowska, A., Jarzyńska, G., Dryżałowska, A., Kojta, A. K., & Zhang, D. (2011). Survey on composition and bioconcentration potential of 12 metallic elements in King Bolete (*Boletus edulis*) mushroom that emerged at 11 spatially distant sites. *Journal of Environmental Science and Health B*, *46*, 231–246.

Falandysz, J., Kojta, A. K., Jarzyńska, G., Drewnowska, M., Dryżałowska, A., Wydmańska, D., ... Szefer, P. (2012). Mercury in bay bolete (*Xerocomus badius*): Bioconcentration by fungus and assessment of element intake by humans eating fruiting bodies. *Food Additives and Contaminants*, *29*, 951–961.

Falandysz, J., Kowalewska, I., Nnorom, I. C., Drewnowska, M., & Jarzyńska, G. (2012). Mercury in Red Aspen Boletes (*Leccinum aurantiacum*) mushrooms and soils. *Journal of Environmental Science and Health A*, *47*, 1695–1700.

Falandysz, J., Krasińska, G., Pankavec, S., & Nnorom, I. C. (2014). Mercury in certain boletus mushrooms from Poland and Belarus. *Journal of Environmental Science and Health B*, *49*, 690–695.

Falandysz, J., Mazur, A., Kojta, A. K., Jarzyńska, G., Drewnowska, M., Dryżałowska, A., & Nnorom, I. C. (2013). Mercury in fruiting bodies of dark honey fungus (*Armillaria solidipes*) and beneath substratum soils collected from spatially distant areas. *Journal of Science of Food and Agriculture*, *93*, 853–858.

Falandysz, J., Nnorom, I. C., Jarzyńska, G., Romińska, D., & Damps, K. (2012). Mercury bioconcentration by Puffballs (*Lycoperdon perlatum*) and evaluation of dietary intake risk. *Bulletin of Environmental Contamination and Toxicology*, *89*, 759–763.

Falandysz, J., & Rizal, L. M. (2016). Arsenic and its compounds in mushrooms: A review. *Journal of Environmental Science and Health C*, *34*, 217–232.

Falandysz, J., Saba, M., Liu, H., Li, T., Wang, J., Wiejak, A., ... Zhang, D. (2016). Mercury in forest mushrooms and topsoil from the Yunnan highlands and the subalpine region of the Minya Konka summit in the Eastern Tibetan Plateau. *Environmental Science and Pollution Research*, *23*, 23730–23741.

Falandysz, J., Sapkota, A., Dryżałowska, A., Mędyk, M., & Feng, X. (2017). Analysis of some metallic elements and metalloids composition and relationships in parasol mushroom *Macrolepiota procera*. *Environmental Science and Pollution Research*, *24*, 15528–15537.

Falandysz, J., Sapkota, A., Mędyk, M., & Feng, X. (2017). Rare earth elements in parasol mushroom *Macrolepiota procera*. *Food Chemistry*, *221*, 24–28.

Falandysz, J., Szymczyk, K., Ichihashi, H., Bielawski, L., Gucia, M., Frankowska, A., & Yamasaki, S. I. (2001). ICP/MS and ICP/AES elemental analysis (38 elements) of edible wild mushrooms growing in Poland. *Food Additives and Contaminants*, *18*, 503–513.

Falandysz, J., Widzicka, E., Kojta, A. K., Jarzyńska, G., Drewnowska, M., Dryżałowska, A., ... Nnorom, I. C. (2012). Mercury in Common Chanterelles mushrooms: *Cantharellus* spp. update. *Food Chemistry*, *133*, 842–850.

Falandysz, J., Zhang, J., Wang, Y., Krasińska, G., Kojta, A., Saba, M., ... Liu, H. (2015). Evaluation of the mercury contamination in mushrooms of genus *Leccinum* from two different regions of the world: Accumulation, distribution and probable dietary intake. *Science of the Total Environment*, *537*, 470–478.

Falandysz, J., Zhang, J., Wang, Y., Saba, M., Krasińska, G., Wiejak, A., & Li, T. (2015). Evaluation of mercury contamination in fungi *Boletus* species from latosols, lateritic red earth, and red and yellow earths in the Circum-Pacific Mercuriferous Belt of southwestern China. *PLoS One*, *10*(11), e0143608.

Falandysz, J., Zhang, J., Wiejak, A., Barałkiewicz, D., & Hanć, A. (2017). Metallic elements and metalloids in *Boletus luridus*, *B. magnificus* and *B. tomentipes* mushrooms from polymetallic soils from SW China. *Ecotoxicology and Environmental Safety*, *142*, 497–502.

Fang, Y., Zhang, Y., Wang, M. Y., Pei, F., Xie, M. H., Li, P., & Hu, Q. (2018). *In vitro* bioaccessibility and speciation changes of selenium in *Pleurotus eryngii* during the growing stage. *Food and Function*, *9*, 4493–4499.

Figueiredo, E., Soares, M. E., Baptista, P., Castro, M., & Bastos, M. L. (2007). Validation of an electrothermal atomization atomic absorption spectrometry method for quantification of total chromium and chromium (VI) in wild mushrooms and underlying soils. *Journal of Agricultural and Food Chemistry*, *55*, 7192–7198.

Fiket, Ž., Medunić, G., Turk, M. F., Ivanić, M., & Kniewald, G. (2017). Influence of soil characteristics on rare earth fingerprints in mosses and mushrooms: Example of a pristine temperate rainforest (Slavonia, Croatia). *Chemosphere*, *179*, 92–100.

Fischer, R. G., Rapsomanikis, S., Andreae, M. O., & Baldi, F. (1995). Bioaccumulation of methylmercury and transformation of inorganic mercury by macrofungi. *Environmental Science and Technology*, *29*, 993–999.

Frankowska, A., Ziółkowska, J., Bielawski, L., & Falandysz, J. (2010). Profile and bioconcentration of minerals in King Bolete (*Boletus edulis*) from the Płocka Dale in Poland. *Food Additives and Contaminants B*, *3*, 1–6.

Gabriel, J., Rychlovský, P., & Krenželok, M. (1995). Beryllium content in some wood-rotting fungi in Czech Republic. *Toxicological and Environmental Chemistry*, *50*, 233–236.

Gabriel, J., Švec, K., Kolihová, D., Tlustoš, P., & Száková, J. (2016). Translocation of mercury from substrate to fruit bodies of *Panellus stipticus*, *Psilocybe cubensis*, *Schizophyllum commune* and *Stropharia rugosoannulata* on oat flakes. *Ecotoxicology and Environmental Safety*, *125*, 184–189.

García, M. Á., Alonso, J., & Melgar, M. J. (2009). Lead in edible mushrooms. Levels and bioaccumulation factors. *Journal of Hazardous Materials*, *167*, 777–783.

Gąsecka, M., Mleczek, M., Siwulski, M., Niedzielski, P., & Kozak, L. (2016). Phenolic and flavonoid content in *Hericium erinaceus*, *Ganoderma lucidum*, and *Agrocybe aegerita* under selenium addition. *Acta Alimentaria*, *45*, 301–309.

Gąsecka, M., Rzymski, P., Mleczek, M., Siwulski, M., Budzyńska, S., Magdziak, Z., ... Sobieralski, K. (2017). The relationship between metal composition, phenolic acid and flavonoid content in *Imleria badia* from non-polluted and polluted areas. *Journal of Environmental Science and Health B*, *52*, 171–177.

Gaur, T., Rao, P. B., & Kushwaha, K. P. S. (2016). Nutritional and anti-nutritional components of some selected edible mushroom species. *Indian Journal of Natural Products and Resources*, *7*, 155–161.

Gdula-Argasińska, J., Grzywacz, A., Krakowska, A., Opoka, W., & Muszyńska, B. (2018). Anti-inflammatory properties of *Cantharellus cibarius* from *in vitro* culture enriched with zinc. *Acta Poloniae Pharmaceutica*, *75*, 423–433.

Georgescu, A. A., Danet, A. F., Radulescu, C., Stihi, C., Dulama, I. D., & Chelarescu, D. E. (2016). Determination of several elements in edible mushrooms using ICP-MS. *Romanian Journal of Physics*, *61*, 1087–1097.

Gezer, K., & Kaygusuz, O. (2014). An assessment of the heavy metal content of various wild edible mushrooms in the Denizli Province, Turkey. *Journal of Environmental Protection and Ecology*, *15*, 425–432.

Gezer, K., Kaygusuz, O., Herken, E. N., Dodurga, Y., Koizhaiganova, M., & Seçme, M. (2016). Evaluation of the nutritional composition of wild edible mushroom *Agaricus lanipes* (F.H. Møller & Jul. Schäff.) Hlaváček. *Bangladesh Journal of Botany*, *45*, 161–166.

Giannaccini, G., Betti, L., Palego, L., Madcia, G., Schmid, L., Lanza, M., ... Lucacchini, A. (2012). The trace element content of top-soil and wild edible mushroom samples collected in Tuscany, Italy. *Environmental Monitoring and Assessment*, *184*, 7579–7595.

Golubkina, N. A., & Mironov, V. E. (2018). Element composition of mushrooms in contrasting anthropogenic loading. *Geochemistry International*, *56*, 1263–1275.

Gonçalves, J. M., de Souza, M. D. C., Rocha, R. C. C., Medeiros, R. J., & do Couto Jacob, S. (2014). Macro and trace elements in edible mushrooms, Shiitake, Shimeji and Cardoncello from Petrópolis, Rio de Janeiro, Brazil. *Ciência Rural*, *44*, 943–949.

Grawunder, A., & Gube, M. (2018). Element distribution in fruiting bodies of *Lactarius pubescens* with focus on rare earth elements. *Chemosphere*, *208*, 614–625.

Gucia, M., Jarzyńska, G., Rafal, E., Roszak, M., Kojta, A. K., Osiej, I., & Falandysz, J. (2012). Multivariete analysis of mineral constituents of edible Parasol Mushroom (*Macrolepiota procera*) and soils beneath fruiting bodies collected from Northern Poland. *Environmental Science and Pollution Research*, *19*, 416–431.

Han, C. C., & Liu, T. J. (2009). A comparison of hypoglycemic activity of three species of basidiomycetes rich in vanadium. *Biological Trace Element Research*, *127*, 177–182.

Harangozo, Ľ., & Stanovič, R. (2016). Heavy metals in edible wild mushrooms collected from former polymetallic ores mining and smelting area (Slovakia). In: *Water resources, forest, marine and ocean ecosystems conference proceedings, SGEM 2016* (Vol. III, pp. 461–468).

Harvey, L. J., Dainty, J. R., Beattie, J. H., Majsak-Newman, G., Wharf, S. G., Reid, M. D., & Fairweather-Tait, S. J. (2005). Copper absorption from foods labelled intrinsically and extrinsically with Cu-65 stable isotope. *European Journal of Clinical Nutrition*, *59*, 363–368.

Huang, J. C., Ben, L. K., Yu, Y. R., Wu, H. W., & Liu, D. L. (2008). Cadmium accumulation in *Agaricus blazei* Murrill. *Journal of the Science of Food and Agriculture*, *88*, 1369–1375.

Huang, Q., Jia, Y., Wan, Y., Li, H., & Jiang, R. (2015). Market survey and risk assessment for trace metals in edible fungi and the substrate role in accumulation of heavy metals. *Journal of Food Science*, *80*, 1612–1618.

Jadán-Piedra, C., Alcántara, C., Monedero, V., Zúñiga, M., Vélez, D., & Devesa, V. (2017). The use of lactic acid bacteria to reduce mercury bioaccessibility. *Food Chemistry*, *228*, 158–166.

Jadán-Piedra, C., Baquedano, M., Puig, S., Vélez, D., & Devesa, V. (2017). Use of *Saccharomyces cerevisiae* to reduce the bioaccessibility of mercury from food. *Journal of Agricultural and Food Chemistry*, *65*, 2876–2882.

Jarzyńska, G., & Falandysz, J. (2012a). Trace elements profile of Slate Bolete (*Leccinum duriusculum*) mushroom and associated upper soil horizon. *Journal of Geochemical Exploration*, *121*, 69–75.

Jarzyńska, G., & Falandysz, J. (2012b). Metallic elements profile of Hazel (Hard) Bolete (*Leccinum griseum*) mushroom and associated upper soil horizon. *African Journal of Biotechnology*, *11*, 4588–4594.

Jarzyńska, G., Chojnacka, A., Dryżalowska, A., Nnorom, I. C., & Falandysz, J. (2012). Concentrations and bioconcentration factors of minerals in Yellow-cracking Bolete (*Xerocomus subtomentosus*) mushroom collected in Noteć Forest, Poland. *Journal of Food Science*, *77*, H202–H206.

Jarzyńska, G., Gucia, M., Kojta, A. K., Rezulak, K., & Falandysz, J. (2011). Profile of trace elements in Parasol Mushroom (*Macrolepiota procera*) from Tucholskie Forest. *Journal of Environmental Science and Health B*, *46*, 741–751.

Jedidi, I. K., Ayoub, I. K., Philippe, T., & Bouzouita, N. (2017). Chemical composition and nutritional value of three Tunisian wild edible mushrooms. *Journal of Food Measurement and Characterization*, *11*, 2069–2075.

Kalač, P. (2010). Trace element contents in European species of wild growing edible mushrooms: A review for the period 2000-2009. *Food Chemistry*, *122*, 2–15.

Kalač, P., Burda, J., & Stašková, I. (1991). Concentrations of lead, cadmium, mercury and copper in mushrooms in the vicinity of a lead smelter. *The Science of the Total Environment*, *105*, 109–119.

Kalač, P., Nižnanská, M., Bevilaqua, D., & Stašková, I. (1996). Concentrations of mercury, copper, cadmium and lead in fruiting bodies of edible mushrooms in the vicinity of a mercury smelter and a copper smelter. *The Science of the Total Environment*, *177*, 251–258.

Kalač, P., & Svoboda, L. (2000). A review of trace element concentrations in edible mushrooms. *Food Chemistry*, *69*, 273–281.

Kalač, P., Wittingerová, M., Stašková, I., Šimák, M., & Bastl, J. (1989). [Contents of mercury, lead and cadmium in mushrooms]. *Československá Hygiena*, *34*, 568–576. (in Czech).

Kaur, G., Kalia, A., & Sodhi, H. S. (2018). Selenium biofortification of *Pleurotus* species and its effects on yield, phytochemical profiles, and protein chemistry of fruiting bodies. *Journal of Food Biochemistry*, *42*, e12467. Available from https://doi.org/10.1111/jfbc.12467.

Khani, R., Moudi, M., & Khojech, V. (2017). Contamination level, distribution and health risk assessment of heavy and toxic metallic and metalloid elements in a cultivated mushroom *Pleurotus florida* (Mont.) singer. *Environmental Science and Pollution Research*, *24*, 4699–4708.

Kivrak, I. (2015). Analytical methods applied to assess chemical composition, nutritional value and in vitro bioactivities of *Terfezia olbiensis* and *Terfezia claveryi* from Turkey. *Food Analytical Methods*, *8*, 1279–1293.

Klán, J., Řanda, Z., Benada, J., & Horyna, J. (1988). Investigation on non-radioactive Rb, Cs, and radiocaesium in higher fungi. *Česká Mykologie*, *42*(3), 158–169.

Klimaszewska, M., Górska, S., Dawidowski, M., Podsadni, P., & Turło, J. (2016). Biosynthesis of Se-methyl-seleno-L-cysteine in *Basidiomycetes* fungus *Lentinula edodes* (Berk.) Pegler. *SpringerPlus*, *5*, Art. Nr. 733, 8 pp.

Kojo, M.-R., & Lodenius, M. (1989). Cadmium and mercury in macrofungi – Mechanisms of transport and accumulation. *Angewandte Botanik*, *63*, 279–292.

Kojta, A. K., & Falandysz, J. (2016a). Metallic elements (Ca, Hg, Fe, K, Mn, Na, Zn) in the fruiting bodies of *Boletus badius*. *Food Chemistry*, *200*, 206–214.

Kojta, A. K., & Falandysz, J. (2016b). Soil-to-mushroom transfer and diversity in total mercury content in two edible Laccaria mushrooms. *Environmental Earth Sciences*, *75*, Art. Nr 1264.

Kojta, A. K., Gucia, M., Jarzyńska, G., Lewandowska, M., Zakrzewska, A., Falandysz, J., & Zhang, D. (2011). Phosphorus and certain metals in Parasol Mushrooms (*Macrolepiota procera*) and soils from the Augustowska Forest and Ełk region in north-eastern Poland. *Fresenius Environmental Bulletin*, *20*, 3044–3052.

Kojta, A. K., Jarzyńska, G., & Falandysz, J. (2012). Mineral composition and heavy metal accumulation capacity of Bay Bolete (*Xerocomus badius*) fruiting bodies collected near a former gold and copper mining area. *Journal of Geochemical Exploration, 121*, 76–82.

Kojta, A. K., Zhang, J., Wang, Y., Li, T., Saba, M., & Falandysz, J. (2015). Mercury contamination of fungi genus *Xerocomus* in the Yunnan province in China and the region of Europe. *Journal of Environmental Science and Health B, 50*, 1342–1350.

Komárek, M., Chrastný, V., & Štíchová, J. (2007). Metal/metalloid contamination and isotopic composition of lead in edible mushrooms and forest soils originating from a smelting area. *Environment International, 33*, 677–684.

Kosanić, M., Ranković, B., Rančić, A., & Stanojković, T. (2017). Evaluation of metal contents and bioactivity of two edible mushrooms *Agaricus campestris* and *Boletus edulis*. *Emirates Journal of Food and Agriculture, 29*, 98–103.

Koutrotsios, G., Danezis, G. P., Georgiou, C. A., & Zervakis, G. I. (2018). Rare earth elements concentration in mushroom cultivation substrate affects the production process and fruit-bodies content of *Pleurotus ostreatus* and *Cyclocybe cylindracea*. *Journal of the Science of Food and Agriculture, 98*, 5418–5427.

Krasińska, G., & Falandysz, J. (2015). Mercury in Hazel Bolete *Leccinum griseum* and soil substratum: Distribution, bioconcentration and dietary exposure. *Journal of Environmental Science and Health A, 50*, 1259–1264.

Krasińska, G., & Falandysz, J. (2016). Mercury in Orange Birch Bolete *Leccinum versipelle* and soil substratum: Bioconcentration by mushroom and probable dietary intake by consumers. *Environmental Science and Pollution Research, 23*, 860–869.

Kubrová, J., Žigová, A., Řanda, Z., Rohovec, J., Gryndler, M., Krausová, I., ... Borovička, J. (2014). On the possible role of macrofungi in the biogeochemical fate of uranium in polluted forest soils. *Journal of Hazardous Materials, 280*, 79–88.

Kułdo, E., Jarzyńska, G., Gucia, M., & Falandysz, J. (2014). Mineral constituents of edible parasol mushroom *Macrolepiota procera* (Scop. ex Fr.) Sing and soils beneath its fruiting bodies collected from a rural forest area. *Chemical Papers, 68*, 484–492.

Larsen, E. H., Hansen, M., & Gössler, W. (1998). Speciation and health risk considerations of arsenic in the edible mushroom *Laccaria amethystina* collected from contaminated and uncontaminated locations. *Applied Organometallic Chemistry, 12*, 285–291.

Lasota, W., & Florczak, J. (1983). [Fluorine content in selected mushroom species collected in Poland.]. *Bromatologia i Chemia Toksykologiczna, 16*, 173–174. (in Polish).

Lavola, A., Aphalo, P. J., & Lehto, T. (2011). Boron and other elements in sporophores of ectomycorrhizal and saprotrophic fungi. *Mycorrhiza, 21*, 155–165.

Lepšová, A., & Král, R. (1988). Lead and cadmium in fruiting bodies of macrofungi in the vicinity of a lead smelter. *The Science of the Total Environment, 76*, 129–138.

Li, M. Y., Wang, P., Wang, J. Y., Chen, X. Q., Zhao, D., Yin, D. X., ... Ma, L. Q. (2019). Arsenic concentrations, speciation, and localization in 141 cultivated market mushrooms: Implications for arsenic exposure to humans. *Environmental Science and Technology, 53*, 503–511.

Li, T., Zhang, J., Shen, T., Shi, Y., Yang, S., Zhang, T., ... Liu, H. (2013). Mineral element content in prized matsutake mushroom (*Tricholoma matsutake*) collected in China. *Chemical Papers, 67*, 672–676.

Lind, Y., Glynn, A. W., Engman, J., & Jorhem, L. (1995). Bioavailability of cadmium from crab hepatopancreas and mushroom in relation to inorganic cadmium – A 9-week feeding study in mice. *Food and Chemical Toxicology, 33*, 667–673.

Liu, H., Zhang, J., Li, T., Shi, Y., & Wang, Y. (2012). Mineral element levels in wild edible mushrooms from Yunnan, China. *Biological Trace Element Research, 147*, 341–345.

Liukkonen-Lilja, H., Kuusi, T., Laaksovirta, K., Lodenius, M., & Piepponen, S. (1986). The effect of lead processing works on the lead, cadmium and mercury contents of fungi. *Zeitschrift für Lebensmittel-Untersuchung und –Forschung, 176*, 120–123.

Llorente-Mirandes, T., Barbero, M., Rubio, R., & López-Sánchez, J. F. (2014). Occurrence of inorganic arsenic in edible Shiitake (*Lentinula edodes*) products. *Food Chemistry, 158*, 207–215.

Llorente-Mirandes, T., Llorens-Muñoz, M., Funes-Collado, V., & Sahuquillo, À. (2016). Assessment of arsenic bioaccessibility in raw and cooked edible mushrooms by a PBET method. *Food Chemistry, 194*, 849–856.

Ma, Z. J., & Fu, Q. (2009). Comparison of hypoglycemic activity and toxicity of vanadium (IV) and vanadium (V) absorbed in fermented mushroom of *Coprinus comatus*. *Biological Trace Element Research, 132*, 278–284.

Maćkiewicz, D., & Falandysz, J. (2012). Total mercury in Yellow Knights (*Tricholoma equestre*) mushrooms and beneath soils. *Bulletin of Environmental Contamination and Toxicology, 89*, 755–758.

Mallikarjuna, S. E., Ranjini, A., Haware, D. J., Haware, J., Vijayalakshmi, M. R., Shashirekha, M. N., & Rajarathnam, S. (2013). Mineral composition of four edible mushrooms. *Journal of Chemistry*, Article ID 805284, 5 pp.

Maseko, T., Callahan, D. L., Dunshea, F. R., Doronila, A., Kolev, S. D., & Ng, K. (2013). Chemical characterisation and speciation of organic selenium in cultivated selenium-enriched *Agaricus bisporus*. *Food Chemistry, 141*, 3681–3687.

Mazurkiewicz, N., & Podlasińska, J. (2014). Bioaccumulation of trace elements in wild-growing edible mushrooms from Lubuskie voivodeship, Poland. *Chemistry and Ecology, 30*, 110–117.

Mędyk, M., Chudzińska, M., Barałkiewicz, D., & Falandysz, J. (2017). Specific accumulation of cadmium and trace elements in *Sarcodon imbricatus* using ICP-MS with a chemometric approach. *Journal of Environmental Science and Health B, 52*, 361–366.

Mędyk, M., Grembecka, M., Brzezicha-Cirocka, J., & Falandysz, J. (2017). Bio- and toxic elements in mushrooms from the city of Umeå and outskirts, Sweden. *Journal of Environmental Science and Health B, 52*, 577–583.

Meisch, H.-U., & Schmitt, J. A. (1986). Characterization studies on cadmium-mycophosphatin from mushroom *Agaricus macrosporus*. *Environmental Health Perspectives, 65*, 29–32.

Melgar, M. J., Alonso, J., & García, M. A. (2009). Mercury in edible mushrooms and underlying soils: Bioconcentration factors and toxicological risk. *Science of the Total Environment, 407*, 5328–5334.

Melgar, M. J., Alonso, J., & García, M. A. (2014). Total contents of arsenic and associated health risk in edible mushrooms, mushroom supplements and growth substrates from Galicia (NW Spain). *Food and Chemical Toxicology, 73*, 44–50.

Melgar, M. J., Alonso, J., & García, M. A. (2016). Cadmium in edible mushrooms fron NW Spain: Bioconcentration factors and consumer health implications. *Food and Chemical Toxicology, 88*, 13–20.

Milovanović, I., Brčeski, I., Stajić, M., Knežević, A., & Vukojević, F. (2013). Potential enrichment of medicinal mushrooms with selenium to obtain new dietary supplements. *International Journal of Medicinal Mushrooms, 15*, 449–455.

Milovanovic, I., Lajin, B., Braeuer, S., Steiner, O., Lisa, F., & Goessler, W. (2019). Simultaneous selenium and sulfur speciation analysis in cultivated *Pleurotus pulmonarius* mushroom. *Food Chemistry, 279*, 231–236.

Minagawa, K., Sasaki, T., Takizawa, Y., Tamura, R., & Oshina, T. (1980). Accumulation route and chemical form of mercury in mushroom species. *Bulletin of Environmental Contamination and Toxicology, 25*, 382–388.

Mitra, A. K., Purkayastha, R. P., Chatterjee, N. B., & Bhattacharyya, B. (1995). Uptake and tissue distribution of cadmium in albino-rat after oral-exposure to cadmium-contaminated edible mushrooms and its effect on blood. *Current Science*, *68*, 1050–1053.

Mleczek, M., Magdziak, Z., Gąsecka, M., Niedzielski, P., Kalač, P., Siwulski, M., ... Sobieralski, K. (2016). Content of selected elements and low-molecular-weight organic acids in fruiting bodies of edible mushroom *Boletus badius* (Fr.) Fr. from unpolluted and polluted areas. *Environmental Science and Pollution Research*, *23*, 20609–20618.

Mleczek, M., Niedzielski, P., Kalač, P., Budka, A., Siwulski, M., Gąsecka, M., ... Sobieralski, K. (2016). Multielemental analysis of 20 mushroom species growing near a heavily trafficked road in Poland. *Environmental Science and Pollution Research*, *23*, 16280–16295.

Mleczek, M., Niedzielski, P., Kalač, P., Siwulski, M., Rzymski, P., & Gąsecka, M. (2016). Levels of platinum group elements and rare-earth elements in wild mushroom species growing in Poland. *Food Additives and Contaminants A*, *33*, 86–94.

Mleczek, M., Niedzielski, P., Rzymski, P., Siwulski, M., Gąsecka, M., & Kozak, L. (2016). Variations pf arsenic species content of edible *Boletus badius* growing at polluted sites. *Journal of Environmental Science and Health B*, *51*, 469–476.

Mleczek, M., Niedzielski, P., Siwulski, M., Rzymski, P., Gąsecka, M., Goliński, P., ... Kozubik, T. (2016). Importance of low substrate arsenic content in mushroom cultivation and safety of final food product. *European Food Research and Technology*, *242*, 355–362.

Mleczek, M., Rzymski, P., Budka, A., Siwulski, M., Jasińska, A., Kalač, P., ... Niedzielski, P. (2018). Elemental characteristics of mushroom species cultivated in China and Poland. *Journal of Food Composition and Analysis*, *66*, 168–178.

Mleczek, M., Siwulski, M., Kaczmarek, Z., Rissmann, I., Sobieralski, K., & Goliński, P. (2013). Concentration of selected trace elements in *Xerocomus badius* mushroom bodies – A health risk for humans?. *Acta Scientiarum Polonorum, Technologia Alimentaria*, *12*, 331–343.

Mleczek, M., Siwulski, M., Mikołajczak, P., Gąsecka, M., Rissmann, I., Goliński, P., & Sobieralski, K. (2015). Differences in Cu content in selected mushroom species growing in the same unpolluted areas in Poland. *Journal of Environmental Science and Health B*, *50*, 659–666.

Mleczek, M., Siwulski, M., Mikołajczak, P., Gąsecka, M., Sobieralski, K., Szymańczyk, M., & Goliński, P. (2015). Content of selected elements in *Boletus badius* fruiting bodies growing in extremely polluted wastes. *Journal of Environmental Science and Health A*, *50*, 767–775.

Mleczek, M., Siwulski, M., Mikołajczak, P., Goliński, P., Gąsecka, M., Sobieralski, K., ... Szymańczyk, M. (2015). Bioaccumulation of elements in three selected mushroom species from southwest Poland. *Journal of Environmental Science and Health B*, *50*, 207–216.

Mleczek, M., Siwulski, M., Rzymski, P., Budka, A., Kalač, P., Jasińska, A., ... Niedzielski, P. (2018). Comparison of elemental composition of mushroom *Hypsizygus marmoreus* originating from commercial production and experimental cultivation. *Scientia Horticulturae*, *236*, 30–35.

Mleczek, M., Siwulski, M., Rzymski, P., Budzyńska, S., Gąsecka, M., Kalač, P., & Niedzielski, P. (2017). Cultivation of mushrooms for production of food biofortified with lithium. *European Food Research and Technology*, *243*, 1097–1104.

Mleczek, M., Siwulski, M., Rzymski, P., Niedzielski, P., Gąsecka, M., Jasińska, A., ... Budka, A. (2017). Multi-elemental analysis of *Lentinula edodes* mushrooms available in trade. *Journal of Environmental Science and Health B*, *52*, 196–205.

Mleczek, M., Siwulski, M., Stuper-Szablewska, K., Rissmann, I., Sobieralski, K., & Goliński, P. (2013). Accumulation of elements by edible mushroom species: I. Problem of trace element toxicity in mushrooms. *Journal of Environmental Science and Health B*, *48*, 69–81.

Mleczek, M., Siwulski, M., Stuper-Szablewska, K., Sobieralski, K., Magdziak, Z., & Goliński, P. (2013). Accumulation of elements by edible mushroom species. II. A comparison of aluminium, barium and nutritional element contents. *Journal of Environmental Science and Health B*, *48*, 308–317.

Muszyńska, B., Piotrowska, J., Krakowska, A., Gruba, A., Kała, K., Sułkowska-Ziaja, K., ... Opoka, W. (2017). Study of physilogically active components in different parts of fruiting bodies of varieties of *Agaricus bisporus* (white mushroom). *European Food Research and Technology*, *243*, 2135–2145.

Muszyńska, B., Rojowski, J., Łazarz, M., Kała, K., Dobosz, K., & Opoka, W. (2018). The accumulation and release of Cd and Pb from edible mushrooms and their biomass. *Polish Journal of Environmental Studies*, *27*, 223–230.

Muszyńska, B., Zając, M., Kała, K., Rojowski, J., & Opoka, W. (2016). Thermal processing can affect zinc bioavailability in some edible mushrooms. *LWT – Food Science and Technology*, *69*, 424–429.

Mutanen, M. (1986). Bioavailability of selenium in mushrooms, *Boletus edulis*, to young women. *International Journal for Vitamin and Nutrition Research*, *56*, 297–301.

Nasr, M., & Arp, P. A. (2011). Hg concentrations and accumulations in fungal fruiting bodies, as influenced by forest soil substrates and moss carpets. *Applied Geochemistry*, *26*, 1905–1917.

Nasr, M., Malloch, D. ,W., & Arp, P. A. (2012). Quantifying Hg within ectomycorrhizal fruiting bodies, from emergence to senescence. *Fungal Biology*, *116*, 1163–1177.

Nearing, M. M., Koch, I., & Reimer, K. J. (2014). Arsenic speciation in edible mushrooms. *Environmental Science and Technology*, *48*, 14203–14210.

Nearing, M. M., Koch, I., & Reimer, K. J. (2015). Uptake and transformation of arsenic during the vegetative life stage of terrestrial fungi. *Environmental Pollution*, *197*, 108–115.

Nearing, M. M., Koch, I., & Reimer, K. J. (2016). Uptake and transformation of arsenic during the reproductive life stage of *Agaricus bisporus* and *Agaricus campestris*. *Journal of Environmental Sciences*, *49*, 140–149.

Niedzielski, P., Mleczek, M., Budka, A., Rzymski, P., Siwulski, M., Jasińska, A., ... Budzyńska, S. (2017). A screening study of elemental composition in 12 marketable mushroom species accessible in Poland. *European Food Research and Technology*, *243*, 1759–1771.

Niedzielski, P., Mleczek, M., Magdziak, Z., Siwulski, M., & Kozak, L. (2013). Selected arsenic species: As(III), As(V) and dimethylarsinic acid (DMAA) in *Xerocomus badius* fruiting bodies. *Food Chemistry*, *141*, 3571–3577.

Niedzielski, P., Mleczek, M., Siwulski, M., Gąsecka, M., Kozak, L., Rissmann, I., & Mikołajczak, P. (2014). Efficacy of supplementation of selected medicinal mushrooms with inorganic selenium salts. *Journal of Environmental Science and Health B*, *49*, 929–937.

Niedzielski, P., Mleczek, M., Siwulski, M., Rzymski, P., Gąsecka, M., & Kozak, L. (2015). Supplementation of cultivated mushroom species with selenium: Bioaccumulation and speciation study. *European Food Research and Technology*, *241*, 419–426.

Nunes, R. G. F. L., Luz, J. M., Freitas, R. B., Higuchi, A., Kasuya, M. C. M., & Vanetti, M. C. D. (2012). Selenium bioaccumulation in shiitake mushrooms: A nutritional alternative source of this element. *Journal of Food Science*, *77*, C983–C986.

Osobová, M., Urban, V., Jedelský, P. L., Borovička, J., Gryndler, M., Ruml, T., & Kotrba, P. (2011). Three metallothionein isoforms and sequestration of intracellular silver in the hyperaccumulator *Amanita strobiliformis*. *New Phytologist*, *190*, 916–926.

Ostos, C., Pérez-Rodríguez, F., Arroyo, B. M., & Moreno-Rojas, R. (2015). Study of mercury content in wild edible mushrooms and its contribution to the Provisional Tolerable Weekly Intake in Spain. *Journal of Food Composition and Analysis*, *37*, 136–142.

Parisis, N. E., & van den Heede, M. A. (1992). Antimony uptake and correlation with other metals in mushroom species. *Toxicological and Environmental Chemistry*, *36*, 205–216.

Petkovšek, A. A. S., & Pokorny, B. (2013). Lead and cadmium in mushrooms from the vicinity of two large emission sources in Slovenia. *Science of the Total Environment*, *443*, 944–954.

Podlasińska, J., Proskura, N., & Szymańska, A. (2015). Content of Pb, Hg, Zn, Mn, Cu and Fe in macrofungi collected from Wkrzanska Forest in northwestern Poland. *Polish Journal of Environmental Studies*, *24*, 651–656.

Poniedziałek, B., Mleczek, M., Niedzielski, P., Siwulski, M., Gąsecka, M., Kozak, L., ... Rzymski, P. (2017). Bio-enriched *Pleurotus* mushrooms for deficiency control and improved antioxidative protection of human platelets?. *European Food Research and Technology*, *243*, 2187–2198.

Popowich, A., Zhang, Q., & Le, X. C. (2016). Arsenobetaine: The ongoing mystery. *National Science Review*, *3*, 451–458.

Proskura, N., Podlasińska, J., & Skopicz-Radkiewicz, L. (2017). Chemical composition and bioaccumulation ability of *Boletus badius* (Fr.) Fr. collected in western Poland. *Chemosphere*, *168*, 106–111.

Radulescu, C., Stihi, C., Busuioc, G., Gheboianu, A. I., & Popescu, I. V. (2010). Studies concerning heavy metals bioaccumulation of wild edible mushrooms from industrial area by using spectrometric techniques. *Bulletin of Environmental Contamination and Toxicology*, *84*, 641–646.

Rashid, M. H., Rahman, M. M., Correll, R., & Naidu, R. (2018). Arsenic and other elemental concentrations in mushrooms from Bangladesh: Health risks. *International Journal of Environmental Research and Public Health*, *15*, Art. No 919.

Rathore, H., Sharma, A., Prasad, S., & Sharma, S. (2018). Selenium bioaccumulation and associated nutraceutical properties in *Calocybe indica* mushroom cultivated on Se-enriched wheat straw. *Journal of Bioscience and Bioengineering*, *126*, 482–487.

Rieder, S. R., Brunner, I., Horvat, M., Jacobs, A., & Frey, B. (2011). Accumulation of mercury and methylmercury by mushrooms and earthworms from forest soils. *Environmental Pollution*, *159*, 2861–2869.

Rossbach, M., Kümmerle, E., Schmidt, S., Gohmert, M., Stieghorst, C., Revay, Z., & Wiehl, N. (2017). Elemental analysis of *Morchella esculenta* from Germany. *Journal of Radioanalytical and Nuclear Chemistry*, *313*, 273–278.

Rudawska, M., & Leski, T. (2005). Trace elements in fruiting bodies of ectomycorrhizal fungi growing in Scots pine (*Pinus sylvestris* L.) stands in Poland. *Science of the Total Environment*, *339*, 103–115.

Ruiz-de-Cenzano, M., López-Salazar, M., Cervera, M. L., & de la Guardia, M. (2016). Non-chromatographic speciation of mercury in mushrooms. *Analytical Methods*, *8*, 1774–1779.

Rzymski, P., Mleczek, M., Niedzielski, P., Siwulski, M., & Gąsecka, M. (2017). Cultivation of *Agaricus bisporus* enriched with selenium, zinc and copper. *Journal of the Science of Food and Agriculture*, *97*, 923–928.

Rzymski, P., Mleczek, M., Siwulski, M., Gąsecka, M., & Niedzielski, P. (2016). The risk of high mercury accumulation in edible mushrooms cultivated on contaminated substrates. *Journal of Food Composition and Analysis*, *51*, 55–60.

Rzymski, P., Mleczek, M., Siwulski, M., Jasińska, A., Budka, A., Niedzielski, P., ... Budzyńska, S. (2017). Multielemental analysis of fruit bodies of three cultivated commercial *Agaricus* species. *Journal of Food Composition and Analysis*, *59*, 170–178.

Rzymski, P., Niedzielski, P., Siwulski, M., Mleczek, M., Budzyńska, S., Gąsecka, M., & Poniedziałek, B. (2017). Lithium biofortification of medicinal mushrooms *Agrocybe cylindracea* and *Hericium erinaceus*. *Journal of Food Science and Technology*, *54*, 2387–2393.

Saba, M., Falandysz, J., & Nnorom, I. C. (2016a). Accumulation and distribution of mercury in fruiting bodies by fungus *Suillus luteus* foraged in Poland, Belarus and Sweden. *Environmental Science and Pollution Research, 23*, 2749–2757.

Saba, M., Falandysz, J., & Nnorom, I. C. (2016b). Mercury bioaccumulation by *Suillus bovinus* mushroom and probable dietary intake with the mushroom meal. *Environmental Science and Pollution Research, 23*, 14549–14559.

Saba, M., Falandysz, J., & Nnorom, I. C. (2016c). Evaluation of vulnerability of *Suillus variegatus* and *Suillus granulatus* mushrooms to sequester mercury in fruiting bodies. *Journal of Environmental Science and Health B, 51*, 540–545.

Salvador, C., Martins, M. R., Vicente, H., & Caldeira, A. T. (2018). A data mining approach to improve inorganic characterization of *Amanita ponderosa* mushrooms. *International Journal of Analytical Chemistry*. Available from https://doi.org/10.1155/2018/5265291, Art. 18 pp.

Sarikurkcu, C., Copur, M., Yildiz, D., & Akata, I. (2011). Metal concentration of wild edible mushrooms in Soguksu National Park, Turkey. *Food Chemistry, 128*, 731–734.

Sarikurkcu, C., Tepe, B., Kocak, M. S., & Uren, M. C. (2015). Metal concentration and antioxidant activity of edible mushrooms from Turkey. *Food Chemistry, 175*, 549–555.

Sarikurkcu, C., Tepe, B., Semiz, D. K., & Solak, M. H. (2010). Evaluation of metal concentration and antioxidant activity of three edible mushrooms from Mugla, Turkey. *Food and Chemical Toxicology, 48*, 1230–1233.

Sarikurkcu, C., Tepe, B., Solak, M. H., & Cetinkaya, S. (2012). Metal concentrations of wild edible mushrooms from Turkey. *Ecology of Food and Nutrition, 51*, 346–363.

Savic, M., Andjekovic, I., Duvnjak, D., Matisajevic, D., Avramovic, A., & Niksic, M. (2012). The fungistatic activity of organic selenium and its application to the production of cultivated mushrooms *Agaricus bisporus* and *Pleurotus* spp. *Archives of Biological Sciences, Belgrade, 64*, 1455–1463.

Schlecht, M. T., & Säumel, I. (2015). Wild growing mushrooms for the Edible City? Cadmium and lead content in edible mushrooms harvested within the urban agglomeration of Berlin, Germany. *Environmental Pollution, 204*, 298–305.

Seeger, R. (1978). [Cadmium in mushrooms]. *Zeitschrift für Lebensmittel Untersuchung und -Forschung, 166*, 23–34. (in German).

Seeger, R., & Gross, M. (1981). [Thallium in mushrooms]. *Zeitschrift für Lebensmittel Untersuchung und -Forschung, 173*, 9–15. (in German).

Seeger, R., Orth, H., & Schweinshaut, P. (1982). [On the strontium content of fungi]. *Zeitschrift für Lebensmittel Untersuchung und –Forschung, 174*, 381–389.

Seeger, R., Schiefelbein, F., Seuffert, R., & Zant, W. (1986). Absorption of cadmium ingested with mushrooms. *Naunyn-Schmiedeberg's Archives of Pharmacology, 332*(Suppl. 110).

Seeger, R., Schleicher, G., & Schweinshaut, P. (1984). [Investigation into the occurrence of beryllium in mushrooms]. *Deutsche Lebensmittel Rundschau, 80*(6), 178–186. (in German).

Seeger, R., & Schweinshaut, P. (1981). [Occurrence of cesium in higher fungi]. *The Science of the Total Environment, 19*, 253–276. (in German).

Şen, I., Alli, H., & Çöl, B. (2012). Boron content of some wild-growing mushrooms collected from the vicinity of boron mines in Balikesir, Turkey. *Biological Trace Element Research, 145*, 233–239.

Severoglu, Z., Sumer, S., Yalcin, B., Leblebici, Z., & Aksoy, A. (2013). Trace metal levels in edible wild fungi. *International Journal of Environmental Science and Technology, 10*, 295–304.

Seyfferth, A. L., McClatchy, C., & Paukett, M. (2016). Arsenic, lead and cadmium in U.S. mushrooms and substrate in relation to dietary exposure. *Environmental Science and Technology, 50*, 9661–9670.

Shimaoka, I., Kodama, J., Nishino, K., & Itokawa, Y. (1993). Purification of a copper binding peptide from the mushroom *Grifola frondosa* and its effect on copper absorption. *Journal of Nutritional Biochemistry, 4*, 33–38.

Silva, M. C. S., Naozuka, J., Luz, J. M., Assunção, L. S., Oliveira, P. V., Vanetti, M. C. D., ... Kasuya, M. C. M. (2012). Enrichment of *Pleurotus ostreatus* mushrooms with selenium on coffee husks. *Food Chemistry, 131*, 558–563.

Silva, M. C. S., Naozuka, J., Oliveira, P. V., Vanetti, M. C. D., Bazzolli, D. M. S., Costa, N. M. B., & Kasuya, M. C. M. (2010). *In vivo* bioavailability of selenium in enriched *Pleurotus ostreatus* mushrooms. *Metallomics, 2*, 162–166.

Širić, I., Humar, M., Kasap, A., Kos, I., Mioč, B., & Pohleven, F. (2016). Heavy metal accumulation by wild edible saprophytic and ectomycorrhizal mushrooms. *Environmental Science and Pollution Research, 23*, 18239–18252.

Širić, I., Kasap, A., Bedeković, D., & Falandysz, J. (2017). Lead, cadmium and mercury contents and bioaccumulation potential of wild edible saprophytic and ectomycorrhizal mushrooms. *Croatia. Journal of Environmental Science and Health B, 52*, 156–165.

Širić, I., Kasap, A., Kos, I., Markota, T., Tomić, D., & Poljak, M. (2016). Heavy metal contents and bioaccumulation potential of some wild edible mushrooms. *Šumarski List, 140*, 29–37.

Širić, I., Kos, I., Bedeković, D., Kaić, A., & Kasap, A. (2014). Heavy metals in edible mushroom *Boletus reticulatus* Schaeff. collected from Zrin mountain, Croatia. *Periodicum Biologorum, 116*, 319–322.

Sithole, S. C., Mugivhisa, L. L., Amoo, S. O., & Olowoyo, J. O. (2017). Pattern and concentration of trace metals in mushrooms harvested from trace metal-polluted soils in Pretoria, South Africa. *South African Journal of Botany, 108*, 315–320.

Siwulski, M., Mleczek, M., Rzymski, P., Budka, A., Jasińska, A., Niedzielski, P., ... Mikolajczak, P. (2017). Screening the multi-element content of *Pleurotus* mushroom species using inductively coupled plasma optical emission spectrometer (ICP-OES). *Food Analytical Methods, 10*, 487–496.

Slekovec, M., & Irgolic, K. J. (1996). Uptake of arsenic by mushrooms from soil. *Chemical Speciation and Bioavailability, 8*(3/4), 67–73.

Šlejkovec, Z., Byrne, A. R., Stijve, T., Goessler, W., & Irgolic, K. J. (1997). Arsenic compounds in higher fungi. *Applied Organometallic Chemistry, 11*, 673–682.

Solovyev, N., Prakash, N. T., Bhatia, P., Prakash, R., Drobyshev, E., & Michalke, B. (2018). Selenium-rich mushrooms cultivation on a wheat straw substrate from seleniferous area in Punjab, India. *Journal of Trace Elements in Medicine and Biology, 50*, 362–366.

Sousa Ferreira, H., Costa Ferreira, S. L., Cervera, M. L., & de la Guardia, M. (2009). Development of a non-chromatographic method for the speciation analysis of inorganic antimony in mushroom samples by hydride generation atomic fluorescence spectrometry. *Spectrochimica Acta B, 64*, 597–600.

Stefanović, V., Trifković, J., Djurdjić, S., Vukojević, V., Tešić, Ž., & Mutić, J. (2016). Study of silver, selenium and arsenic concentration in wild edible mushroom *Macrolepiota procera*, health benefit and risk. *Environmental Science and Pollution Research, 23*, 22084–22098.

Stijve, T. (1977). Selenium content of mushrooms. *Zeitschrift für Lebensmittel Untersuchung und Forschung, 164*, 201–203.

Stijve, T., Andrey, D., Lucchini, G. F., & Goessler, W. (2002). Lanthanides and other less common metals in mushrooms. *Deutsche Lebensmittel-Rundschau, 98*(3), 82–87.

Stijve, T., & Besson, R. (1976). Mercury, cadmium, lead and selenium content of mushroom species belonging to the genus *Agaricus*. *Chemosphere, 5*, 151–158.

Stijve, T., & Bourqui, B. (1991). Arsenic in edible mushrooms. *Deutsche Lebensmittel-Rundschau, 87*(10), 307–310.

Stijve, T., Diserens, H., Oberson, J. M., & de Meijer, A. A. R. (1998). The natural bromide content of edible mushrooms. *Deutsche Lebensmittel-Rundschau, 94*(4), 112–117.

Stijve, T., Goessler, W., & Dupuy, G. (2004). Influence of soil particles on concentrations of aluminium, iron, calcium and other metals in mushrooms. *Deutsche Lebensmittel-Rundschau, 100*(1), 10–13.

Stijve, T., Noorloos, T., Byrne, A. R., Šlejkovec, Z., & Goessler, W. (1998). High selenium levels in edible *Albatrellus* mushrooms. *Deutsche Lebensmittel-Rundschau, 94*(8), 275–279.

Sun, L., Chang, W., Bao, C., & Zhuang, Y. (2017). Metal contents, bioaccumulation, and health risk assessment in wild edible *Boletaceae* mushrooms. *Journal of Food Science, 82*, 1500–1508.

Svoboda, L., Kalač, P., Špička, J., & Janoušková, D. (2002). Leaching of cadmium, lead and mercury from fresh and differently preserved edible mushroom, *Xerocomus badius*, during soaking and boiling. *Food Chemistry, 79*, 41–45.

Svoboda, L., Havlíčková, B., & Kalač, P. (2006). Contents of cadmium, mercury and lead in edible mushrooms growing in a historical silver-mining area. *Food Chemistry, 96*, 580–585.

Svoboda, L., Zimmermannová, K., & Kalač, P. (2000). Concentrations of mercury, cadmium, lead and copper in fruiting bodies of edible mushrooms in an emission area of a copper smelter and a mercury smelter. *The Science of the Total Environment, 246*, 61–67.

Szubstarska, J., Jarzyńska, G., & Falandysz, J. (2012). Trace elements in Variegated Bolete (*Suillus variegatus*) fungi. *Chemical Papers, 66*, 1026–1031.

Tel-Çayan, G., Öztürk, M., Duru, M. E., Yabanli, M., & Türkoğlu, A. (2017). Content of minerals and trace elements determined by ICP-MS in eleven mushroom species from Anatolia, Turkey. *Chiang Mai Journal of Science, 44*, 939–945.

Thomet, U., Vogel, E., & Krähenbühl, U. (1999). The uptake of cadmium and zinc by mycelia and their accumulation in mycelia and fruiting bodies of edible mushrooms. *European Food Research and Technology, 209*, 317–324.

Tsivileva, O., & Perfileva, A. (2017). Selenium compounds biotransformed by mushrooms: Not only dietary sources, but also toxicity mediators. *Current Nutrition and Food Science, 13*, 1–15.

Turfan, N., Pekşen, A., Kibar, B., & Ünal, S. (2018). Determination of nutritional and bioactive properties in some selected wild growing and cultivated mushrooms from Turkey. *Acta Scientiarum Polonorum Hortorum Cultus, 17*(3), 57–72.

Vahdani, M., Rastegar, S., Rahimzadeh, M., Ahmadi, M., & Karmostaji, A. (2017). Physicochemical characteristics, phenolic profile, mineral and carbohydrate contents of two truffle species. *Journal of Agricultural Science and Technology, 19*, 1091–1101.

Vetter, J. (1995). [Boron content of edible mushrooms of Hungary]. *Zeitschrift für Lebensmittel-Untersuchung und –Forschung, 201*, 524–527.

Vetter, J. (2004). Arsenic content of some edible mushroom species. *European Food Research and Technology, 219*, 71–74.

Vetter, J. (2005). Lithium content of some common edible wild-growing mushrooms. *Food Chemistry, 90*, 31–37.

Vetter, J. (2010). Inorganic iodine content of common, edible mushrooms. *Acta Alimentaria, 39*, 424–430.

Vieira, P. A. F., Gontijo, D. C., Vieira, B. C., Fontes, E. A. F., de Assunção, L. S., Leite, J. P. V., ... Kasuya, M. C. M. (2013). Antioxidant activities, total phenolics and metal contents in *Pleurotus ostreatus* mushrooms enriched with iron, zinc or lithium. *LWT – Food Science and Technology, 54*, 421–425.

Vinichuk, M. M. (2013). Copper, zinc, and cadmium in various fractions of soil and fungi in a Swedish forest. *Journal of Environmental Science and Health A, 48*, 980–987.

Wang, J., Wang, B., Zhang, D., & Wu, Y. (2016). Selenium uptake, tolerance and reduction in *Flammulina velutipes* supplied with selenite. *Peer Journal, 4*, e1993, 17 pp.

Wang, X., Liu, H., Li, T., & Wang, Y. (2017). Evaluation of heavy metal concentrations of edible wild-grown mushrooms from China. *Journal of Environmental Science and Health B*, *52*, 178–183.

Wang, X., Zhang, J., Li, T., Li, J., Wang, Y., & Liu, H. (2015a). ICP-AES determination of mineral content in *Boletus tomentipes* collected from different sites of China. *Spectroscopy and Spectral Analysis*, *35*, 1398–1403.

Wang, X., Zhang, J., Li, T., Li, J., Wang, Y., & Liu, H. (2015b). Variations in element levels accumulated in different parts of *Boletus edulis* collected from Central Yunnan Province, China. *Journal of Chemistry*, Article ID 372152, 7 pp.

Wang, X., Zhang, J., Li, T., Wang, Y., & Liu, H. (2015). Content and bioaccumulation of nine mineral elements in ten mushroom species of the genus *Boletus*. *Journal of Analytical Methods in Chemistry*, Article ID 165412, 7 pp.

Wang, X., Zhang, J., Wu, L., Zhao, Y., Li, T., Li, J., ... Liu, H. (2014). A mini-reiew of chemical composition and nutritional value of edible wild-grown mushroom from China. *Food Chemistry*, *151*, 279–285.

Wiejak, A., Wang, Y., Zhang, J., & Falandysz, J. (2014). Bioconcentration potential and contamination with mercury of pantropical mushroom *Macrocybe gigantea*. *Journal of Environmental Science and Health B*, *49*, 811–814.

Wu, L., Taylor, M. P., Handley, H. K., & Gulson, B. L. (2016). Insight into past atmospheric lead emissions using lead concentrations and isotopic compositions in historic lichens and fungi (1852-2008) from central and southern Victory, Australia. *Atmospheric Environment*, *139*, 46–55.

Wu, L., Taylor, M. P., Handley, H. K., & Wu, M. (2016). Australian atmospheric lead deposition reconstructed using lead concentrations and isotopic compositions of archival lichen and fungi. *Environmental Pollution*, *208*, 678–687.

Wuilloud, R. G., Kannamkumarath, S. S., & Caruso, J. A. (2004). Speciation of essential and toxic elements in edible mushrooms: Size-exclusion chromatography separation with on-line UV-inductively coupled plasma mass spectrometry detection. *Applied Organometallic Chemistry*, *18*, 156–165.

Yamaç, M., Yildiz, D., Sarikürkcü, C., Çelikkollu, M., & Solak, M. H. (2007). Heavy metals in some edible mushrooms from the Central Anatolia, Turkey. *Food Chemistry*, *103*, 263–267.

Yokota, M. E., Frison, P. S., Marcante, R. C., Jorge, L. F., Valle, J. S., Dragunski, D. C., ... Linde, G. A. (2016). Iron translocation in *Pleurotus ostreatus* basidiocarps: Production, bioavailability and antioxidant activity. *Genetics and Molecular Research*, *15*, gmr. 15017888, 10pp.

Yoshida, S., & Muramatsu, Y. (1997). Determination of major and trace elements in mushroom, plant and soil samples collected from Japanese forests. *International Journal of Environmental Analytical Chemistry*, *67*, 49–58.

Zajac, M., Muszynska, B., Kala, K., Sikora, A., & Opoka, W. (2015). Popular species of edible mushrooms as a good source of zinc to be released to artificial digestive juices. *Journal of Physiology and Pharmacology*, *66*, 763–769.

Zavastin, D. E., Biliută, G., Dodi, G., Macsim, A.-M., Lisa, G., Gherman, S. P., ... Coseri, S. (2018). Metal content and crude polysaccharide characterization of selected mushrooms growing in Romania. *Journal of Food Composition and Analysis*, *67*, 149–158.

Zeng, X., Suwandi, J., Fuller, J., Doronila, A., & Ng, K. (2012). Antioxidant capacity and mineral contents of edible wild Australian mushrooms. *Food Science and Technology International*, *18*, 367–379.

Zhang, D., Frankowska, A., Jarzyńska, G., Kojta, A. K., Drewnowska, M., Wydmańska, D., ... Falandysz, J. (2010). Metals of King Bolete (*Boletus edulis*) Bull.:Fr. collected at the same site over two years. *African Journal of Agricultural Research*, *5*, 3050–3055.

Zhang, J., Li, T., Yang, Y. L., Liu, H. G., & Wang, Y. Z. (2015). Arsenic concentrations and associated health risks in *Laccaria* mushrooms from Yunnan (SW China). *Biological Trace Element Research, 164*, 261–266.

Zhang, J., Liu, H. G., Li, S. J., Wang, Y. Z., & Li, T. (2015). Arsenic in edible and medicinal mushrooms from Southwest China. *International Journal of Medicinal Mushrooms, 17*, 601–605.

Zhou, F., Yang, W., Wang, M., Miao, Y., Cui, Z., Li, Z., & Liang, D. (2018). Effects of selenium application on Se content and speciation in *Lentinula edodes*. *Food Chemistry, 265*, 182–188.

Zhu, F., Qu, L., Fan, W., Qiao, M., Hao, H., & Wang, X. (2011). Assessment of heavy metals in some wild edible mushrooms collected from Yunnan Province, China. *Environmental Monitoring and Assessment, 179*, 191–199.

Zocher, A. L., Kraemer, D., Merschel, G., & Bau, M. (2018). Distribution of major and trace elements in the bolete mushroom *Suillus luteus* and the bioavailability of rare earth elements. *Chemical Geology, 483*, 491–500.

Zou, Y., Du, F., Zhang, H., & Hu, Q. (2018). Selenium speciation and biological characteristics of selenium-rich Bailing mushroom, *Pleurotus tuoliensis*. *Emirates Journal of Food and Agriculture, 30*, 704–708.

Zsigmond, A. R., Varga, K., Kántor, I., Urák, I., May, Z., & Héberger, K. (2018). Elemental composition of wild growing *Agaricus campestris* mushroom in urban and peri-urban regions of Transylvania (Romania). *Journal of Food Composition and Analysis, 72*, 15–21.

Further reading

Cejpková, J., Gryndler, M., Hršelová, H., Kotrba, P., Řanda, Z., Synková, I., & Borovička, J. (2016). Bioaccumulation of heavy metals, metalloids, and chlorine in ectomycorrhizae from smelter-polluted area. *Environmental Pollution, 218*, 176–185.

Svoboda, L., & Chrastný, V. (2008). Levels of eight trace elements in edible mushrooms from a rural area. *Food Additives and Contaminants, 25*, 51–58.

Chungu, D., Mwanza, A., Ńgandwe, P., Chungu, B. C., & Maseka, K. (2019). *Variation of heavy metal contamination between mushroom species in the Copperbelt province, Zambia: are people at risk? Journal of the Science of Food and Agriculture* (99, pp. 3410–3416).

Oliveira, A. P., & Naozuka, J. (2019). Preliminary results on the feasibility of producing selenium-enriched pink (*Pleurotus djamor*) and white (*Pleurotus ostreatus*) oyster mushrooms: Bioaccumulation, bioaccessibility, and Se-proteins distribution. *Microchemical Journal, 145*, 1143–1150.

Rasalanavho, M., Moodley, R., & Jonnalagadda, S. B. (2019). Elemental distribution including toxic elements in edible and inedible wild growing mushrooms from South Africa. *Environmental Science and Pollution Research, 26*, 7913–7925.

Šíma, J., Vondruška, J., Svoboda, L., Šeda, M., & Rokos, L. (2019). The accumulation of risk and essential elements in edible mushrooms *Chlorophyllum rhacodes, Suillus grevillei, Imleria badia*, and *Xerocomellus chrysenteron* growing in the Czech Republic. *Chemistry and Biodiversity, 16*, e1800478.

Siwulski, M., Rzymski, P., Budka, A., Kalač, P., Budzyńska, S., Dawidowicz, L., ... Niedzielski, P. (2019). The effect of different substrates on the growth of six cultivated mushroom species and composition of macro and trace elements in their fruiting bodies. *European Food Research and Technology, 245*, 419–431.

Zou, H., Zhou, C., Li, Y., Yang, X., Wen, J., Hu, X., & Sun, C. (2019). Occurrence, toxicity, and speciation analysis of arsenic in edible mushrooms. *Food Chemistry, 281*, 269–284.

Chapter 5

Radioactivity*

Contamination of the environment with anthropogenic radionuclides has originated from the global fallout following atmospheric nuclear weapons testing during the 1950s–1960s, operation of nuclear energy industries, accidents involving nuclear materials, and from other uses of radioisotopes in medical or industrial applications. Fungi, both filamentous and mushrooms, have been found to be very efficient in absorption of radionuclides. They are an important component of long-term accumulation of radionuclides due to their long-living and huge mycelial network and biomass in the upper horizon of forest soils.

Limited information on wild mushroom radioactivity was available prior to Chernobyl Nuclear Power Plant (CNPP) disaster in 1986. Knowledge greatly expanded after this event, resulting in several hundreds of papers. The topic was reviewed in several articles citing numerous references. The reviews focused either on the environmental aspects and transfer chiefly of radiocesium to fungi (both microfungi and mushrooms) (Dighton, Tugay, & Zhdanova, 2008; Duff & Ramsey, 2008; Gillett & Crout, 2000), or on viewpoints of the intake of radionuclides after consuming contaminated mushrooms (Falandysz & Borovička, 2013; Guillén & Baeza, 2014; Kalač, 2001, 2012).

Similarly as in Chapter 3, Major essential elements, and Chapter 4, Trace elements, particularly the latest information since 2010 will be given with references, while only the weightiest older papers will be cited in this chapter. The used literature data are largely mean values expressed per kg of mushroom dry matter (DM). For a simplified recalculation to fresh matter (FM), DM content of $100\,g\,kg^{-1}$ FM (i.e., 10%) is used if actual DM is unknown. Only data for at least five fruiting bodies per species are inserted into the tables. Superscripts C and S are used in the tables for the radioactivity of caps and stipes, respectively. The superscripts are given in order of increasing activity concentrations (e.g., $X^{C,S}$ if the level is higher in stipes than in caps).

* *The chapter was written in collaboration with Dr. Javier Guillén Gerada from the University of Extremadura, Cáceres, Spain.*

Mineral Composition and Radioactivity of Edible Mushrooms.
DOI: https://doi.org/10.1016/B978-0-12-817565-1.00005-4

5.1 Radioactivity units and legislation

Decay of some elements results in the emission of dangerous subatomic particles, alpha (α, helium nuclei formed by two protons), beta minus (β^-, electrons), beta plus (β^+, positrons), and gamma (photons). The half-life ($T_{1/2}$) of a radionuclide is the time required to elapse in order to decay by half. It varies extremely widely from minutes to millions of years, but it is a constant for a given radionuclide. Characteristics of the main radionuclides reported in mushrooms are given in Table 5.1.

One becquerel (Bq) is the unit of a radioactive source activity in which, on average, one atom decays per second. Activity concentration, that is, activity per DM unit (Bq kg^{-1} DM) will be used in this chapter.

Maximum permitted levels in terms of ^{134}Cs and ^{137}Cs in foods are 600 and 370 Bq kg^{-1} FM for adults and infants, respectively, in the European Union (EU; Regulation EEC No 737/90). Thus the derived limit for adults would be 6000 Bq kg^{-1} DM for mushrooms. However, the considerable increase of foodstuff radioactivity following the Chernobyl disaster elicited within the EU series of legislative provisions and recommendations. Under the regulation from 1987, the maximum permitted level of ^{137}Cs in mushrooms was 1250 Bq kg^{-1} FM, that is, 12,500 Bq kg^{-1} DM. A similar limit of 1000 Bq kg^{-1} FM (i.e., 10,000 Bq kg^{-1} DM) was recommended by the International Atomic Energy Agency (IAEA) in 1994. Codex Alimentarius (FAO/WHO, 1991) explicitly defined the intervention level for foodstuffs

TABLE 5.1 Characteristics of main radionuclides reported in mushrooms.

Element	Isotope	Detection method	Half-life ($T_{1/2}$)	Dose coefficient (Conversion factor) for adults (Sv Bq^{-1})
Lead	^{210}Pb	γ, LSC, GFPC	22.2 years	6.9×10^{-7}
Polonium	^{210}Po	α	138.4 days	1.2×10^{-6}
Potassium	^{40}K	γ	1.25×10^{9} years	6.2×10^{-9}
Radium	^{226}Ra	α, γ, LSC, GFPC	1600 years	2.8×10^{-7}
	^{228}Ra	γ	5.75 years	6.9×10^{-7}
Cesium	^{134}Cs	γ	2.06 years	1.9×10^{-8}
	^{137}Cs	γ	30.17 years	1.3×10^{-8}
Strontium	^{90}Sr	LSC, GFPC	28.79 years	2.8×10^{-8}

Detection methods: α, α-spectrometry; γ, γ-spectrometry; *GFPC*, gas-flow proportional counter; *LSC*, liquid scintillation counting.

being 1000 Bq kg^{-1} FM for ^{137}Cs. This level can be used only under situations related to nuclear accidents or radiological events. Thus the reference limits of the European Union, IAEA, Codex Alimentarius, and Japan (see Section 5.3.5) differ.

Effective dose (E) given in millisieverts (mSv) per year is a unit expressing a possible risk of radioactivity for human health. Under the recommendation of the IAEA (1996), the acceptable yearly burden for an adult of the public is 1 mSv above natural background excluding medical treatments.

Various emitters have different risk levels for human health. This is expressed by dose coefficient (or conversion factor) defined as the dose received by a person of a given age group per unit intake of radioactivity (Sv Bq^{-1}) for a given exposure time (50 years for adults and 70 years for infants). The values of dose coefficients are given in Table 5.1. For instance, 1 Bq emitted by lead radionuclide ^{210}Pb is potent by two orders of magnitude more than 1 Bq originating from potassium isotope ^{40}K.

A contribution to the yearly effective ingestion dose (D) for an adult from mushroom consumption can be calculated as:

$$D\left(\text{Sv year}^{-1}\right) = \sum Y \times A_i \times e_i(g),$$

where Y = annual intake of mushrooms (kg DM per person),

A_i = activity concentration for radionuclide i (Bq kg^{-1} DM),
$e_i(g)$ = dose coefficient for radionuclide i and group population g (Sv Bq^{-1}).

5.2 Methods of radioactivity measurement

The appropriate method for the determination of radioactivity concentration in environmental samples depends on the decay scheme of a radionuclide and its decay chain (Guillén, Baeza, Salas, Corbacho, & Rodríguez, 2017). The gamma-spectrometry method is mainly used for the determination of γ-emitting radionuclides, such as ^{137}Cs, ^{134}Cs, and ^{40}K, among others. Sample preparation is relatively simple for mushrooms as it merely consists in grinding to make the sample homogeneous. Fresh and dried mushroom samples can be used. When considering low activity levels, samples can also be ashed in order to reduce the volume and to lower the detection limit. In this case, ashing temperature is important, because there can be loss of radiocesium at temperatures higher than 400°C. Detectors are usually HPGe (hyperpure germanium) or NaI(Tl), and they must be calibrated with the same geometries and matrix as the samples. The main advantage of γ-spectrometry is that it is a multielemental method, although some precautions have to be taken. Radium determination via secular equilibrium with its daughters, ^{214}Pb and ^{214}Bi, requires a really good sealed sample in order to avoid radon losses until equilibrium is reached (usually after 21 days).

Radioiodine determinations require that samples were not heated at 100°C to avoid losses during the drying process. For low-energy γ-emitting radionuclides, such as ^{210}Pb or ^{241}Am, corrections due to sample autosorption may be necessary to be considered, depending on sample composition.

The determination of α- and/or β-emitting radionuclides (U, Th, ^{226}Ra, ^{210}Po, ^{90}Sr, etc.) require sample digestion and radiochemical separation procedures. For most radionuclides, calcination (usually at 600°C) is a good option to remove organic matter. However, it cannot be applied for ^{210}Po determination due to its volatility. Then the sample is acid digested. Radiochemical procedures are mainly based on the use of ion exchange resins, either general or specific, in order to isolate the corresponding radionuclide. Due to the great interaction of alpha particles with the matter, sources for α-spectrometry (U, Th, ^{226}Ra, ^{210}Po, etc.) must be as thin as possible. Therefore electrodeposition and microprecipitation are mostly used. Polonium radionuclide ^{210}Po is spontaneously deposited on silver and nickel (autodeposition). Regarding β-emitting radionuclides, such as ^{90}Sr, determinations are usually carried out by liquid scintillation counting (LSC) or by gas-flow proportional counters. In LSC, the sample after separation is mixed with the scintillation cocktail, which is usually specific for radionuclide and detection equipment, and a β-spectrum is obtained. On the contrary, gas-flow proportional counter have no spectrometric abilities and only reports α- and β-events. It can be used for measuring radionuclides after the appropriate chemical separation. Depending on the radionuclide to be determined, it may be necessary for it to reach equilibrium with its daughters.

5.3 Radionuclide concentration in mushrooms

Information on high radioactivity of some wild-growing mushroom species in years following the Chernobyl disaster aroused qualm within the European public. Such fear was ascribed to anthropogenic (artificial) radionuclides. Nevertheless, some mushroom species have relatively high activity concentrations of natural radioactive isotopes.

5.3.1 Naturally occurring radionuclides

Mushrooms contain considerably higher levels of potassium than most foods of plant origin. Potassium is highly bioaccumulated in fruiting bodies from the underlying substrate (for more information see Section 3.5). Natural potassium is a mixture of several isotopes with prevailing ^{39}K. However, there also occurs radionuclide ^{40}K at the constant level of 0.012% of all isotopes. Its half-life is extremely long, over one billion years. It is primarily a beta-emitter with stable ^{40}Ca as the final product.

Data on activity concentrations of ^{40}K in numerous mushroom species published during the past decade are given in Table 5.2. The values are very

TABLE 5.2 Data on mean activity concentrations of natural isotope ^{40}K (Bq kg^{-1} dry matter) in wild-growing and cultivated mushrooms published since 2010.

Species	Activity concentration	Country	References
Wild growing			
Agaricus campestris	130, 500	Turkey	Yilmaz et al. (2016)
Boletus appendiculatus	1200^{C}, 1600^{C}; 830^{S}, 870^{S}	China	Falandysz, Zhang, and Zalewska (2017)
	720^{m}	China	Tuo et al. (2017)
Boletus auripes	1100^{C}, 1400^{C}; 620^{S}, 840^{S}	China	Falandysz et al. (2017)
Boletus bicolor	$630–1300^{C}$; $470–1400^{S}$	China	Falandysz et al. (2017)
Boletus bruneissimus	620^{m}	China	Tuo et al. (2017)
Boletus edulis	830^{C}	Poland	Falandysz, Zalewska et al. (2015)
	$740–1500^{C}$; $360–1200^{S}$	China	Falandysz et al. (2017)
	760^{m}	China	Tuo et al. (2017)
Boletus impolitus	1100^{C}, 1400^{C}; 880^{S}, 930^{S}	China	Falandysz et al. (2017)
Boletus luridus	$1,000–1500^{C}$; $240–1300^{S}$	China	Falandysz et al. (2017)
Boletus luridiformis	1300, 1600	Czech Republic	Čadová, Havránková, Havránek, and Zölzer (2017)
Boletus magnificus	$830–1500^{C}$; $400–1100^{S}$	China	Falandysz et al. (2017)
Boletus pinophilus	760^{C}	Poland	Falandysz, Zalewska et al. (2015)
Boletus purpureus	$1,200–1900^{C}$; $840–1700^{S}$	China	Falandysz et al. (2017)
Boletus sinicus	1400^{C}, 1500^{C}; 1100^{S}, 1200^{S}	China	Falandysz et al. (2017)
Boletus speciosus	$1000–1500^{C}$; $730–1000^{S}$	China	Falandysz et al. (2017)
Boletus tomentipes	$1100–1800^{C}$; $940–1800^{S}$	China	Falandysz et al. (2017)

(*Continued*)

TABLE 5.2 Data on mean activity concentrations of natural isotope ^{40}K (Bq kg^{-1} dry matter) in wild-growing and cultivated mushrooms published since 2010. (Continued)

Species	Activity concentration	Country	References
Boletus umbriniporus	$910–1500^{C}$; $660–1300^{S}$	China	Falandysz et al. (2017)
Cantharellus cibarius	1550	Poland	Falandysz, Zalewska, Apanel, Drewnowska, and Kluza (2016)
	1500, 2100	Czech Republic	Čadová et al. (2017)
Laccaria amethystina	2900	Czech Republic	Čadová et al. (2017)
Leccinum chromapes	$950–1300^{C}$; $690–1300^{S}$	China	Falandysz et al. (2018)
Leccinum griseum	$1300–1800^{C}$; $1200–1700^{S}$	China	Falandysz et al. (2017)
	1200^{C}, 1300^{C}; 700^{S}, 810^{S}	China	Falandysz et al. (2018)
Leccinum rugosiceps	$770–1200^{C}$; $460–900^{S}$	China	Falandysz et al. (2018)
Leccinum scabrum	730	Norway	Gwynn, Nalbandyan, and Rudolfsen (2013)
	1200	Czech Republic	Čadová et al. (2017)
	2000^{C}, 900^{S}	China	Falandysz et al. (2018)
Leccinum variicolor	1700^{C}, 1700^{S}	China	Falandysz et al. (2018)
Leccinum versipelle	790	Norway	Gwynn et al. (2013)
	1100^{C}, 710^{S}	China	Falandysz et al. (2018)
Lentinula edodes	630^{m}	China	Tuo et al. (2017)
Macrocybe gigantea	1260^{C}, 990^{S}	China	Falandysz, Zhang et al. (2015)
Morchella esculenta	1070	Germany	Rossbach et al. (2017)
Russula decolorans	990	Norway	Gwynn et al. (2013)

(Continued)

TABLE 5.2 Data on mean activity concentrations of natural isotope ^{40}K (Bq kg^{-1} dry matter) in wild-growing and cultivated mushrooms published since 2010. (Continued)

Species	Activity concentration	Country	References
Russula grisea	3600^C, 2700^S	China	Falandysz et al. (2018)
Russula integra	1200	Czech Repubic	Čadová et al. (2017)
Russula paludosa	960	Norway	Gwynn et al. (2013)
Tricholoma matsutake	$960–1900^C$; $1200–1500^S$	China	Falandysz et al. (2018)
Xerocomu badius	1200^C	Poland	Falandysz, Zalewska et al. (2015)
Xerocomus spadiceous	$420–1200^C$; $520–1000^S$	China	Falandysz et al. (2017)
70 Species (including inedible)	mostly 1000–2500	Poland	Mietelski et al. (2010)
49 Species	1030 (12–2400)	Japan	Fujii et al. (2014)
50 Samples (species unspecified)	570	Turkey	Türkekul et al. (2018)
Cultivated			
Agaricus bisporus	750	Brazil	De Castro, Maihara, Silva, and Figueira (2012)
Lentinula edodes	750	Brazil	De Castro et al. (2012)

C, caps; *m*, median value; *S*, stipes.

similar to those published previously as collated in the reviews of Kalač (2001) and Guillén and Baeza (2014). The most common activity concentrations are 800–1500 Bq kg^{-1} DM. The range of variation is relatively narrow, only three orders of magnitude. The frequency distribution is of the Gaussian type (Baeza et al., 2004). An extremely high-activity concentration of ^{40}K, nearly 12,000 Bq kg^{-1} DM, was observed in *Laccaria laccata* growing in a site in southern Poland (Mietelski, Dubchak, Błażej, Anielska, & Turnau, 2010).

Unlike ^{137}Cs from radioactive fallout, natural ^{40}K is usually distributed evenly in the vertical profile of forest soils. Knowledge on the transfer factor for ^{40}K from underlying soil to fruiting bodies has been very limited, the available information gives values exceeding 10. It seems that the incorporation of the stable potassium and, hence, also ^{40}K is self-regulated by physiological requirements of a mushroom. No correlation between ^{40}K and ^{137}Cs was observed despite cesium being a chemical analog of potassium (Baeza et al., 2004).

In mushrooms collected in the vicinity of uranium mines there were determined higher levels of isotopes ^{226}Ra, ^{210}Pb, and ^{210}Po from the uranium ^{238}U decay chain, than in those growing in unaffected sites. Another radium isotope, ^{228}Ra, belongs to the natural series, parent of which is thorium ^{232}Th. Limited data on both the radium isotopes are given in Table 5.3. The ^{226}Ra concentrations in mushrooms were reported in the range of 0.02–87 Bq kg^{-1} DM (Guillén & Baeza, 2014). Radioisotopes of uranium and thorium in mushrooms are of limited significance (Baeza & Guillén, 2006; Tuo et al., 2017). Recent results for ^{238}U from Turkey report mean values in *Agaricus campestris* 12.1 Bq kg^{-1} DM (Yilmaz, Yildiz, Çelik, & Çevik, 2016) and 84 Bq kg^{-1} DM in 50 unspecified mushroom samples (Türkekul, Yeşilkanat, Ciriş, Kölemen, & Çevik, 2018). The respective values for ^{232}Th are 11.7 and 45 Bq kg^{-1} DM.

TABLE 5.3 Data on mean activity concentrations of natural isotopes ^{226}Ra and ^{228}Ra (Bq kg^{-1} dry matter) in wild-growing and cultivated mushrooms published since 2010.

Species	^{226}Ra	^{228}Ra	Country	Reference
Wild growing				
Boletus appendiculatus	0.24^{m}	0.81^{m}	China	Tuo et al. (2017)
Boletus brunneissimus	0.75^{m}	2.56^{m}	China	Tuo et al. (2017)
Boletus edulis	0.35^{m}	1.72^{m}	China	Tuo et al. (2017)
Lentinula edodes	0.29^{m}	0.38^{m}	China	Tuo et al. (2017)
30 species ^{FM}	mostly <0.3		Greece	Kioupi, Florou, Kapsanaki-Gotsi, and Gonou-Zagou (2016)
Cultivated				
Agaricus bisporus	<7.3	<3.1–27.0	Brazil	De Castro et al. (2012)
L. edodes	<7.3–23	<3.1–35.6	Brazil	De Castro et al. (2012)

FM, fresh matter; *m*, median value.

The ^{226}Ra decays via radon to ^{210}Pb. Radon is a gas emanating from soils into the atmosphere, thus ^{210}Pb may be deposited onto fruiting bodies. Nevertheless, the main uptake of ^{210}Pb into fruiting bodies is directly from soil. A correlation has been observed between ^{210}Pb and stable lead in fruiting bodies. Saprobic species had a somewhat higher level of ^{210}Pb than mycorrhizal ones (Guillén, Baeza, Ontalba, & Míguez, 2009). Some recent data on activity concentrations of ^{210}Pb are given in Table 5.4. Higher ranges of 0.75–202 Bq kg^{-1} DM were reported in Spanish mushrooms (Guillén et al., 2009) and mushrooms from Finnish boreal forests, namely, 1.4–16.2 Bq kg^{-1} DM (Vaaramaa, Solatie, & Aro, 2009).

^{210}Po (half-life 138.4 days) is produced by the decay of ^{210}Pb via ^{210}Bi with a short half-life of 5.0 days. Therefore data on ^{210}Po in mushrooms should be accompanied by the corresponding ^{210}Pb content such as in results

TABLE 5.4 Data on mean activity concentrations of natural isotopes ^{210}Po and ^{210}Pb (Bq kg^{-1} dry matter) in fruiting bodies of wild-growing mushrooms published since 2010.

Species	^{210}Po	^{210}Pb	Year(s) of collection	Country	References
Leccinum aurantiacum	0.8–4.9	0.4–1.5	2006–10	Poland	Strumińska-Parulska et al. (2016)
	1.0–1.8	0.5–1.3	2006–10	Poland	Szymańska et al. (2018)
Leccinum duriusculum	1.3–2.1	1.2–2.3	2006–10	Poland	Szymańska et al. (2018)
Leccinum scabrum	94	2.5	2010	Norway	Gwynn et al. (2013)
Leccinum versipelle	198	3.1	2010	Norway	Gwynn et al. (2013)
Leccinum vulpinum	0.6–2.3	1.3–2.6	2006–10	Poland	Szymańska et al. (2018)
Macrolepiota procera	9.0–14.1	5.4–8.4	2016	Poland	Strumińska-Parulska, Olszewski, and Falandysz (2017)
Russula decolorans	7.4	3.2	2010	Norway	Gwynn et al. (2013)
Russula paludosa	4.7	3.3	2010	Norway	Gwynn et al. (2013)

given in Table 5.4. Most mushroom species accumulate ^{210}Po preferentially over ^{210}Pb. Vaaramaa et al. (2009) reported activity concentration of ^{210}Po from 7.1 to 1174 Bq kg^{-1} DM in *Russula paludosa* and *Leccinum vulpinum*, respectively. The highest level was recorded in the *Boletaceae* family. Lower values were determined by Skwarzec and Jakusik (2003) in 20 edible and inedible species from Poland. The highest mean activity concentration of about 40 Bq kg^{-1} DM was found in *Boletus edulis* and *Leccinum scabrum*, while the lowest, 2.1–4.3 Bq kg^{-1} DM, was observed in *Xerocomus badius* and *Xerocomus subtomentosus*. This is interesting because all these species are taxonomically closely related. In both the articles, caps were richer in ^{210}Po than stipes. Strumińska-Parulska, Szymańska, Krasińska, Skwarzec, and Falandysz (2016) and Szymańska, Falandysz, Skwarzec, and Strumińska-Parulska (2018) determined very low activity concentrations of both the isotopes in three species of genus *Leccinum* (Table 5.4). Moreover, they observed very low bioconcentration factors for both the isotopes and high correlation between their concentrations in underlying soil and fruiting bodies.

The cosmogenic radioisotope beryllium ^{7}Be is deposited from the atmosphere by rainfall. It was detectable only in a few of 72 samples of various species from Spain (Baeza et al., 2004).

In conclusion, natural radioactivity of mushrooms is higher than that of foods of plant origin, ^{40}K occurs in the highest concentration. Nevertheless, ^{210}Po and ^{210}Pb should be taken under consideration in regions with low contamination with anthropogenic radionuclides.

5.3.2 Anthropogenic radionuclides other than radiocesium

Mushrooms did not accumulate ^{90}Sr, a chemical analog of calcium (see Sections 3.1 and 4.3.15), or radioisotopes of plutonium at toxicologically momentous levels. Saniewski et al. (2016) determined ^{90}Sr in several mushroom species collected during the period 1996–2013 both from regions contaminated by the fallout from the Chernobyl disaster and from distant China. Activity concentrations were low, generally below 2 Bq kg^{-1} DM. According to Lehto, Vaaramaa, and Leskinen (2013), activity concentrations of $^{239,240}Pu$ in *Russula decolorans* from Finland were negligibly low, being only 0.002 Bq kg^{-1} DM.

5.3.3 Anthropogenic radiocesium until 1985

Several radionuclides were discharged into the global environment through atmospheric nuclear weapons testing. The total release of the most important radionuclide, ^{137}Cs, for the global fallout was estimated as 9.6×10^{17} Bq (UNSCEAR, 1982).

High radioactivity levels of some wild-growing mushroom species originated from ^{137}Cs have been reported in the 1960s (Grüter, 1964). Limited data have been available for mushroom radioactivity until 1985, usual values of ^{137}Cs activity concentrations have been below 1000 Bq kg^{-1} DM. *X. badius* and *Xerocomus chrysenteron* were already then identified as accumulating species.

Most mushroom species take up nonradioactive isotopes of cesium in a low extent. The reported bioaccumulation factors fruiting body/underlying soil are not significantly different from vascular plants. Nevertheless, the observed values for radiocesium from the fallout were higher for at least one order of magnitude.

5.3.4 Mushroom radioactivity after the Chernobyl disaster

5.3.4.1 Chernobyl disaster

The main radionuclides produced during an explosive fission reaction are ^{137}Cs and ^{90}Sr with long half-lives of 30.2 and 28.8 years, respectively. The ^{134}Cs with half-life of 2.06 years, also participating in mushroom contamination, is produced in reactors during long-term fission.

The disaster of the CNPP (Ukraine, former Soviet Union) on April 26, 1986, was caused by inappropriate reactor operations by the staff. It released into the environment in total about 5.3×10^{18} Bq (excluding noble gases), including approximately 3.8×10^{16} Bq from ^{137}Cs decay (UNSCEAR, 1988). The ratio ^{137}Cs to ^{134}Cs was approximately 2:1. Moreover, ^{144}Ce, ^{131}I, ^{95}Nb, ^{239}Pu, ^{240}Pu, ^{103}Ru, ^{106}Ru, ^{230}Th, ^{232}Th, and ^{95}Zr were detected in mushrooms early after the accident (Mietelski et al., 2002; Zarubina, 2004). Their toxicological risk through mushroom consumption was, however, limited.

The contamination level of an area was affected by the direction and speed of the radioactive cloud, distance from the CNPP, and notably by wet or dry deposition during passage of the clouds. The levels of fallout were, thus, very different, even in adjacent sites. Contamination varied very widely in the orders of magnitude of 10^1-10^5 Bq m^{-2}. Radioactivity of ^{137}Cs may be of a health concern for up to the next three centuries in the most heavily polluted areas adjacent to the CNPP.

Both the radiocesium isotopes participated in mushroom radioactivity during the initial years after the accident. Since about the mid-1990s ^{137}Cs remains the crucial radionuclide.

5.3.4.2 Mushroom radioactivity between 1986 and 2000

Data on mushroom radioactivity during the years following the CNPP disaster were reviewed by Gillett and Crout (2000), Kalač (2001), Duff and Ramsey (2008), and Guillén and Baeza (2014). Numerous references are available therein. Most of the data from that period deal with European countries, primarily those affected by the radioactive fallout.

Overall, activity concentrations have varied very widely. In mycorrhizal species from several hundreds to above 100,000 Bq kg^{-1} DM, in saprobic and parasitic species between a few hundreds and a few thousands Bq kg^{-1} DM. The provisional EU statutory limit for mushrooms of 12,500 Bq kg^{-1} DM was often significantly surpassed (overall Kalač, 2001). Commonly consumed species with different rates of radiocesium accumulation are given in Table 5.5. Nearly all highly and medium accumulating species are of mycorrhizal nutritional strategy, whereas saprobic species prevail in the group with low levels of radiocesium accumulation.

Very wide differences, however, occur within a species, up to three orders of magnitude. A unique survey was carried out in Poland in 1991 with 278 samples of highly accumulating and widely consumed *X. badius*, covering systematically the whole area of the country. Maps of ^{137}Cs, ^{134}Cs, and ^{40}K activity concentrations were prepared. The most frequent levels were 2000–10,000 and 200–600 Bq kg^{-1} DM for ^{137}Cs and ^{134}Cs, respectively (Mietelski, Jasińska, Kubica, Kozak, & Macharski, 1994).

Maximum levels of mushroom radioactivity were found in 1987 and notably in 1988. This lag was caused by a subsequent supply of radionuclides to the upper soil horizon through dropped needles and leaching from needles and bark. As observed by Bem, Lasota, Kuśmierek, and Witusik (1990), activity concentration of ^{137}Cs increased about 10 times in several species collected in a Polish site about 500 km west of the CNPP in 1986

TABLE 5.5 Some edible mushroom species with different rates of radiocesium accumulation.

High	Medium	Low
Cantharellus lutescens	*Agaricus sylvaticus*	*Amanita rubescens*
Cantharellus tubaeformis	*Boletus edulis*	*Armillariella mellea*
Cortinarius caperatus	*Cantharellus cibarius*	*Calocybe gambosa*
Hydnum repandum	*Leccinum aurantiacum*	*Laccaria laccata*
Laccaria amethystina	*Leccinum scabrum*	*Lepista nuda*
Russula cyanoxantha	*Russula xerampelina*	*Lycoperdon perlatum*
Russula vesca		*Macrolepiota procera*
Suillus luteus		
Suillus variegatus		
Xerocomus badius		
Xerocomus chrysenteron		

Categorization results from numerous reports published after the Chernobyl Nuclear Power Station disaster.

compared with levels below 500 Bq kg^{-1} DM in 1984 and 1985. For instance, the concentrations were 40, 45, 650, 227, and 2110 Bq kg^{-1} DM in *L. scabrum* sampled yearly between 1984 and 1988.

Data on activity concentrations of ^{134}Cs were reported until the mid-1990s due to the relatively short half-life of the radioisotope. However, traces were still detected in some mushroom species in Poland even in 2006 and 2007 (Mietelski et al., 2010).

5.3.4.3 Mushroom radioactivity since 2001

The frequency of data on radioactivity of mushrooms collected after 2000 markedly decreased compared with the period just after the CNPP disaster. All values in this section deal with ^{137}Cs activity concentrations. The latest reported data are collated in Table 5.6. As results show from the table, and generally from trends in mushroom radioactivity since 1986, two main factors have affected levels of radioactivity, that are, mushroom species and level of contamination of a site by the fallout from the CNPP disaster. The importance of the time factor whittles away due to the decreasing ^{137}Cs activity concentrations with the prolonging period since 1986.

Mascanzoni (2009) published an interesting long-term series of activity concentrations determined from 1986 to 2007 in a site of southern Sweden with high contamination of 35,000 Bq m^{-2} from the CNPP fallout. The activity concentration in accumulating *Suillus luteus* remained stable at a level around 120,000 Bq kg^{-1} DM likewise for the aggregated transfer factor. Surprisingly, both the parameters increased about three times in an unspecified *Cantharellus* spp. during the same period. A possible elucidation is location of the mycelia in various depths and gradual migration of deposited radiocesium downward toward the soil profile.

Another study on long-term changes of activity concentrations of several mushroom species collected from an area in central France was carried out Daillant, Boilley, Josset, Hetwig, and Fischer (2013) during 1986–2011. The activity decreased considerably in litter-decomposing (i.e., saprobic) as well as in wood-inhabiting species. Different changes were observed in mycorrhizal mushrooms. The decrease followed only after the initial increase lasting 5–6 years in *Hydnum repandum* and even 9–16 years in *Rozites caperatus*.

The mean activity concentration of 10 mushroom species collected in 8 European countries from Ukraine to Belgium during 2004, was 834 Bq kg^{-1} DM; however, the range was extremely wide from 0.6 to 4300 Bq kg^{-1} DM. Also in this report, *X. badius* sampled in Poland showed the highest determined activity (Szántó, Hult, Wätjen, & Altzitzoglou, 2007).

Activity concentration of ^{137}Cs in *B. edulis* from the Balkan countries of Macedonia and Kosovo analyzed yearly between 2008 and 2017, decreased from 20 to 5 Bq kg^{-1} FM. Thus the extrapolated ecological half-life of ^{137}Cs was about 7.7 years (Chiaravalle et al., 2018).

TABLE 5.6 Data on mean activity concentrations of radioisotope ^{137}Cs (Bq kg^{-1} dry matter) in wild-growing and cultivated mushrooms published since 2010.

Species	Activity concentration	Year(s) of collection	Country	References
Wild growing				
Albatrellus confluens	40^{mFM}	2015	Japan, near Fukushima	Orita et al. (2017)
Amanita caesarea	1.8^{FM}	2008–17	Macedonia, Kosovo	Chiaravalle et al. (2018)
Armillariella mellea	7	2012	Croatia Japan, near Fukushima	Tucaković, Barišić, Grahel, Kasap, and Širić (2018)
	70^{mFM}	2013		Nakashima et al. (2015)
	70^{mFM}	2015		Orita et al. (2017)
Boletus aestivalis	1090^{C}, 500^{S}	2006	Poland	Falandysz, Zalewska et al. (2015)
	8	2010	Spain	García, Alonso, and Melgar (2015)
	13–1210 (mostly <30)	2012	Croatia	Tucaković et al. (2018)
Boletus auripes	8^{C}, 6^{S},11^{C}, 9^{S}	2011–14	China	Falandysz et al. (2017)
Boletus bicolor	$5–21^{C}$, $5–10^{S}$	2011–14	China	Falandysz et al. (2017)
Boletus edulis	330	1993	Italy	Cocchi, Kluza, Zalewska, Apanel, and Falandysz (2017)
	270^{C}, 160^{S}	1995	Poland	Cocchi et al. (2017)
	88	2010	Spain	García et al. (2015)
	220 (2–710)	2012	Croatia	Tucaković et al. (2018)

(*Continued*)

TABLE 5.6 Data on mean activity concentrations of radioisotope ^{137}Cs (Bq kg^{-1} dry matter) in wild-growing and cultivated mushrooms published since 2010. (Continued)

Species	Activity concentration	Year(s) of collection	Country	References
	<5–14^{C}, <2–13^{S}	2011–14	China	Falandysz et al. (2017)
	8^{C}, 5^{S}	2014	China	Falandysz, Zalewska et al. (2015)
	51^{C}, 61^{S}	2015	Poland	Cocchi et al. (2017)
	580$^{m\ FM}$	2015	Ukraine	Orita et al. (2018)
	8.8^{FM}	2008–17	Macedonia, Kosovo	Chiaravalle et al. (2018)
Boletus ferrugineus	<3–15^{C}, <3–20^{S}	2011–14	China	Falandysz et al. (2017)
Boletus impolitus	280^{C}, 150^{S}	2003	Poland	Falandysz, Zalewska et al. (2015)
Boletus luridiformis	0.40, 0.76	2014	Czech Republic	Čadová et al. (2017)
Boletus luridus	7–36^{C}, 9–11^{S}	2011–14	China	Falandysz et al. (2017)
Boletus magnificus	<5–9^{C}, <4–10^{S}	2011–14	China	Falandysz et al. (2017)
Boletus pinophilus	960^{C}, 470^{S}	2000	Poland	Falandysz, Zalewska et al. (2015)
	11	2010	Spain	García et al. (2015)
Boletus purpureus	6–12^{C}, 6–12^{S}	2011–14	China	Falandysz et al. (2017)
Boletus speciosus	6–21^{C}, <3–10^{S}	2011–14	China	Falandysz et al. (2017)
Boletus tomentipes	<4–14^{C}, 3–11^{S}	2011–14	China	Falandysz et al. (2017)
Boletus umbriniporus	5–14^{C}, <4–16^{S}	2011–14	China	Falandysz et al. (2017)

(*Continued*)

TABLE 5.6 Data on mean activity concentrations of radioisotope ^{137}Cs ($Bq\ kg^{-1}$ dry matter) in wild-growing and cultivated mushrooms published since 2010. (Continued)

Species	Activity concentration	Year(s) of collection	Country	References
Cantharellus cibarius	380–800	2000	Poland	Falandysz et al. (2016)
	84–1400	2007	Poland	Falandysz et al. (2016)
	73	2010	Spain	García et al. (2015)
	370, 1000	2014	Czech Republic	Čadová et al. (2017)
Cantharellus tubaeformis	45	2007	Poland	Falandysz et al. (2016)
	289	2010	Spain	García et al. (2015)
Cortinarius caperatus	13,000^{C}, 4200^{S}	1996	Poland	Zalewska, Cocchi, and Falandysz (2016)
	19,900^{C}, 7130^{S}	2006–07	Finland	Lehto et al. (2013)
	5600^{C}, 1900^{S}	2010	Poland	Zalewska et al. (2016)
Hydnum repandum	1020	2010	Spain	García et al. (2015)
Hygrophorus russula	1300^{mFM}	2015	Japan, near Fukushima	Orita et al. (2017)
Laccaria amethystina	80	2014	Czech Republic	Čadová et al. (2017)
Leccinum aurantiacum	250$^{m\ FM}$	2015	Ukraine	Orita et al. (2018)
Leccinum chromapes	5–9^{C}, 8–11^{S}	2011–12	China	Falandysz et al. (2018)
Leccinum griseum	<5–15^{C}, <4–15^{S}	2011–14	China	Falandysz et al. (2017)
Leccinum rugosiceps	<4–38^{C}, <3–19^{S}	2011–12	China	Falandysz et al. (2018)

(Continued)

TABLE 5.6 Data on mean activity concentrations of radioisotope ^{137}Cs (Bq kg^{-1} dry matter) in wild-growing and cultivated mushrooms published since 2010. (Continued)

Species	Activity concentration	Year(s) of collection	Country	References
Leccinum scabrum	220	2010	Norway	Gwynn et al. (2013)
	770	2014	Czech Republics	Čadová et al. (2017)
	$290^{m\ FM}$	2015	Ukraine	Orita et al. (2018)
Leccinum versipelle	380	2010	Norway	Gwynn et al. (2013)
Lyophyllum fumosum	100^{mFM}	2015	Japan, near Fukushima	Orita et al. (2017)
Macrocybe gigantea	6^{C}, 6^{S}	2012–13	China	Falandysz, Zhang et al. (2015)
Macrolepiota procera	8	2012	Croatia	Tucaković et al. (2018)
Morchella esculenta	13	2016	Germany	Rossbach et al. (2017)
Pholiota nameko	653^{mFM}	2013	Japan, near Fukushima	Nakashima et al. (2015)
Russula decolorans	7700^{C}, 2600^{S}	2006–07	Finland	Lehto et al. (2013)
	170	2010	Norway	Gwynn et al. (2013)
Russula integra	470	2014	Czech Republics	Čadová et al. (2017)
Russula paludosa	9500^{C}, 3800^{S}	2006–07	Finland	Lehto et al. (2013)
	180	2010	Norway	Gwynn et al. (2013)
Sarcodon aspratus	668^{mFM}	2013	Japan, near Fukushima	Nakashima et al. (2015)
	620^{mFM}	2015		Orita et al. (2017)
Suillus variegatus	$16{,}500^{C}$	2006–07	Finland	Lehto et al. (2013)

(Continued)

TABLE 5.6 Data on mean activity concentrations of radioisotope ^{137}Cs (Bq kg^{-1} dry matter) in wild-growing and cultivated mushrooms published since 2010. (Continued)

Species	Activity concentration	Year(s) of collection	Country	References
Tricholoma equestre	200^{mFM}	2015	Japan, near Fukushima	Nakashima et al. (2015)
Tricholoma matsutake	$9-19^{C}$, $5-7^{S}$	2011–12	China	Falandysz et al. (2018)
	300^{mFM}	2013	Japan, near Fukushima	Nakashima et al. (2015)
Tricholoma portentosum	016	2010	Spain	García et al. (2015)
Xerocomus badius	5110^{C}, 4610^{S}	2000	Poland	Falandysz, Zalewska et al. (2015)
	1430^{C}, $20{,}760^{C}$; 1370^{S}, $14{,}800^{S}$	2010	Belarus	Falandysz, Zalewska et al. (2015)
58 Samples (unspecified species)	300, 25^{m} (1–4,100)	2006–10	Japan	Fujii et al. (2014)
Cultivated				
Agaricus bisporus	<1	–	Brazil	De Castro et al. (2012)
Lentinula edodes	4	–	Brazil	De Castro et al. (2012)

C, caps; *FM*, fresh matter; *m*, median value; *S*, stipes.
Source: Data from Lehto, J., Vaaramaa, K., & Leskinen, A. (2013). 137Cs, 239,240Pu and 241Am in boreal forest soil and their transfer into wild mushrooms and berries. *Journal of Environmental Radioactivity*, 116, 124–132 deal with mushrooms from a site with mean deposition 20,000 Bq m^{-2} and 95% fraction of the Chernobyl fallout. Data from Orita, M., Kimura, Y., Taira, Y., Fukuda, T., Takahashi, J., Gutevych, O., ... Takamura, N. (2018). Activities concentration of radiocesium in wild mushrooms collected in Ukraine 30 years after the Chernobyl power plant accident. *Peer Journal*, 6, e4222, doi:10.7717/perj.4222 are expressed as Bq kg^{-1} fresh matter; the values expressed in dry matter would be approximately ten times higher.

A specific situation was observed in a very contaminated site in southern Poland, where contamination from the fallout was up to >60,000 Bq m^{-2} in 1993. A very wide range between 30 and 54,070 Bq kg^{-1} DM was determined in over 70 species of both edible and inedible mushroom species collected in the site during 2006 and 2007. Extraordinary high means nearly 12,000 and about 10,000 Bq kg^{-1} DM were found in *Suillaceae* families and in mycorrhizal species of *Tricholomataceae*, respectively (Mietelski et al., 2010).

Analysis of 82 fruiting bodies of highly valuable *Tuber aestivum* (Burgundy truffles) from five European countries, in particular Switzerland, both wild-growing and cultivated, collected between 2010 and 2014, revealed minute ^{137}Cs activity concentrations below 2 Bq kg^{-1} FM. Such low levels are surprising in the underground species. The reasons have not yet been explained (Büntgen et al., 2016).

5.3.5 Mushroom radioactivity after the Fukushima disaster

The Fukushima Daiichi Nuclear Power Plant (FNPP; Honshu Island, Japan) disaster was caused by the devastating tsunami following the East Japan earthquake of magnitude 9.0 on March 11, 2011. Three of six reactors exploded due to the formed hydrogen. In contrast to the CNPP disaster, only gas phase radionuclides were released. Approximately 80% of the radionuclides were transported offshore and deposited into the Pacific Ocean. The total activity of the released radionuclides has been estimated to be 5.2×10^{17} Bq (with a range of $3.4–8.0 \times 10^{17}$ Bq), that is, about 10 times lower than that from the Chernobyl disaster. The FNPP did not cause any casualties due to acute radiation. Radiological consequences in countries other than Japan appear negligible (Steinhauser, Brandl, & Johnson, 2014).

The Japanese Ministry of Health, Labor, and Welfare conducted a comprehensive food monitoring study including mushrooms. During the period March 2011–March 2016 almost 20,000 edible mushroom samples were tested for radioactivity. Only 2.6% were found to exceed Japanese regulatory limit for adults, namely 500 Bq kg^{-1} FM, during the first year after the FNPP accident and 100 Bq kg^{-1} FM afterward. However, the proportion of exceeding samples was higher, over 7%, during the first year. Mycorrhizal species took up considerably more radionuclides than saprobic species. *Lentinula edodes* (shiitake), a widely consumed species in Japan, belongs to the latter group. Due to low consumption, mushrooms participate only in a limited extent at ingestion dose (Prand-Stritzko & Steinhauser, 2018).

L. edodes is cultivated in bed-logs and mushroom beds under outdoor or indoor conditions. Its radioactivity has been higher than that of other agricultural products and some batches produced open-air on raw logs were restrained from sale. Tagami, Uchida, and Ishii (2017) found similar geometric means of ^{137}Cs activity concentration from an area within the Fukushima prefecture and seven prefectures outside Fukushima in mushrooms cultivated both outdoors and indoors. Ohnuki et al. (2016) reported, for the first time, the direct accumulation pathway from radioactive-Cs-contaminated wood logs to fruiting bodies of *L. edodes* through the basal part of the stipe. Radioactive cesium was not transported through the hyphae.

Data on ^{137}Cs activity concentrations of several mushroom species collected in a village 30 km from the FNPP in 2013 and 2015 are given in Table 5.6 (Nakashima et al, 2015; Orita et al., 2017).

5.4 Paramaters affecting radiocesium transfer from soils to mushrooms

Edible mushrooms have been collected mostly in forests, which form semi-natural ecosystems. As reviewed by Calmon, Thiry, Zibold, Rantavaara, and Fesenko (2009), forest soils differ from agricultural cultivated land. Temperate forest soils are multilayered with forest floor, hemiorganic, and mineral layers. Fungal and microbial activities likely contribute, in a great extent, to long-term radionuclides retention in organic layers. High variability is, thus, usually observed in radionuclide transfers and redistribution patterns in contaminated forests. Soil compartments constitute the major pool of radionuclides, which can cause long-term contamination of the food chain. Mineral components of forest soils, especially clays, have a higher affinity for cesium than organic matter. Cesium is, thus, more available for mushroom mycelium located in organic layers. Generally, mycelium of saprobic species is located mainly in surface organic layers, while that of mycorrhizal species lies in deeper layers. Overall, long-lasting availability of some radionuclides was shown to be the source of their much higher transfer in forest ecosystems than in agricultural lands.

There exists a consensus from numerous researchers that mushrooms of different nutritional strategy accumulate ^{137}Cs in the order of mycorrhizal > saprobic > or ≈ parasitic (overall in Gillett & Crout, 2000). Transfer factors of ^{137}Cs for mushrooms from coniferous forests usually have exceeded those factors for mushrooms in deciduous woods (Vinichuk & Johanson, 2003).

Zarubina (2016) reported considerable changes in ^{137}Cs activity concentrations of *Cantharellus cibarius* during the fructification period. There were observed two peaks in the seasonal dynamics of ^{137}Cs activity concentrations - in mid-summer, but not every year and in mid-October. The growth of mycelium induce an elevated uptake of minerals including ^{137}Cs into hyphae followed by heightened level of the radionuclide activity in fruiting bodies.

Cultivated mushrooms, commonly grown on wood, sawdust, straw, or various agricultural by-products have lower levels of anthropogenic radionuclides as compared to wild species, mainly due to the lower contents of the radionuclides in the substrates than in forest soils.

5.5 Distribution of radiocesium in fruiting bodies

Several articles (e.g., Baeza, Guillén, Salas, & Manjón, 2006; Bakken & Olsen, 1990) from various European countries have reported uneven distribution of radiocesium within fruiting bodies. Flesh and skin had very similar activity concentrations, whereas spore-bearing parts (gills or tubes) had 50%–250% higher levels. Maximum values of ^{134}Cs were found in mature fruiting bodies.

Repeatedly observed high accumulation of radiocesium in *X. badius*, particularly in caps including tubes, has been ascribed to pigments badione and norbadione causing chocolate brown or golden yellow coloration of this and related species (Aumann, Clooth, Steffan, & Steglich, 1989). The pigments have, in their structure, numerous acid–base functional groups, which are able to bind monovalent cations including Cs^{+}. In contrast, Neukom and Gisler (1991) did not find any significant enrichment of radiocesium activity concentrations in the surface layer of caps (epicutis) of *X. badius*. About 12% of the total radiocesium observed in the epicutis were in proportion to its weight.

5.6 Decrease of mushroom radioactivity by culinary treatments

Fresh mushrooms are either cooked in various ways or preserved for later consumption. They are not generally eaten raw. Changes in the level of radioactivity caused by various preservation or cooking methods were reviewed in articles by Beresford et al. (2001), Guillén and Baeza (2014), and Beňová, Dvořák, Tomko, and Falis (2016).

The extraction of radiocesium from intact fruiting bodies into soaking water or table salt solutions is low due to the lipophilic, gel-like surface of mushrooms. On the contrary, shrinkage between 36%–87% of the initial levels has been reported from boiled slices of several species of mushrooms (Klán, Řanda, Benada, & Horyna, 1988; Neukom & Gisler, 1991; Skibniewska & Smoczyński, 1999). Another way is by cooking mushrooms in a table salt solution. Steger, Burger, Ziegler, and Wallnöfer (1987) boiled *Stropharia rugosoannulata* in a 2% solution of NaCl for 15 min. The total activity of ^{134}Cs and ^{137}Cs decreased to 37%–64% of the initial level. Neukom and Gisler (1991) reported a higher decrease in total activity of ^{134}Cs and ^{137}Cs in *X. badius* boiled in water than in a 0.5% table salt solution. The experiments showed considerably higher efficiency of radiocesium extraction from mushrooms with cell tissues destroyed by deep freezing or drying compared to fresh mushrooms. Obviously, the used bathes have to be discarded.

Tagami and Uchida (2013) found that parameters describing the retention of ^{137}Cs and ^{40}K during cooking of various vegetables, including mushrooms, highly correlate. Therefore ^{40}K can be an analog to estimate the removal rates of radiocesium. The mean removal of ^{40}K was 32% for the five mushrooms species mostly consumed in Japan.

Steinhauser and Steinhauser (2016) reported a decrease of ^{137}Cs by up to about 30% of the initial level in pieces of *C. cibarius*, and only 9% of *B. edulis*, following pan-frying in vegetable oil for 4 min. Radiocesium removal into released juices was more effective in the mushrooms washed before frying.

Air-drying at ambient temperature is an ancient preservation method; however, drying under elevated temperatures using various dryers is also applied in households. Drying increases the contents of radionuclides due to water loss of up to 10 times. Mushrooms dried, usually as slices, are commonly soaked before cooking.

Deep freezing of fresh-sliced, cubed, or complete fruiting bodies to about −20°C is an easy preservation method, nevertheless consistency is damaged. A decrease of radioactivity can be supposed due to the release of the cell sap during thawing. This sap has to be discarded.

Salting is a preservation method traditionally used in households. Mushrooms are usually sliced and then repeatedly blanched, that is, shortly boiled in a water bath, left to drain, and then canned in brine. Pickling is another common preservation method. Mushrooms, usually cut to cubes, are blanched and then canned in vinegar. In model experiments with three wild species immersed in a solution of 2% acetic acid at 10°C for up to 168 h, Dvořák, Kunová, and Beňová (2006) observed an exponential drop of ^{137}Cs activity. The reduction was, in average, 59% for fresh mushrooms and 73% for air-dried counterparts. The used pickle has to be discarded.

5.7 Radioactivity burden due to mushroom consumption

As results from the previous sections, calculations of believable radioactivity dose from ingested mushrooms have been complicated. Imperfect input data burden the credibility of the calculations. The activity concentrations of individual radionuclides both among and within mushroom species vary widely. Tabular data can be therefore misleading. Moreover, information on wild mushroom intake, both on weight and species composition, is usually fragmentary. The reported calculations were carried out on fresh or dried mushrooms and did not take into consideration the possible decrease of radionuclides during culinary treatments. Thus the literature data should be perceived as qualified estimations. The dose calculations for radiological protection of the population are very conservative. The worst case scenario is considered, so no correction for culinary treatments is used.

A review of Guillén and Baeza (2014), evaluating numerous reports, assessed body burden with radioactivity originating from consumed mushrooms. The calculated yearly internal dose from mushrooms ranged from 10^{-7} to 480 μSv. As mentioned before, the permissible yearly dose limit is 1000 μSv for adults.

5.8 Radiocesium in meat of game feeding mushrooms

The reports on considerable increase of radioactivity in tissues of both wild and domestic animals foraging mushrooms appeared particularly from Scandinavia in the years following the CNPP disaster. These regions were affected by the extensive fallout and had a high density of wild-growing mushrooms. The contamination was observed both in grazing goats and sheep, and in wild animals, roe deer (*Capreolus capreolus*), red deer (*Cervus elaphus*), reindeer (*Rangifer tarandus*), and wild boar (*Sus scrofa*). Generally, the meat of roe deers and wild boars were more contaminated than that of red deer. The limit of 600 Bq kg^{-1} was often, and highly, surpassed. The effective ^{137}Cs half-life of 2.9 and 3.2 years was determined for red deer and roe deer, respectively, while 38 years, however with high uncertainty, was determined for wild boars showing repeated intake of the radionuclide in their digestive tracts (Škrkal, Rulík, Fantínová, Mihalík, & Timková, 2015).

The time course of game meat radioactivity has been different in ruminating deers and in monogastric wild boars. Roe deer usually live in a relatively small territory, feeding mostly on less-contaminated herbal plants, apart from during the mushroom season. Activity concentrations are, thus, rather low (except for the mushroom season in fall) and continually decrease with time following the Chernobyl fallout. Wild boars are capable to move over long distances. They belong to omnivores and consume a variety of food, including an underground inedible mushroom *Elaphomyces granulatus*, with the common name "deer truffle." The species highly accumulates ^{137}Cs, often at levels of thousands Bq per kg FM. In a very comprehensive set of 2433 wild boars shot in southwest Germany during 2001–03, 21%–26% and 1%–9.3% of the tested meats exceeded the limit of 600 Bq kg^{-1} during summer and winter, respectively (Hihmann & Huckschlag, 2005). As reported by Strebl and Tataruch (2007), the mean ^{137}Cs activity in wild-boar meat fluctuated around 2000 Bq kg^{-1} in the Austrian region during the yearly monitoring between 1990 and 2003. The fat tissues of wild boars are not a reservoir for radiocesium (Steinhauser, Knecht, & Sipos, 2017).

The impact of the CNPP disaster on the ^{137}Cs activities found in the meat of wild boars in Europe has been much higher than the impact of the FNPP fallout on wild boars in Japan (Steinhauser & Saey, 2016).

Overall, a steady decrease of meat contamination with ^{137}Cs via mushrooms is expected in roe deer and red deer. However, in wild-boar meat there is anticipated great variability and in some regions the preservation of recent levels exceeding the permissible limit is predicted for a long time, probably a few decades.

5.9 Conclusions

Several general conclusions can be drawn:

- Contamination of cultivated mushrooms with anthropogenic radionuclides is significantly lower than that of wild-growing species. Mushrooms cultivated outdoors, for example, *Pleurotus ostreatus* on logs, can be an exception if they remained outdoors when radioactive fallout occurred.

- A serious situation can occur in regions heavily contaminated with radioactive fallout if combined with high local consumption of wild-growing species, particularly of radiocesium accumulating species of the family *Boletaceae*, in the period following the fallout. Such situation concerned some regions of Ukraine, Russia, Belarus, and Poland after the CNPP disaster.
- The body burden decreases as time lag from the one-shot contamination prolongs. For instance, total dose estimates were 80 and 2 μSv in 1986 and 2015, respectively, in the Czech population (Škrkal, Fojtík, Malátová, & Bartusková, 2017).
- However, some mushroom species from heavily contaminated areas will be an important source of ingested radionuclides for many decades.
- In countries which were not affected by the disasters of the two nuclear power plants, mushrooms (both wild-growing and cultivated) participate in the intake of natural radionuclides, particularly ^{40}K.

References

Aumann, D. C., Clooth, G., Steffan, B., & Steglich, W. (1989). Complexation of ^{137}Cs by cap pigments of *Xerocomus badius*. *Angewandte Chemie*, *101*, 495–496. (in German).

Baeza, A., & Guillén, J. (2006). Influence of the soil bioavailability of radionuclides on the transfer of uranium and thorium to mushrooms. *Applied Radiation and Isotopes*, *64*, 1020–1026.

Baeza, A., Guillén, J., Salas, A., & Manjón, J. L. (2006). Distribution of radionuclides in different parts of a mushroom: Influence of the degree of maturity. *Science of the Total Environment*, *359*, 255–266.

Baeza, A., Hernández, S., Guillén, F. J., Moreno, G., Manjón, J. L., & Pascual, R. (2004). Radiocaesium and natural gamma emitters in mushrooms collected in Spain. *Science of the Total Environment*, *318*, 59–71.

Bakken, L. R., & Olsen, R. A. (1990). Accumulation of radicaesium in fungi. *Canadian Journal of Microbiology*, *36*, 704–710.

Bem, H., Lasota, W., Kuśmierek, E., & Witusik, M. (1990). Accumulation of ^{137}Cs by mushrooms from Rogozno area of Poland over the period 1984–1988. *Journal of Radioanalytical and Nuclear Chemistry*, *145*, 39–46.

Beňová, K., Dvořák, P., Tomko, M., & Falis, M. (2016). Artificial environmental radonuclides in Europe and methods of lowering their food stuff contamination – A review. *Acta Veterinaria Brno*, *85*, 105–112.

Beresford, N. A., Voigt, G., Wright, S. M., Howard, B. J., Barnett, C. L., Prister, B., et al. (2001). Self-help countermeasure strategies for populations living within contaminated areas of Belarus, Russia and Ukraine. *Journal of Environmental Radioactivity*, *56*, 215–239.

Büntgen, U., Jäggi, M., Stobbe, U., Tegel, W., Sproll, L., Eikenberg, J., & Egli, S. (2016). All-clear for gourmets: Truffles not radioactive. *Biogeosciences*, *13*, 1145–1147.

Čadová, M., Havránková, R., Havránek, J., & Zölzer, F. (2017). Radioactivity in mushrooms from selected locations in the Bohemian Forest, Czech Republic. *Radiation and Environmental Biophysics*, *56*, 167–175.

Calmon, P., Thiry, Y., Zibold, G., Rantavaara, A., & Fesenko, S. (2009). Transfer parameter values in temperate forest ecosystems: A review. *Journal of Environmental Radioactivity, 100*, 757–766.

Chiaravalle, A. E., Mangiacotti, M., Marchesani, G., Bortone, N., Tomaiuolo, M., & Trotta, G. (2018). A ten-year survey of radiocontamination of edible Balkan mushrooms: Cs-137 activity levels and assessed dose to the population. *Food Control, 94*, 263–267.

Cocchi, L., Kluza, K., Zalewska, T., Apanel, A., & Falandysz, J. (2017). Radioactive caesium (^{134}Cs and ^{137}Cs) in mushrooms of the genus *Boletus* from the Reggio Emilia in Italy and Pomerania in Poland. *Isotopes in Environmental and Health Studies, 53*, 620–627.

Daillant, O., Boilley, D., Josset, M., Hetwig, B., & Fischer, H. W. (2013). Evolution of radiocaesium contamination in mushrooms and influence of treatment after collection. *Journal of Radioanalytical and Nuclear Chemistry, 297*, 437–441.

De Castro, L. P., Maihara, V. A., Silva, P. S. C., & Figueira, R. C. L. (2012). Artificial and natural radioactivity in edible mushrooms from Sao Paulo, Brazil. *Journal of Environmental Radioactivity, 113*, 150–154.

Dighton, J., Tugay, T., & Zhdanova, N. (2008). Fungi and ionizing radiation from radionuclides. *FEMS Microbiology Letters, 281*, 109–120.

Duff, M. C., & Ramsey, M. L. (2008). Accumulation of radiocesium by mushrooms in the environment: A literature review. *Journal of Environmental Radioactivity, 99*, 912–932.

Dvořák, P., Kunová, V., & Beňová, K. (2006). Exponential drop of radicesium activity in mushrooms due to the effect of acetic acid. *European Food Research and Technology, 222*, 139–143.

Falandysz, J., & Borovička, J. (2013). Macro and trace mineral constituents and radionuclides in mushrooms: Health benefits and risks. *Applied Microbiology and Biotechnology, 97*, 477–501.

Falandysz, J., Saniewski, M., Zhang, J., Zalewska, T., Liu, H. G., & Kluza, K. (2018). Artificial ^{137}Cs and natural ^{40}K in mushrooms from the subalpine region of the Minya Konka summit and Yunnan Province in China. *Environmental Science and Pollution Research, 25*, 615–627.

Falandysz, J., Zalewska, T., Apanel, A., Drewnowska, M., & Kluza, K. (2016). Evaluation of the activity concentrations of ^{137}Cs and ^{40}K in some *Chantarelle* mushrooms from Poland and China. *Environmental Science and Pollution Research, 23*, 20039–20048.

Falandysz, J., Zalewska, T., Krasińska, G., Apanel, A., Wang, Y., & Pankavec, S. (2015). Evaluation of the radioactive contamination in fungi genus *Boletus* in the region of Europe and Yunnan Province in China. *Applied Microbiology and Biotechnology, 99*, 8217–8224.

Falandysz, J., Zhang, J., & Zalewska, T. (2017). Radioactive artificial ^{137}Cs and natural ^{40}K activity in 21 edible mushrooms from the genus *Boletus* species from SW China. *Environmental Science and Pollution Research, 24*, 8189–8199.

Falandysz, J., Zhang, J., Zalewska, T., Apanel, A., Wang, Y., & Wiejak, A. (2015). Distribution and possible dietary intake of radioactive ^{137}Cs, ^{40}K and ^{226}Ra with the pantropical mushroom *Macrocybe gigantea* in SW China. *Journal of Environmental Science and Health A, 50*, 941–945.

FAO/WHO (1991). Food Standards Programme. *Levels for radionuclides*. Codex Alimentarius, Vol. 1, Section 6.1.

Fujii, A., Koura, T., Yoshimoto, T., Kawabata, T., Nakamura, Y., Hamamichi, K., … Hayakawa, K. (2014). Concentrations of ^{137}Cs and ^{40}K in wild mushrooms collected in a forest on Noto Peninsula, Japan. *Journal of Radioanalytical and Nuclear Chemistry, 300*, 707–717.

García, M. A., Alonso, J., & Melgar, M. J. (2015). Radiocaesium activity concentrations in macrofungi from Galicia (NW Spain): Influence of environmental and genetic factors. *Ecotoxicology and Environmental Safety*, *115*, 152–158.

Gillett, A. G., & Crout, N. M. J. (2000). A review of ^{137}Cs transfer to fungi and consequences for modelling environmental transfer. *Journal of Environmental Radioactivity*, *48*, 95–121.

Grüter, H. (1964). Accumulation of a fission product ^{137}Cs in mushrooms. *Naturwissenschaften*, *51*(7), 161–162. (in German).

Guillén, J., & Baeza, A. (2014). Radioactivity in mushrooms: A health hazard? *Food Chemistry*, *154*, 14–25.

Guillén, J., Baeza, A., Ontalba, M. A., & Míguez, M. P. (2009). ^{210}Pb and stable lead content in fungi: Its transfer from soil. *Science of the Total Environment*, *407*, 4320–4326.

Guillén, J., Baeza, A., Salas, A., Corbacho, J. A., & Rodríguez, A. (2017). *Radiochemical procedures applied to low-level environmental samples*. Environmental science and engineering. *Vol. 7:* Instrumentation, modelling and analysis. USA: Studium Press LLC.

Gwynn, J. P., Nalbandyan, A., & Rudolfsen, G. (2013). ^{210}Po, ^{210}Pb, ^{40}K and ^{137}Cs in edible wild berries and mushrooms and ingestion doses to man from high consumption rates of these wild foods. *Journal of Environmental Radioactivity*, *116*, 34–41.

Hihmann, U., & Huckschlag, D. (2005). Investigations on the radiocaesium contamination of wild boar (*Sus scrofa*) meat in Rhineland-Palatinate: A stomach content analysis. *European Journal of Wildlife Research*, *51*, 263–270.

IAEA Safety Series No 115 (1996). International Basic Safety Standards for Protection against Ionizing Radiation and for the Safety of Radiation Sources, 370 pp.

Kalač, P. (2001). A review of edible mushroom radioactivity. *Food Chemistry*, *75*, 29–35.

Kalač, P. (2012). Radioactivity of European wild growing edible mushrooms. In S. Andres, & N. Baumann (Eds.), *Mushrooms: Types, properties and nutrition* (pp. 215–230). New York: Nova Science Publication.

Kioupi, V., Florou, H., Kapsanaki-Gotsi, E., & Gonou-Zagou, Z. (2016). Bioaccumulation of the artificial Cs-137 and the natural radionuclides Th-234, Ra-226, and K-40 in the fruit bodies of *Basidiomycetes* in Greece. *Environmental Science and Pollution Research*, *23*, 613–624.

Klán, J., Řanda, Z., Benada, J., & Horyna, J. (1988). Investigation of non-radioactive Rb, Cs, and radiocesium in higher fungi. *Česká Mykologie*, *42*, 158–169. (in Czech).

Lehto, J., Vaaramaa, K., & Leskinen, A. (2013). ^{137}Cs, $^{239,240}Pu$ and ^{241}Am in boreal forest soil and their transfer into wild mushrooms and berries. *Journal of Environmental Radioactivity*, *116*, 124–132.

Mascanzoni, D. (2009). Long-term transfer of ^{137}Cs from soil to mushrooms in a semi-natural environment. *Journal of Radioanalytical and Nuclear Chemistry*, *282*, 427–431.

Mietelski, J. W., Baeza, A. S., Guillén, J., Buzinny, M., Tsigankov, N., Gaca, P., ... Tomankiewicz, E. (2002). Plutonium and other alpha emitters in mushrooms from Poland, Spain and Ukraine. *Applied Radiation and Isotopes*, *56*, 717–729.

Mietelski, J. W., Dubchak, S., Błażej, S., Anielska, T., & Turnau, K. (2010). ^{137}Cs and ^{40}K in fruiting bodies of different fungal species collected in a single forest in southern Poland. *Journal of Environmental Radioactivity*, *101*, 706–711.

Mietelski, J. W., Jasińska, M., Kubica, B., Kozak, K., & Macharski, P. (1994). Radioactive contamination of Polish mushrooms. *Science of the Total Environment*, *157*, 217–226.

Nakashima, K., Orita, M., Fukuda, N., Taira, Y., Hayashida, N., Matsuda, N., & Takamura, N. (2015). Radiocesium concentration in wild mushrooms collected in Kawauchi Village after the accident at the Fukushima Daiichi Nuclear Power Plant. *Peer Journal*, *3*, e1427. Available from https://doi.org/10.7717/peerj.1427.

Neukom, H. P., & Gisler, E. (1991). Extraction of radioactive caesium from mushrooms with *Xerocomus badius* as an example. *Lebensmittel Wissenschaft und Technologie, 24*, 442–444.

Ohnuki, T., Aiba, Y., Sakamoto, F., Kozai, N., Niizato, T., & Sasaki, Y. (2016). Direct accumulation pathway of radioactive cesium to fruit-bodies of edible mushroom from contaminated wood logs. *Scientific Reports, 6*, 29866. Available from https://doi.org/10.1038/srep29866.

Orita, M., Nakashima, K., Taira, Y., Fukuda, T., Fukushima, Y., Kudo, T., ... Takamura, N. (2017). Radiocesium concentrations in wild mushrooms after the accident at the Fukushima Daiichi Nuclear Power Station: Follow-up study in Kawauchi village. *Scientific Reports, 7*, 6744. Available from https://doi.org/10.1038/s41598-017-05963-0.

Orita, M., Kimura, Y., Taira, Y., Fukuda, T., Takahashi, J., Gutevych, O., ... Takamura, N. (2018). Activities concentration of radiocesium in wild mushrooms collected in Ukraine 30 years after the Chernobyl power plant accident. *Peer Journal, 6*, e4222. Available from https://doi.org/10.7717/perj.4222.

Prand-Stritzko, B., & Steinhauser, G. (2018). Characteristics of radiocesium contaminations in mushroom after the Fukushima nuclear accident: Evaluation of the food monitoring data from March 2011 to March 2016. *Environmental Science and Pollution Research, 25*, 2409–2416.

Rossbach, M., Kümmerle, E., Schmidt, S., Gohmert, M., Stieghorst, C., Revay, Z., & Wiehl, N. (2017). Elemental analysis of *Morchella esculenta* from Germany. *Journal of Radioanalytical and Nuclear Chemistry, 313*, 273–278.

Saniewski, M., Zalewska, T., Krasińska, G., Szylke, N., Wang, Y., & Falandysz, J. (2016). ^{90}Sr in King Bolete *Boletus edulis* and certain other mushrooms consumed in Europe and China. *Science of the Total Environment, 543*, 287–294.

Skibniewska, K. A., & Smoczyński, S. S. (1999). Influence of cooking on radiocaesium contamination of edible mushrooms. *Roczniki Państwowego Zakladu Higieny, 50*(2), 157–162.

Škrkal, J., Rulík, P., Fantínová, K., Mihalík, J., & Timková, J. (2015). Radiocaesium levels in game in the Czech Republic. *Journal of Environmental Radioactivity, 139*, 18–23.

Škrkal, J., Fojtík, P., Malátová, I., & Bartusková, M. (2017). Ingestion intakes of ^{137}Cs by the Czech population: Comparison of different approaches. *Journal of Environmental Radioactivity, 171*, 110–116.

Skwarzec, B., & Jakusik, A. (2003). ^{210}Po accumulation by mushrooms from Poland. *Journal of Environmental Monitoring, 5*, 791–794.

Steger, U., Burger, A., Ziegler, W., & Wallnöfer, P. R. (1987). Distribution of Cs-134 and Cs-137 in culinary processed foodstuffs. *Deutsche Lebensmittel Rundschau, 83*, 85–88. (in German).

Steinhauser, G., Brandl, A., & Johnson, T. E. (2014). Comparison of the Chernobyl and Fukushima nuclear accidents: A review of the environmental impacts. *Science of the Total Environment, 470–471*, 800–817.

Steinhauser, G., Knecht, C., & Sipos, W. (2017). Fat tissue is not a reservoir for radiocesium in wild boars. *Journal of Radioanalytical and Nuclear Chemistry, 312*, 705–709.

Steinhauser, G., & Saey, P. R. J. (2016). ^{137}Cs in the meat of wild boars: A comparison of the impacts of Chernobyl and Fukushima. *Journal of Radioanalytical and Nuclear Chemistry, 307*, 1801–1806.

Steinhauser, G., & Steinhauser, V. (2016). A simple and rapid method for reducing radiocesium concentrations in wild mushrooms (*Cantharellus* and *Boletus*) in the course of cooking. *Journal of Food Protection, 79*, 1995–1999.

Strebl, F., & Tataruch, F. (2007). Time trends (1986–2003) of radiocesium transfer to roe deer and wild boar in two Austrian forest regions. *Journal of Environmental Radioactivity*, *98*, 137–152.

Strumińska-Parulska, D. I., Olszewski, G., & Falandysz, J. (2017). ^{210}Po and ^{210}Pb bioaccumulation and possible related dose assessment in parasol mushroom (*Macrolepiota procera*). *Environmental Science and Pollution Research*, *24*, 26858–26864.

Strumińska-Parulska, D. I., Szymańska, K., Krasińska, G., Skwarzec, B., & Falandysz, J. (2016). Determination of ^{210}Po and ^{210}Pb in red-capped scaber (*Leccinum aurantiacum*): Bioconcentration and possible related dose assessment. *Environmental Science and Pollution Research*, *23*, 22606–22613.

Szántó, Z., Hult, M., Wätjen, U., & Altzitzoglou, T. (2007). Current radioactivity content of wild edible mushrooms: A candidate for an environmental reference material. *Journal of Radioanalytical and Nuclear Chemistry*, *273*, 167–170.

Szymańska, K., Falandysz, J., Skwarzec, B., & Strumińska-Parulska, D. (2018). ^{210}Po and ^{210}Pb in forest mushrooms of genus *Leccinum* and topsoil from northern Poland and its contribution to the radiation dose. *Chemosphere*, *213*, 133–140.

Tagami, K., & Uchida, S. (2013). Comparison of food processing retention factors of ^{137}Cs and ^{40}K in vegetables. *Journal of Radioanalytical and Nuclear Chemistry*, *295*, 1627–1634.

Tagami, K., Uchida, S., & Ishii, N. (2017). Effects of indoor and outdoor cultivation conditions on Cs-137 concentrations in cultivated mushrooms produced after the Fukushima Daichii Nuclear Power Plant accident. *Journal of the Science of Food and Agriculture*, *97*, 600–605.

Tucaković, I., Barišić, D., Grahel, Ž., Kasap, A., & Širić, I. (2018). ^{137}Cs in mushrooms from Croatia sampled 15–30 years after Chernobyl. *Journal of Environmental Radioactivity*, *181*, 147–151.

Tuo, F., Zhang, J., Li, W., Yao, S., Zhou, Q., & Li, Z. (2017). Radionuclides in mushrooms and soil-to-mushroom transfer factors in certain areas of China. *Journal of Environmental Radioactivity*, *180*, 59–64.

Türkekul, I., Yeşilkanat, C. M., Ciriş, A., Kölemen, U., & Çevik, U. (2018). Interpolated mapping and investigation of environmental radioactivity levels in soils and mushrooms in the Middle Black Sea Region of Turkey. *Isotopes in Environmental and Health Studies*, *54*, 262–273.

UNSCEAR. (1982). *Ionizing radiation source and biological effects*. New York: United Nations.

UNSCEAR. (1988). *Source, effects and risks of ionizing radiation*. New York: United Nations.

Vaaramaa, K., Solatie, D., & Aro, L. (2009). Distribution of ^{210}Pb and ^{210}Po concentrations in wild berries and mushrooms in boreal forest ecosystems. *Science of the Total Environment*, *408*, 84–91.

Vinichuk, M. M., & Johanson, K. J. (2003). Accumulation of ^{137}Cs by fungal mycelium in forest ecosystems of Ukraine. *Journal of Environmental Radioactivity*, *64*, 27–43.

Yilmaz, A., Yildiz, S., Çelik, A., & Çevik, U. (2016). Determination of heavy metal and radioactivity in *Agaricus campestris* mushroom collected from Kahramanmaraş and Erzuzum provinces. *Turkish Journal of Agriculture – Food Science and Technology*, *4*, 208–215.

Zalewska, T., Cocchi, L., & Falandysz, J. (2016). Radiocesium in *Cortinarius* spp. mushrooms in the regions of Reggio Emilia in Italy and Pomerania in Poland. *Environmental Science and Pollution Research*, *23*, 23169–23174.

Zarubina, N. E. (2004). The content of accidental radionuclides in mushrooms from the 30-km zone of Chernobyl Nuclear Power Station. *Mikologiya i Fitopatologiya*, *38*(3), 36–40. (in Russian).

Zarubina, N. (2016). The influence of biotic and abiotic factors on ^{137}Cs accumulation in higher fungi after the accident at Chernobyl NPP. *Journal of Environmental Radioactivity*, *161*, 66–72.

Chapter 6

Conclusion

This book deals with the nutritional and health benefits, as well as the risks, of the mineral constituents and radionuclides of edible mushrooms. Food chemistry and human nutrition are, thus, the prevailing points of view.

The term "mushroom" in this text relates to the fleshy fruiting bodies of edible, particularly culinary species of macrofungi, both freshly harvested and processed. Over 2000 species are estimated to be safe for consumption. Mushrooms, formerly only wild-growing, have been traditionally consumed worldwide as a delicacy appreciated for their specific aroma and texture. The consumption of cultivated and wild-growing mushrooms has recently been recognized as promoting a healthy lifestyle due to their low-energy level, convenient fiber content, and nutraceuticals.

Some 100 species can be cultivated commercially, but only about 20 of these on an industrial scale. The total global production of cultivated mushrooms was nearly 11 million metric tons in 2016, with China being the leading producer by far. *Agaricus bisporus* (white or button mushrooms, brown mushrooms, portobello, crimini) is the most produced species, followed by *Lentinula edodes* (shiitake), several species of the genus *Pleurotus* (particularly *P. ostreatus*, oyster mushroom), *Flammulina velutipes* (golden needle mushroom), *Grifola frondosa* (ram's head), *Volvariella volvacea* (straw mushroom), and *Hericium erinaceus* (lion's mane mushroom).

In the Slavic countries of Central and East Europe, wild-growing species have been preferred over cultivated mushrooms for consumption due to their more savorous properties and species diversity. Information on wild-mushroom consumption, both on weight and species proportions, has been very scarce. The published data have been more or less qualified estimates.

Medicinal mushrooms have an established history of use in traditional ancient therapies, mainly in China, Japan, and Korea. Recent extensive research of many effective components, polysaccharides in particular, revealed numerous medicinal actions. However, there are many mushroom species that are inedible, deleterious, or toxic. These groups are beyond the scope of this book.

The nutritional benefits of edible mushrooms have been generally overrated. Overall, the dry matter (DM) of mushrooms is low, usually

Mineral Composition and Radioactivity of Edible Mushrooms.
DOI: https://doi.org/10.1016/B978-0-12-817565-1.00006-6

8–14 g 100 g^{-1} of fresh matter (FM). DM of 10 g 100 g^{-1} FM (10%) has been commonly used for the conversion between DM and FM if the actual DM is unknown. Usual proximal compositions are 20–25, 2–3, and 5–12 g 100 g^{-1} DM for crude protein, crude fat, and ash (minerals), respectively, with various carbohydrates forming the rest. The level of dietary fiber ranges around 25–30 g 100 g^{-1} DM with about half being in an insoluble form. Due to their very low DM and fat content, mushrooms are a low-energy food item. The calculated energy value mostly ranges between 300 and 400 kcal (1250–1670 kJ) kg^{-1} FM. Nevertheless, such data are overestimated because a considerable proportion of polysaccharides is indigestible.

The crude ash of mushrooms consists of seven major mineral elements (see Section 6.2), quantitatively highly prevailing, and numerous trace elements generally occurring at levels up to 5 mg 100 g^{-1} FM (i.e., about up to 50 mg 100 g^{-1} DM) for each of them. Mushrooms' ash content is generally higher than, or comparable to, that of most vegetables. Available information on particularly toxic and essential trace elements has expanded greatly during the past few decades.

Information on radioactivity in edible mushrooms has become widely diffused within the population of European countries during years following the disaster of the Chernobyl Nuclear Power Plant (CNPP), Ukraine, in 1986. The elevated level in mushrooms continues in the stricken regions until now and will be in existence for the next decades.

Most data on minerals and radioactivity deal with fresh fruiting bodies, whereas information on changes in mineral content and composition and in radioactivity during preservation, storage, and various culinary treatments has been limited until now.

6.1 Overall outline of mineral composition

The content of individual minerals, particularly trace elements, within a mushroom species ranges in one and seldom even two orders of magnitude. Such variability is notably higher than that in crops. Generally, element contents in fruiting bodies are species-dependent. Substrate composition is an important factor, but great differences exist in the uptake of individual metals. Many elements are distributed unevenly within fruiting bodies. The highest levels are observed in many species in the spore-forming parts (hymenophore), less in the flesh of caps, and the lowest in stipes.

Many papers have reported that contents of various elements increase in fruiting bodies from anthropogenically polluted areas compared with those from unpolluted, pristine or rural sites, which have been taken as background values. Moreover, geologically specific substrates can affect the mineral composition of the mushrooms. Considerably increased levels of the main deleterious metals (i.e., cadmium, mercury, and lead) occur in mushrooms growing within towns and notably in the vicinity of both former and operating metal smelters or mining areas and also in metal-ore–rich areas and landfills of sewage sludge. Different proportions of various forms (e.g., exchangeable, absorbable, organic-matter-bound, etc.) of the elements present in underlying soils seem to be an important factor affecting the level of bioaccumulation in fruiting bodies. The ability to accumulate an element from substrate to fruiting body is expressed by the bioconcentration factor (BCF, also bioaccumulation factor or transfer factor), which is the ratio of an element's content in the fruiting body to the content in the underlying substrate, both values given in DM. If the BCF value is >1, an element is bioaccumulated, at value <1 it is bioexcluded.

According to numerous research works, no mushroom species can be considered as an exact indicator of environmental pollution with deleterious elements. Such attitude remains valid in spite of from time to time emerging suggestion of a species.

Only limited information is available from which substrate horizons individual mushroom species take their nutrients. Mycelium of saprobic species, nutrients of which originate from the organic matter, is generally located in the litter layers rich in humus, usually at or very close to the substrate surface. On the contrary, mycelium of mycorrhizal species is dispersed in the mineral layer where roots of the host plant are growing, that is, at lower horizons.

The mycorrhizal mushrooms participate in crucial symbiotic relationships with plants that grow on contaminated sites and alleviate metal toxicity for their host plants. A great proportion of some metals, particularly zinc, copper, and cadmium, was found to be fixed in mycorrhizas, thus forming a biological barrier that reduces movement of the metals to the tissues of host plants. The participating mechanisms can be described as extracellular and intracellular.

The available data on various mineral element contents in fruiting bodies mostly report the total level of an element. Nevertheless, for the evaluation of biological effects in human nutrition and health information on chemical species is needed, which can differ considerably in their effects. For instance, methylmercury cation is much more dangerous for human health than inorganic mercury compounds.

The statutory limits of 0.2 and 0.3 mg kg^{-1} FM for total cadmium and lead, respectively, are now valid for mushrooms in the European Union.

Information on changes in mineral composition of mushrooms during various preservation methods and cooking treatments has been very limited. It may be deduced from the available data that both blanching and pickling of mushrooms can effectively decrease the levels of most detrimental metals, but, at the same time, also deprive the meal from a proportion of the essential elements in discarded extracts.

While hundreds of papers have reported data on mineral element contents in various species of wild-growing and cultivated edible mushrooms, only minimal information has been published until now on the bioavailability of these elements. Bioavailability is defined as the degree to which an element becomes available for the body use or deposition after oral exposure.

As mentioned, mineral element levels in fruiting bodies are affected by numerous factors and usually vary widely within a species. Representative sampling is, therefore, necessary. The low number of fruiting bodies analyzed either separately or as a pool sample cannot provide sufficient data on mineral composition. Optimally, as many as 15 fruiting bodies should be used. The samples are dried and powdered. Wet mineralization usually follows. Various variants of atomic absorption spectrometry and inductively coupled plasma prevail among measurement techniques.

Over the next three sections, the elements discussed in this book are presented in alphabetical order.

6.2 Major essential elements

The major mineral elements are calcium, chlorine, magnesium, phosphorus, potassium, sodium, and sulfur. The last element is included in food chemistry among minerals even though it occurs in mushrooms mostly in organic forms. All these elements are essential for the normal functioning of various physiological processes in humans.

The most frequently reported *calcium* levels are 0.05–0.75 g kg^{-1} DM in cultivated and wild-growing fruiting bodies. Its distribution between caps and stipes differs in various reports. The element does not belong among accumulated elements; however, differences probably exist among species. The calcium content in mushrooms is considerably lower than that in most of vegetables.

Data on *chlorine* content in mushrooms have been virtually lacking. The sporadic values are lower, or comparable, with vegetables.

The usual range of *magnesium* content is $<0.5–1.5$ g kg^{-1} DM. Similarly as for calcium, wide ranges in numerous reports were determined in various species, which most probably have different abilities to bioaccumulate magnesium. Distribution of magnesium seems to be either even or a somewhat higher level is observed in caps than in stipes. Magnesium content in mushrooms is lower than that in most vegetables.

Phosphorus contents range widely between <2.5 and >10 g kg^{-1} DM, although levels above 10 g kg^{-1} DM often occur in cultivated species. The reported contents in caps are mostly higher than the levels in stipes. Mushrooms are able to bioaccumulate phosphorus extensively in their fruiting bodies from the underlying substrates. Mushroom meals can be evaluated as a relatively rich source of phosphorus, and more potent than numerous vegetables.

Potassium comprises the prevailing part of ash in mushrooms. The most frequent contents are between <10 and 35 g kg^{-1} DM in wild-growing and cultivated species. Distribution of potassium between caps and stipes seems to be balanced in some species, while in others the contents are higher in caps than in stipes. Potassium is highly bioaccumulated in fruiting bodies from the underlying substrate and usual BCF values are in the tens and hundreds. Potassium content in mushrooms is comparable with most vegetables (e.g. cabbage, lettuce, carrot or tomato). Mushrooms can, thus, be included in diets of patients with chronic potassium deficiency. On the contrary, detrimental effects should be taken into consideration for some individuals, particularly in the case of renal insufficiency.

The usual *sodium* levels of mushrooms are 0.05–0.75 $g\ kg^{-1}$ DM, that is, the same as for calcium. Sodium distribution in caps and stipes varies among species. There are species with balanced content and those with differences. The element is bioaccumulated in fruiting bodies from the underlying substrates. Sodium content is lower, or comparable, with most vegetables. Its intake should be kept down in human nutrition, thus, mushrooms are an advantageous food item.

Data for *sulfur* are insufficient for generalization. Mostly reported contents are 2–3 $g\ kg^{-1}$ DM. Such values are comparable with vegetables, but lower than those in pulses.

Overall, potassium and phosphorus are the highly prevailing elements in mushrooms, whereas calcium and sodium comprise only a very low proportion of ash. When compared with most vegetables, mushrooms are richer in potassium and phosphorus and lower in magnesium, sodium, and calcium. Unfortunately, information on the major elements' bioavailability from mushroom meals remains lacking.

6.3 Essential trace elements

Up to 12 trace elements are classified as essential for humans. For instance, the European Food Safety Authority provided average daily requirements of eight trace elements (copper, fluorine, iodine, iron, manganese, molybdenum, selenium, and zinc), whereas no requirements have been approved for boron, cobalt, nickel, and silicon. Nevertheless, even the essential trace elements intake is limited. The upper intake is determined for chromium (Cr^{III}), copper, iron, nickel, and zinc.

The data on *boron* are limited. The contents vary widely between <1 and >20 $mg\ kg^{-1}$ DM. The highest levels occur primarily in cultivated species. No data are available either on boron distribution within fruiting bodies, or on bioaccumulation/bioexclusion.

Cobalt contents in wild-growing species vary from <0.2 to 10 $mg\ kg^{-1}$ DM; however, considerably higher levels have also been reported. The element is not bioaccumulated in fruiting bodies.

Usual *copper* contents from <10 to 75 $mg\ kg^{-1}$ DM have been determined in wild-growing species, whereas lower levels of up to

30 mg kg^{-1} DM were reported in cultivated ones. Nevertheless, considerably higher contents were observed in mushrooms growing in polluted sites. The element is distributed within fruiting bodies either evenly or with higher levels in caps than in stipes. Literature data on BCF values vary widely, from values around 1 to 10s. Copper contents were effectively elevated in fruiting bodies of several species cultivated in substrates fortified with copper salts.

The US Institute of Medicine considers *chromium* as an essential mineral, while the European Food Safety Authority does not. Usual contents of total chromium in mushrooms range between 0.5 and 10 mg kg^{-1} DM. The element is not bioaccumulated in fruiting bodies and its distribution within caps and stipes is even. Available literature data refer to total chromium content in mushrooms. However, whereas trivalent chromium Cr^{III} is necessary for the normal human metabolism, hexavalent chromium Cr^{VI} is toxic. Information on the proportion of the chemical species is, thus, needed.

Reports on *fluorine* content in edible mushrooms have been virtually lacking.

According to a single report, mushrooms seem to be a very limited source of dietary *iodine*. Nevertheless, this data originated from inland Hungary, thus, it would be useful to obtain information from coastal sites.

Iron belongs among frequently determined trace elements in mushrooms. The usual contents in wild species vary widely, between <50 and 1000 mg kg^{-1} DM, while levels in cultivated species are lower, namely <50–300 mg kg^{-1} DM. Nevertheless, considerably higher contents were reported in several wild-growing species. Distribution of the element within fruiting bodies seems to be even in many species, while the contents in others are usually higher in caps than in stipes. Iron belongs among trace elements bioexcluded by mushrooms. Dietary iron shortage is the most prevalent nutritional deficiency worldwide, occurring primarily in developing countries. Recent research, therefore, have been searching for ways to fortify cultivated mushroom species with the element.

Usual contents of *manganese* range between <25–75 and <25 mg kg^{-1} DM in wild-growing and cultivated fruiting bodies, respectively. Values of BCF are commonly <0.5, that is, manganese is bioexcluded. Data on its distribution within fruiting bodies differ. Manganese is distributed evenly in a part of the tested species; however, in the others the contents are higher in stipes than in caps.

Data on *molybdenum* have been limited. Usual contents vary from undetectable levels to 1 mg kg^{-1} DM in both wild-growing and cultivated species. Therefore its nutritional asset from mushrooms appears to be marginal.

The contents of *nickel* in mushrooms vary widely, from levels below 0.5 mg kg^{-1} DM, occurring particularly in cultivated fruiting bodies, to more than 20 mg kg^{-1} DM. The most frequent contents seem to be within the range of 0.5–5 mg kg^{-1} DM. The distribution of nickel within fruiting bodies differs among species. Nickel does not belong among the elements bioaccumulated in mushroom fruiting bodies.

Selenium is a hugely important essential metalloid involved in the human Se–antioxidant defense system. It is insufficient in food chains in many world regions. The usual selenium contents in cultivated and wild-growing mushrooms range between <0.5 and 5 mg kg^{-1} DM. Higher contents are not, however rare, for example, in "true boletes." Reports on selenium distribution within fruiting bodies vary as does information on BCFs in various species. The element occurs in mushrooms in several chemical species, both inorganic (e.g., selenites and selenates) and organic (e.g., several selenoamino acids). There exists consensus that organic selenium highly prevails over inorganic forms. Selenates (Se^{VI}) and, particularly, prevailing selenites (Se^{IV}) show detrimental effects.

Cultivated mushroom species appear to be a promising source of organic selenium species via several ways of biofortification. The most common experimentally tested procedure is supplementation of growing substrates with sodium selenite, sodium selenate, or selenized yeast. Such fortification seems to be successful, nevertheless, more data on selenium bioavailability from the fortified fruiting bodies are necessary.

Data on *silicon* in mushrooms have been very scarce with usual values in tens and hundreds mg kg^{-1} DM. Such contents are comparable with numerous vegetables.

Zinc belongs among the most reported elements in edible mushrooms. The most common levels vary between <25 and 125 mg kg^{-1} DM; however, higher contents are not rare. Considerably elevated zinc contents were observed in mushrooms from the vicinity of a zinc smelter. Caps usually have somewhat higher zinc levels than stipes and the BCF for the element is mostly <10. Zinc ranks among essential trace elements often deficient in human nutrition. The possibility to enrich fruiting bodies of cultivated species has been tested, but only to a limited extent until now. The initial research on the bioavailability of zinc from mushrooms reports a nutritional benefit.

6.4 Detrimental trace elements

This section deals with eight trace elements assessed as noxious. Within the European Union, only the limits of 0.2 and 0.3 mg kg^{-1} FM (i.e., approximately 2 and 3 mg kg^{-1} DM) for cadmium and lead, respectively, are now valid for mushrooms. According to the WHO materials, values of provisional tolerable weekly intake are 0.015, 0.0058, 0.004, and 0.025 mg kg^{-1} bodyweight of an adult for deleterious arsenic, cadmium, total mercury, and lead, respectively.

The usual levels of total *arsenic* range from undetectable to 2 mg kg^{-1} DM. Nevertheless, considerably higher, and even extremely high contents over 100 mg kg^{-1} DM, were repeatedly reported mainly in several species of the genus *Laccaria*. *Cyanoboletus pulverulentus* can be classified as a hyperaccumulator. According to the limited data, the ability to bioaccumulate arsenic from the underlying substrate varies widely among individual mushroom species. Arsenic is present in mushrooms as organic and inorganic compounds. Inorganic arsenites (As^{III}) and arsenates (As^{V}) are toxic to humans. Organoarsenic compounds are of low toxicity. The proportion of inorganic and organic As–containing compounds differs widely among mushroom species. A very high proportion of inorganic forms was observed in mushrooms growing in soils contaminated with inorganic arsenic substances from various industrial activities. Arsenobetaine is usually the main compound within the group of organoarsenic species. Mushroom blanching or boiling seem to be efficient for the release of arsenic compounds due to their good solubility in water. High in vitro bioaccessibility of arsenic was observed in raw and cooked mushrooms. Thus an elevated content of arsenic in fruiting bodies has to be prevented.

The most frequent levels of *barium* in both cultivated and wild-growing species are below 2 mg kg^{-1} DM. No accumulating species was proved until now.

Beryllium does not belong among the elements often determined in fruiting bodies. The usual contents <0.5 mg kg^{-1} DM in mushrooms are comparable with those in vegetables and have no toxicological significance.

On the contrary, *cadmium* belongs among the most frequently determined elements in mushrooms. The usual levels range between <1 and 5 mg kg^{-1} DM in wild-growing species, whereas contents >1 mg kg^{-1} DM are sparse within cultivated species. Some species of the genus *Agaricus* show to be highly accumulative, mainly yellowing after mechanical damage of tissues (group *flavescentes*). Although mushrooms bioaccumulate cadmium, the reported values of BCF differ widely among species and within a species. Even medium-accumulating species can, thus, reach figures in the tens and highly accumulating species in the hundreds mg kg^{-1} DM in polluted areas. Commonly, cadmium contents are higher in caps than in stipes. Information on chemical forms of cadmium in mushrooms has been very limited. Cadmium was leached during blanching to a greater extent from partially destroyed deep-frozen cut tissues than from fresh or freeze-dried counterparts. No generalizing conclusion can be given at this stage of the research on the bioavailability of the element due to very limited data.

Lead also belongs among the widely determined elements. Contents up to 5 mg kg^{-1} DM are common in cultivated and wild-growing species. Very high levels occur mainly in mushrooms growing in polluted sites such as around lead smelters or highways. Some species, however, have been repeatedly found to contain elevated contents. The reported BCFs are very low, often ≤ 0.1. The initial information on isotopic ratio of $^{206}Pb/^{207}Pb$ in fruiting bodies enables to identify possible lead sources. Similarly as cadmium, soaking and boiling leached lead to a greater extent from deep-frozen slices of *Xerocomus badius* than from fresh, air-dried, or freeze-dried counterparts. Information on lead bioavailability from mushroom meals remains entirely insufficient.

The usual contents of total *mercury* range in wild-growing species between <0.5 and 5 mg kg^{-1} DM. Considerably higher levels were observed in fruiting bodies growing in soils highly contaminated with mercury. The reported contents in cultivated species are low. Mercury levels in caps are generally higher than in stipes. According to the available data, mushroom species can be classified into groups of weak, medium, and extensive bioaccumulators of mercury. Some species of genera *Agaricus* and *Boletus*, *Lepista nuda*, *Macrolepiota procera*, and others belong to the third group. Mercury-containing compounds are highly toxic. Methylmercury $CH_3Hg^{(+)}$ is more toxic than the inorganic counterparts; recent values of tolerable weekly intake are 4 and 1.3 μg kg^{-1} bodyweight for inorganic mercury and methylmercury, respectively. Fortunately, the mostly reported proportions of methylmercury from total mercury in mushrooms are $<10\%$. Similarly as in cadmium and lead, mercury leaching during soaking and blanching of cut mushrooms was more effective from deep-frozen tissues than from fresh or air-dried counterparts. The information on mercury bioavailability from mushrooms has been virtually lacking.

The most frequent *silver* contents are up to 2 and <0.5 mg kg^{-1} DM in wild-growing and cultivated species, respectively. Considerably higher levels have been reported for fruiting bodies from polluted sites. Generally, silver belongs among the elements bioaccumulated in fruiting bodies. Several species were proven to be strong silver bioaccumulators, for example, some species of the genus *Agaricus*. *Amanita strobiliformis* is known as a hyperaccumulator. The element is distributed evenly in caps and stipes.

So far limited data report low levels of *thallium* in fruiting bodies, commonly below 0.3 mg kg^{-1} DM.

Overall, the contents of the deleterious elements, particularly in wild-growing mushrooms, vary widely. The consideration of a possible health hazard is, therefore, rather speculative. As a worst-case scenario, the only one mushroom serving of 25 g DM (i.e., about 250 g FM) would fulfill the provisional tolerable weekly intake values of arsenic, cadmium, total mercury, and lead at contents of 36, 13.9, 9.6, and 60 mg kg^{-1} DM, respectively, calculated for an adult weighing 60 kg. Mushrooms are not, however, the only source of detrimental elements in diet. Generally, cultivated mushrooms are of a low risk.

6.5 Nutritionally nonessential elements

There occur in mushrooms *tens of further mineral trace elements* considered recently as nutritionally unimportant. Nevertheless, several can be potentially detrimental if entering the environment from various human activities, for example, the platinum group elements. On the contrary, some of these trace elements can have curative properties, for example, lithium. Generally, data for most are very limited, originating from a few articles and dealing with only several species. Such data are available mostly for wild-growing species sampled from unpolluted sites.

Only two elements, aluminum and rubidium, occur at usual contents between <25 and 500 mg kg^{-1} DM. Bromine, cesium, gallium, tin, and titanium levels were reported to be up to 10 mg kg^{-1} DM, while contents of indium, lithium, strontium, and uranium were up to about 2 mg kg^{-1} DM. Many further elements are present at very low levels, often <0.5 and even <0.1 mg kg^{-1} DM, including platinum group elements and rare earth elements (with prevailing cerium, lanthanum, and neodymium). Nevertheless, the contents can be multifold elevated in mushrooms growing in highly polluted soils, as was observed for antimony or gold, for example. Surprisingly, higher levels of several elements were reported in cultivated species than in those growing wildly. Such findings need to be elucidated by further research.

Overall, nutritional and health effects of this group of trace elements seem to be marginal due to their usually very low contents. There are experiments in progress with the aim to fortify some cultivated species with lithium for use in psychiatry.

6.6 Radioactivity

Information on high radioactivity of some wild-growing mushroom species in years following the fallout of Chernobyl Nuclear Power Plant (CNPP) accident in 1986 aroused qualm within the European public. Such fear was ascribed to artificial (anthropogenic) radionuclides. Nevertheless, some mushroom species have relatively high activity concentrations of natural radioactive isotopes. Mushrooms contain considerably higher levels of potassium, including radionuclide ^{40}K at the constant level of 0.012% of all isotopes, than other foods of plant origin. The most common activity concentrations are 800–1500 Bq kg^{-1} DM. The natural radioactivity of mushrooms is, thus, relatively high. Among further natural radionuclides, ^{210}Po and ^{210}Pb should be taken under consideration in regions with low contamination with anthropogenic radionuclides.

Several artificial radionuclides were discharged into the global environment through nuclear-weapons testing until the 1960s. The total release of the most important radionuclide ^{137}Cs was estimated as 9.6×10^{17} Bq (becquerel, the unit of a radioactive source activity in which, on average, one atom decays per second). Mushrooms accumulated neither ^{90}Sr or radioisotopes of plutonium at toxicologically momentous levels.

The extensive radioactivity contamination of a great part of Europe was brought about after the disaster of the CNPP (Ukraine, former Soviet Union) on April 26, 1986. It released into the environment in total about 5.3×10^{18} Bq (excluding noble gases), including approximately 3.8×10^{16} Bq from ^{137}Cs decay. Two cesium radioisotopes, ^{134}Cs (half-life 2.06 years) and particularly ^{137}Cs (half-life 30.17 years), have been the main vehicles of following radioactivity.

Mushrooms were early detected as radiocesium bioaccumulators. Activity concentrations have varied very widely. In mycorrhizal species from several hundreds to above 100,000 Bq kg^{-1} DM, in saprobic and parasitic species between a few hundreds and a few thousands Bq kg^{-1} DM. Very wide differences occurred among species and within a species, up to three orders of magnitude. The provisional statutory limit of the European Union at 12,500 Bq kg^{-1} DM for mushrooms was often significantly surpassed. Maximum levels of mushroom radioactivity were found between 1987 and 1989. Data on the activity concentrations of ^{134}Cs were reported until the mid-1990s due to the relatively short half-life of the radioisotope. Two main factors have affected the level of radioactivity in the subsequent period, namely the mushroom species and level of contamination of a site by the fallout from the CNPP disaster. The time factor since 1986 shows to be of lower importance as the decrease of activity concentrations becomes slower as the period prolongs.

The Fukushima Daiichi Nuclear Power Plant (FNPP; Honshu Island, Japan) disaster was caused by the devastating tsunami following an earthquake on March 11, 2011. Total activity of the released radionuclides has been estimated to be 5.2×10^{17} Bq, that is, about ten times lower than that from the Chernobyl disaster. Moreover, about 80% of the radionuclides were transported offshore and deposited in the Pacific Ocean. Within a comprehensive governmental monitoring, only 2.6% of the tested mushrooms were found to exceed Japanese regulatory limits until 2016. The limits for adults were 500 Bq kg^{-1} FM (i.e., about 5000 Bq kg^{-1} DM) during the first year after the FNPP accident and 100 Bq kg^{-1} FM afterward. Radioactivity of cultivated *L. edodes* (shiitake), the widely consumed species in Japan, has been higher than that of other agricultural products and some batches produced open-air on raw logs were restrained from sale.

Several general conclusions can be drawn from the periods following the two disasters:

- A serious situation can occur in regions heavily contaminated with radioactive fallout if combined with high-local consumption of wild-growing mushrooms, particularly of radiocesium accumulating species of family *Boletaceae*, in the period following a nuclear fallout.

- The burden decreases with the prolonged time from the one-shot contamination; however, some mycorrhizal species from heavily contaminated areas will be an important source of ingested radionuclides for many decades.
- The contamination of cultivated mushrooms with anthropogenic radionuclides is significantly lower than that of wild-growing species. Mushrooms cultivated outdoors, for example, *P. ostreatus* on logs, can be an exception.
- In countries which were not affected by the two disasters, mushrooms (wild-growing and cultivated) participate in the intake of natural radionuclides, particularly ^{40}K.
- Soaking, blanching, and boiling mushrooms decrease their radioactivity. The extracts must be discarded.

A possible risk of radioactivity for human health is expressed by a unit effective dose given in millisieverts (mSv) per year. The acceptable yearly burden for an adult of the public is 1 mSv above natural background, and excluding medical treatments.

Various emitters have different risk levels for human health. This is expressed by dose coefficient (or conversion factor) defined as the dose received by an adult per unit intake of radioactivity (Sv Bq^{-1}). The calculations of believable radioactivity dose from ingested mushrooms have been complicated due to imperfect input data. The reported yearly internal effective dose from consumed mushrooms ranged extremely widely from 10^{-10} to 0.48 mSv.

Reports on a considerable increase of radioactivity in tissues of wild and domestic animals foraging mushrooms appeared in years following the CNPP accident. The steady decrease of meat contamination with ^{137}Cs via mushrooms is expected in roe deer and red deer. However, in wild-boar meat there is anticipated great variability and in some regions the preservation of recent levels exceeding the permissible limit is supposed for a long time, probably a few decades, due to feeding on highly contaminated underground *Elaphomyces granulatus*, known by their common name as deer truffles.

6.7 Prospects

There exist wide differences among individuals in mushroom consumption. Numerous species of wild-growing mushrooms are accepted in certain countries as a widely consumed and valued delicacy. On the contrary, some individuals do not eat mushrooms at all. The nutritional and health benefits or risks resulting from mushroom ingestion furthermore depend on the species and rate of contamination of growing substrate, which affects levels of numerous elements in fruiting bodies.

Research on the mineral composition of edible mushrooms has provided over five decades comprehensive knowledge, primarily for widely consumed species and nutritionally and toxicologically important elements. The data deal mostly with the total contents of individual elements in fresh fruiting bodies. Information on chemical species with different biological effects, for example, selenium, arsenic, mercury, or chromium, has been insufficient, as are results on the effects of various preservation and culinary treatments. Knowledge on bioaccessibility and bioavailability, notably of the detrimental elements, remains the weakest segment. Nearly all reports on the level of detrimental elements in wild-growing species originate from developed countries. Nevertheless, searching for accumulating species and contaminated sites would be desirable also in developing countries with tradition in wild-growing mushrooms consumption.

A promising field of research is the potential biofortification of cultivated species with required elements, particularly selenium, zinc, iron, and lithium.

Great knowledge on mushroom radioactivity collected since the considerable contamination of the environment following the disasters of nuclear power plants seems to be sufficient for precautions in case of further similar accidents.

Appendix I

List of abbreviations

Abbreviation	Expansion	See page
AAS	Atomic absorption spectrometry	20
AB	Arsenobetaine	190
ASV	Anodic stripping voltammetry	20
BCF	Bioconcentration factor	65
CNPP	Chernobyl Nuclear Power Plant	299
CRM	Certified reference material	21
CV-AAS	Cold vapor atomic absorption spectrometry	20
DM	Dry matter (or dry weight)	3
DMA	Dimethylarsinic acid	189
DNA	Deoxyribonucleic acid	14
EFSA	European Food Safety Authority	–
EU	European Union	–
FAO	Food and Agriculture Organization	–
FM	Fresh matter (or fresh weight)	3
FNPP	Fukushima Nuclear Power Plant	317
HG-AAS	Hydrid generation atomic absorption spectrometry	20
HPLC	High-performance liquid chromatography	282
HREEs	Heavy rare-earth elements	258
IAEA	International Atomic Energy Agency	–
ICP-AES	Inductively coupled plasma–atomic emission spectroscopy	20
ICP-MS	Inductively coupled plasma–mass spectrometry	20
ICP-OES	Inductively coupled plasma–optical emission spectroscopy	67
IMEP	International Measurement Evaluation Program	–
LREEs	Light rare-earth elements	258
LSC	Liquid scintillation counting	302
MMA	Monomethylarsonic acid	189
NAA	Neutron activation analysis	20
NMR	Nuclear magnetic resonance	67
PGEs	Platinum group elements	75
PMTDI	Provisional maximum tolerable daily intake	76
PTWI	Provisional tolerable weekly intake	241
RDA	Recommended daily allowance	154
REEs	Rare earth elements	258
TDI	Tolerable daily intake	18

(Continued)

(Continued)

Abbreviation	Expansion	See page
TETRA	Tetramethylarsonium ion	19
TMAO	Trimethylarsine oxide	189
UNSCEAR	United Nations Scientific Committee on the Effects of Atomic Radiation	–
WHO	World Health Organization	–

Appendix II

Commonly used Japanese names of mushrooms

Japanese common name (in English transcription)	Scientific name
Agitake	*Pleurotus eryngii* var. *ferulae*
Aragekikurage	*Auricularia polytricha*
Buna shimeji	*Hypsizygus marmoreus*
Enokitake	*Flammulina velutipes*
Eringi	*Pleurotus eryngii*
Hanabiratake	*Sparassis crispa*
Hatakeshimeji	*Lyophyllum decastes*
Himarayahiratake	*Pleurotus sajor-caju*
Himematsutake	*Agaricus subrufescens* (syn. *A. brasiliensis* or *A. blazei*)
Hiratake	*Pleurotus ostreatus*
Houbitake	*Pleurotus sajor-caju*
Honshimeji	*Lyophyllum shimeji*
Kawaratake	*Trametes versicolor*
Kikurage	*Auricularia auricula-judae*
Maitake	*Grifola frondosa*
Mannentake	*Ganoderma lucidum*
Nameko	*Pholiota nameko*
Reishi	*Ganoderma lucidum*
Shiitake	*Lentinula edodes*
Shimeji	*Hypsizygus tessulatus*
Shirokikurage	*Tremella fuciformis*
Tokiirohiratake	*Pleurotus salmoneostramineus*
Tsukuritake	*Agaricus bisporus*
Yamabushitake	*Hericium erinaceus*

Appendix III

List of images

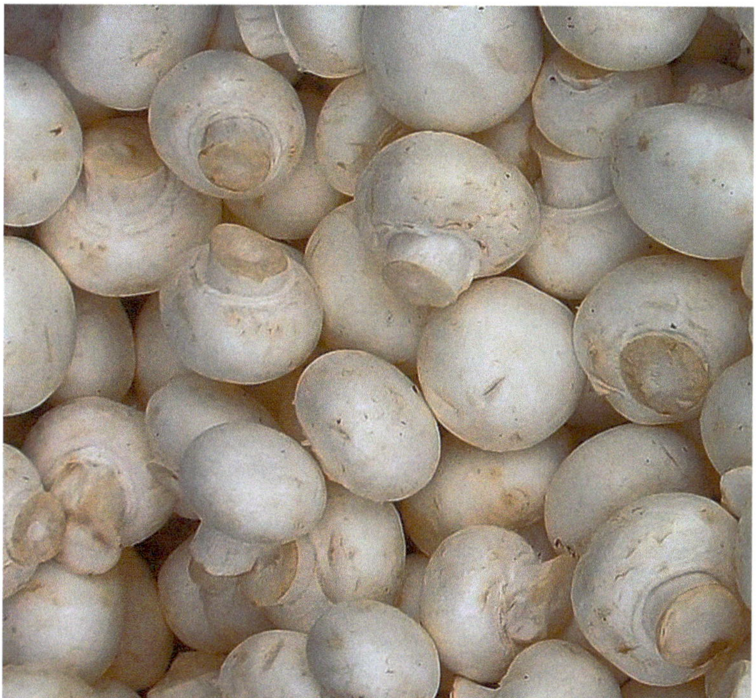

PHOTO 1 *Agaricus bisporus* white. *https://commons.wikimedia.org/wiki/Category:Edible_mushrooms.*

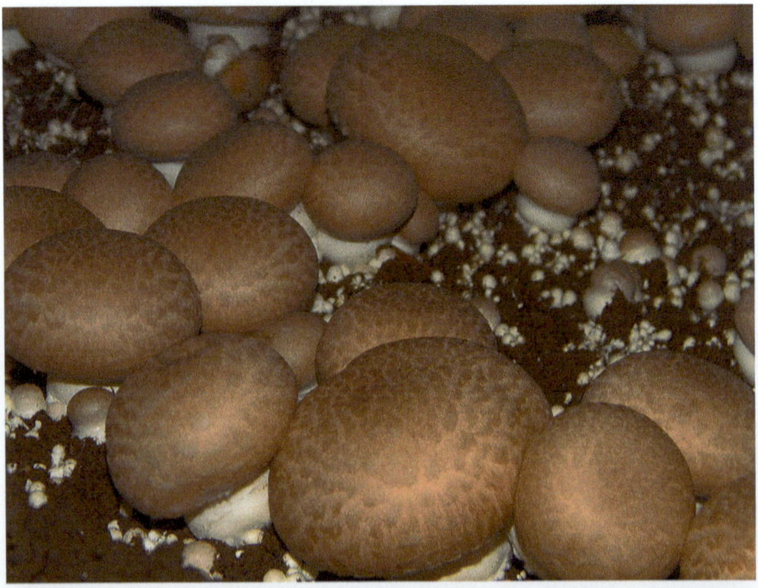

PHOTO 2 *Agaricus bisporus* brown (cremini). *https://commons.wikimedia.org/wiki/Category:Edible_mushrooms.*

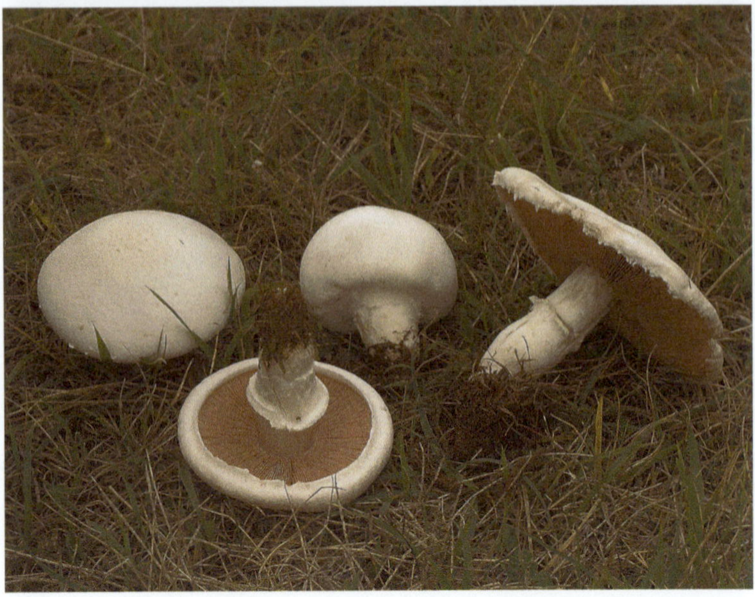

PHOTO 3 *Agaricus campestris. https://commons.wikimedia.org/wiki/Category:Edible_mushrooms.*

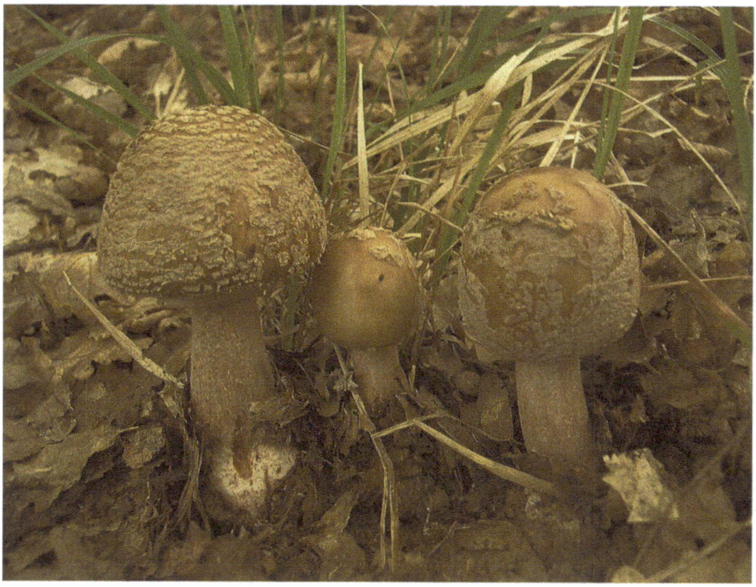

PHOTO 4 *Amanita rubescens. https://commons.wikimedia.org/wiki/Category:Edible_mushrooms.*

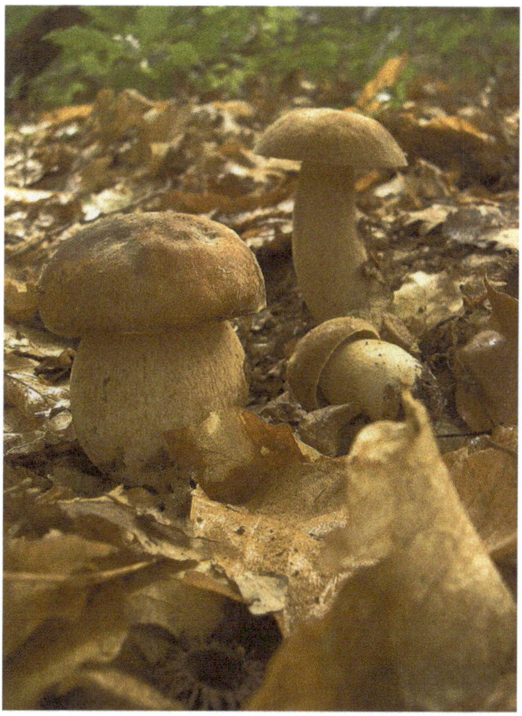

PHOTO 5 *Boletus aestivalis. https://commons.wikimedia.org/wiki/Category:Edible_mushrooms.*

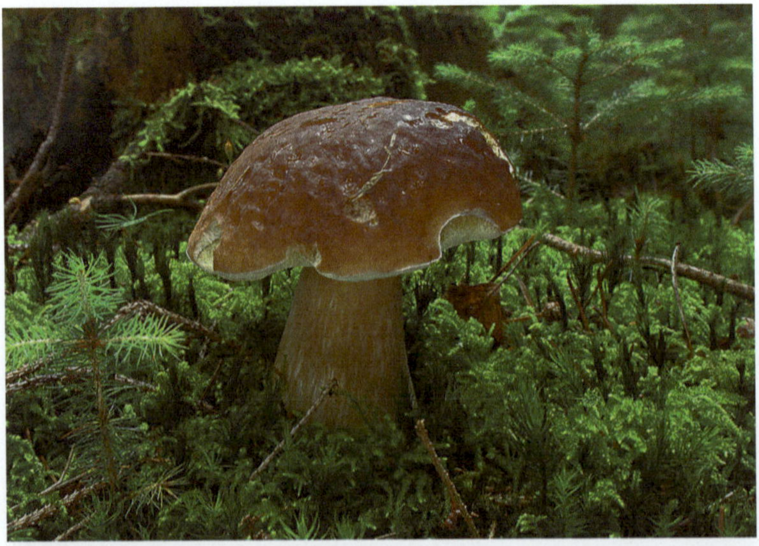

PHOTO 6 *Boletus edulis. https://commons.wikimedia.org/wiki/Category:Edible_mushrooms.*

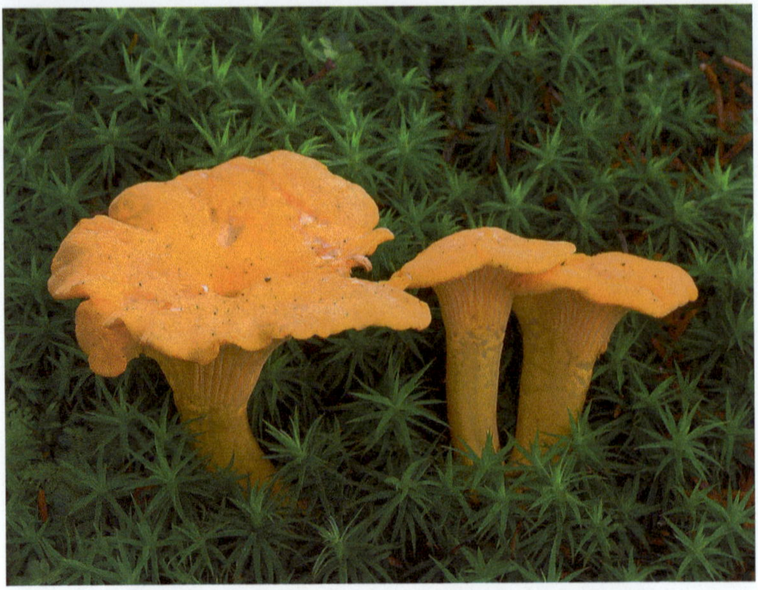

PHOTO 7 *Cantharellus cibarius. https://commons.wikimedia.org/wiki/Category:Edible_mushrooms.*

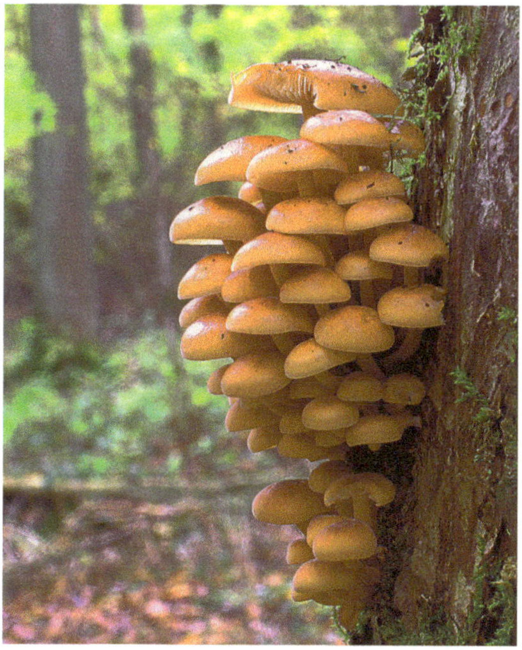

PHOTO 8 *Flammulina velutipes. https://commons.wikimedia.org/wiki/Category:Edible_mushrooms.*

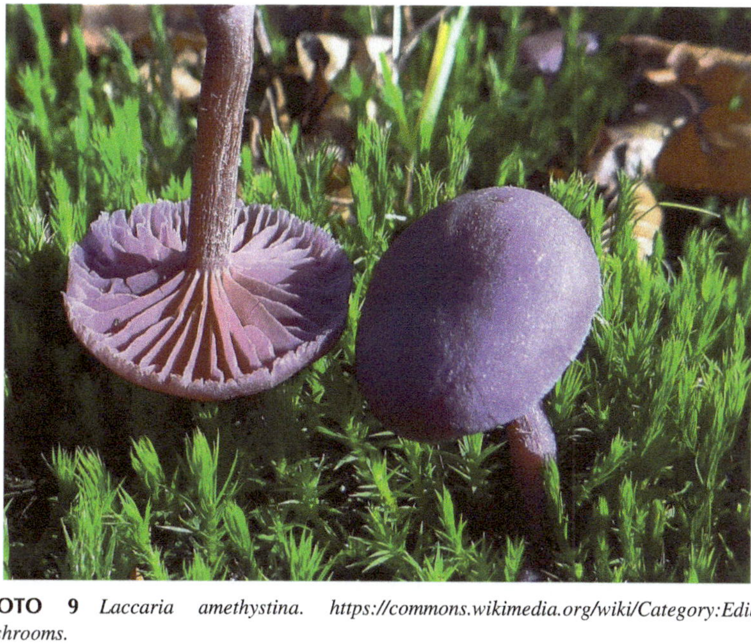

PHOTO 9 *Laccaria amethystina. https://commons.wikimedia.org/wiki/Category:Edible_mushrooms.*

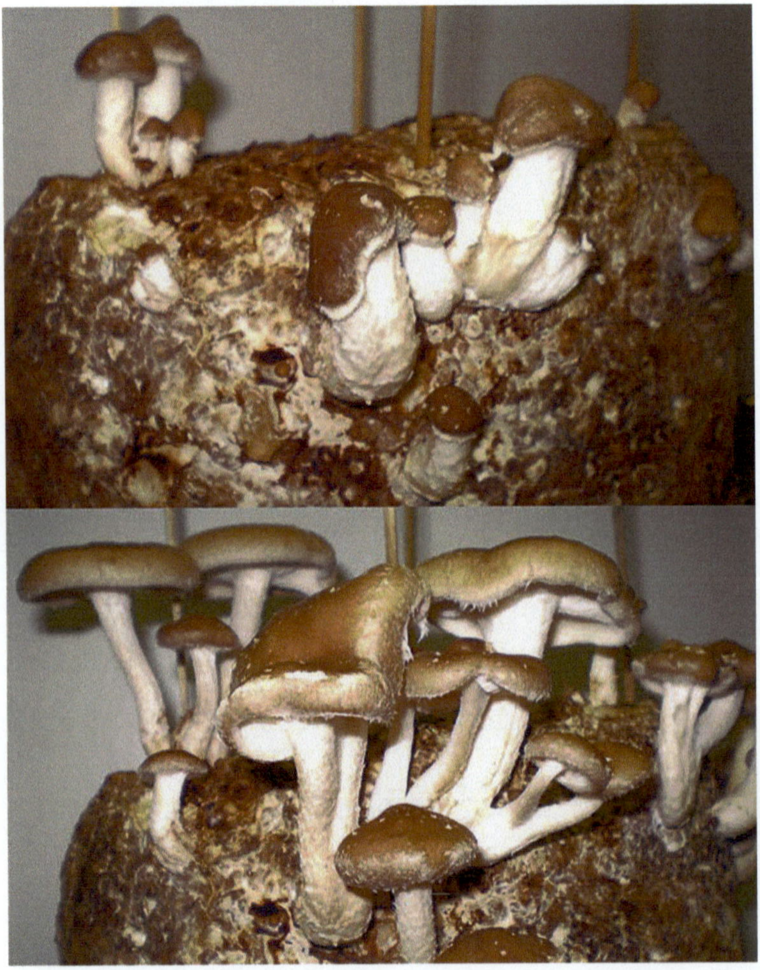

PHOTO 10 *Lentinula edodes. https://commons.wikimedia.org/wiki/Category:Edible_mushrooms.*

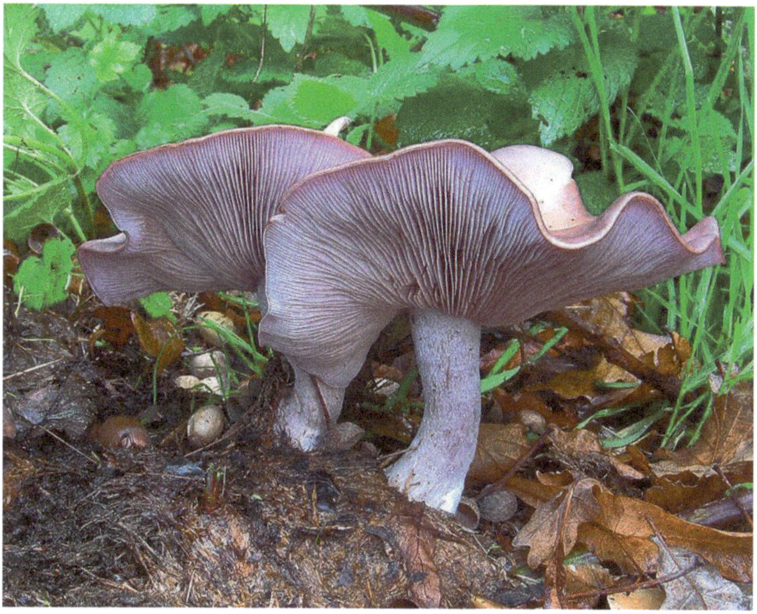

PHOTO 11 *Lepista nuda. https://commons.wikimedia.org/wiki/Category:Edible_mushrooms.*

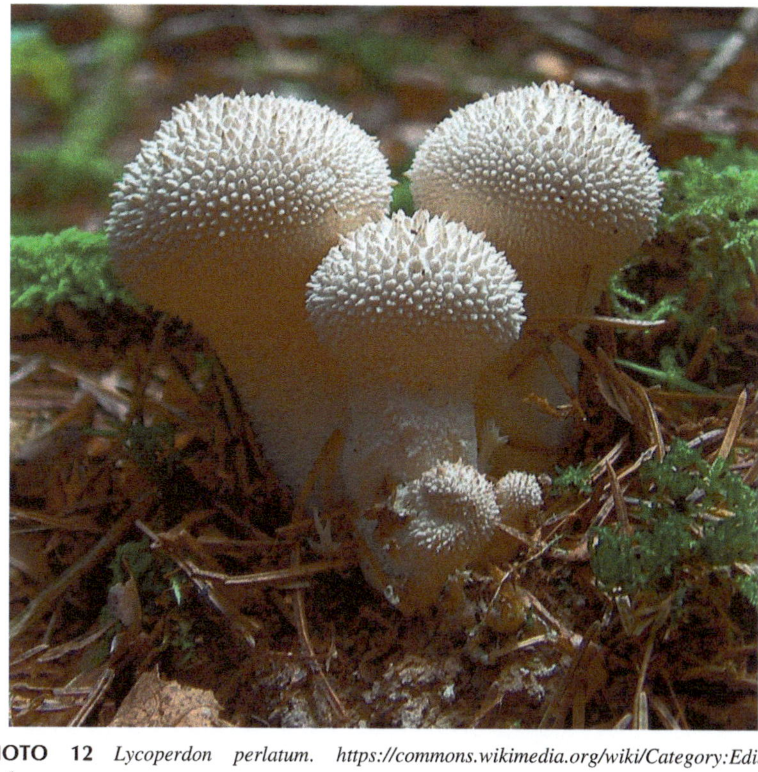

PHOTO 12 *Lycoperdon perlatum. https://commons.wikimedia.org/wiki/Category:Edible_mushrooms.*

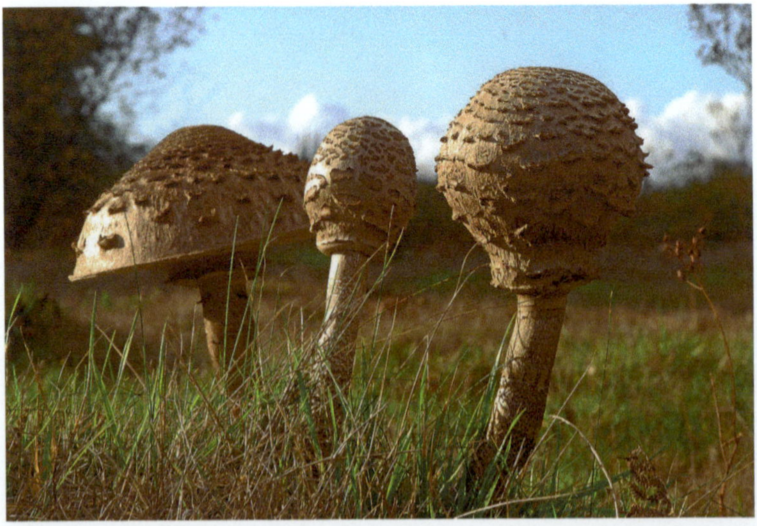

PHOTO 13 *Macrolepiota procera. https://commons.wikimedia.org/wiki/Category:Edible_mushrooms.*

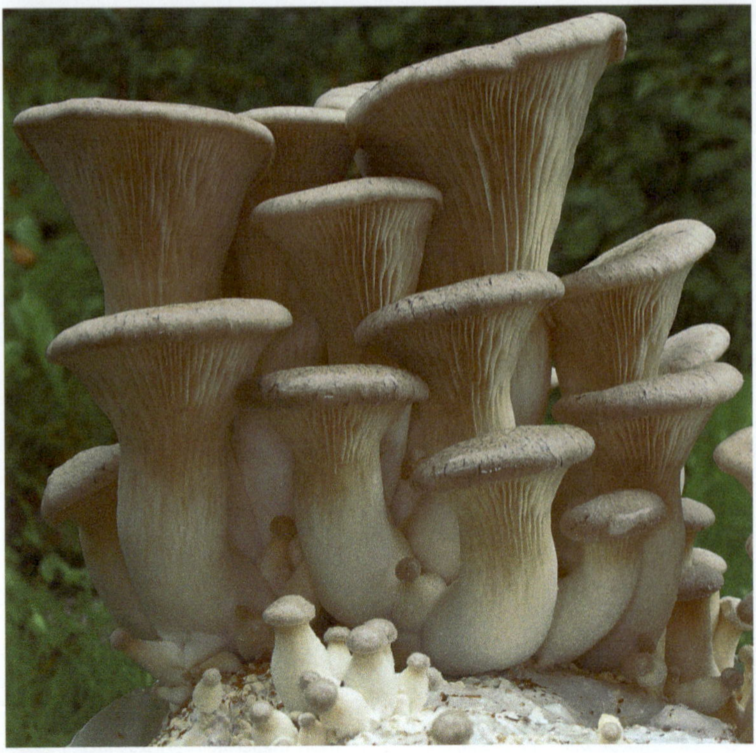

PHOTO 14 *Pleurotus eryngii. https://commons.wikimedia.org/wiki/Category:Edible_mushrooms.*

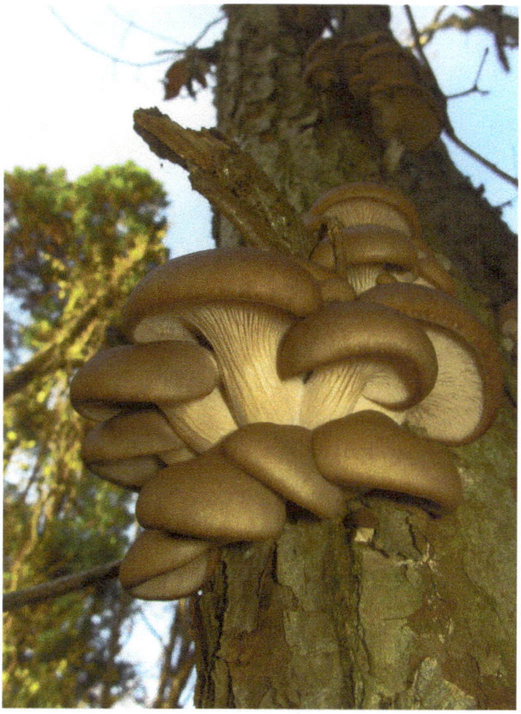

PHOTO 15 *Pleurotus ostreatus* wild growing. *https://commons.wikimedia.org/wiki/Category:Edible_mushrooms.*

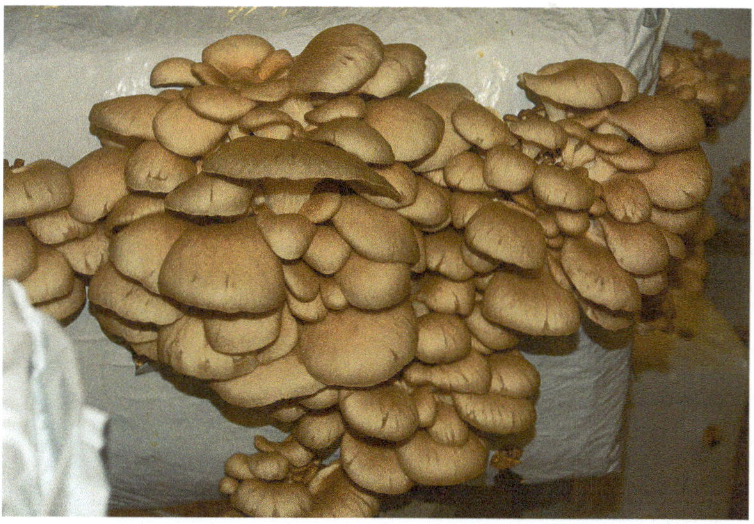

PHOTO 16 *Pleurotus ostreatus* cultivated. *https://commons.wikimedia.org/wiki/Category:Edible_mushrooms.*

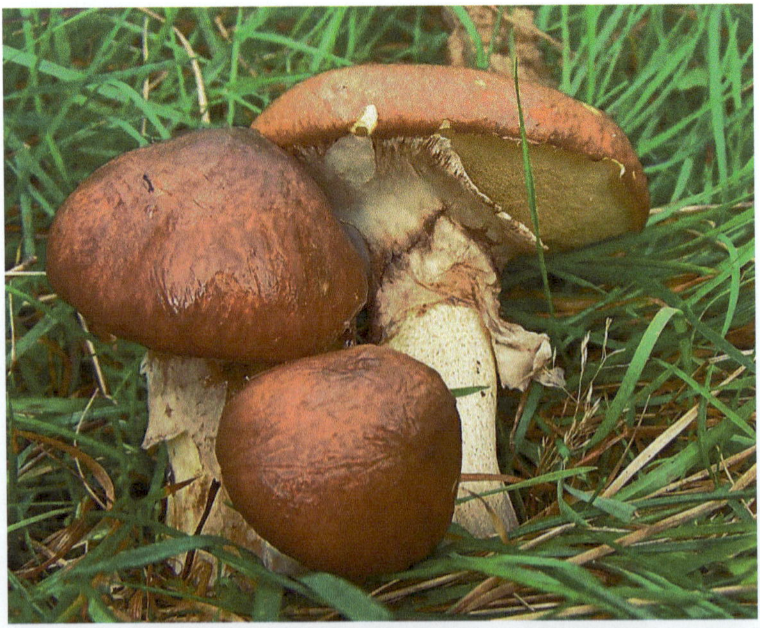

PHOTO 17 *Suillus luteus. https://commons.wikimedia.org/wiki/Category:Edible_mushrooms.*

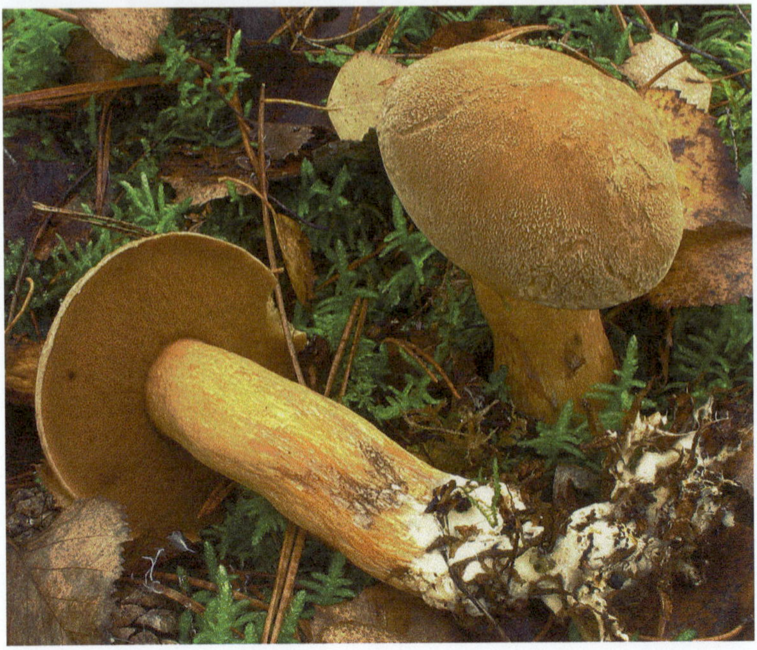

PHOTO 18 *Suillus variegatus. https://commons.wikimedia.org/wiki/Category:Edible_mushrooms.*

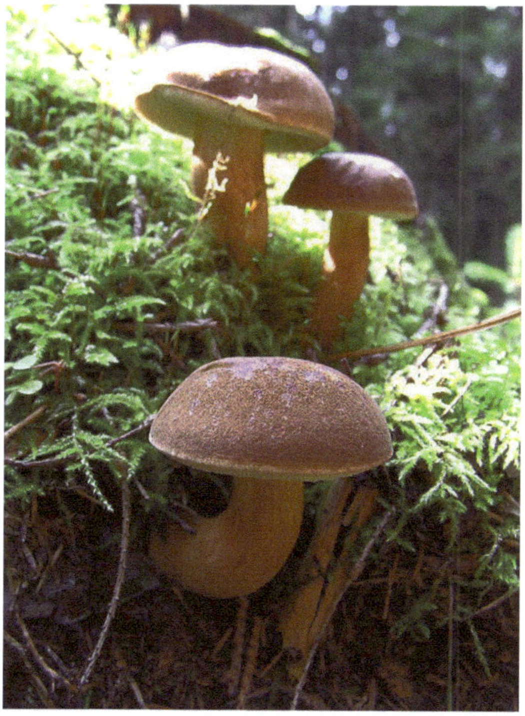

PHOTO 19 *Xerocomus badius. https://commons.wikimedia.org/wiki/Category:Edible_mushrooms.*

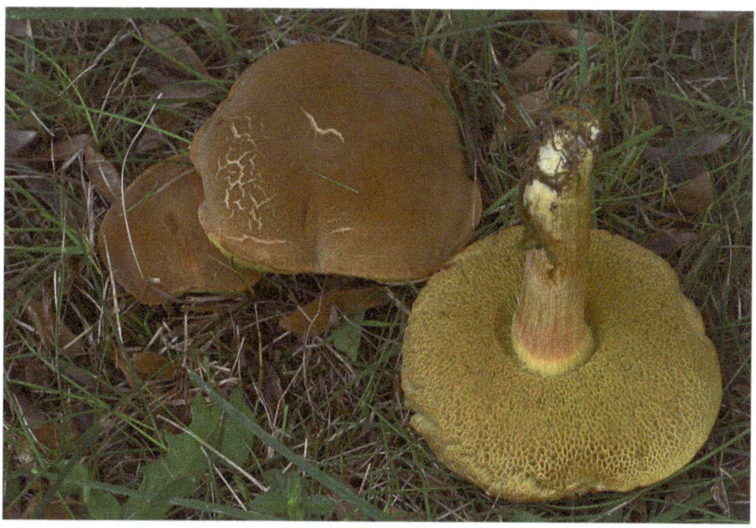

PHOTO 20 *Xerocomus chrysenteron. https://commons.wikimedia.org/wiki/Category:Edible_mushrooms.*

Index of Mushroom Species

Note: Page numbers followed by "*f*" and "*t*" refer to figures and tables, respectively.

M

P

R

S

T

V

X

Subject Index

Note: Page numbers followed by "*f*" and "*t*" refer to figures and tables, respectively.

C

D

E

U

V

W

X

Y

Z

Kolibri 360 GmbH
Ferdinand-Jühlke-Straße 7
99095 Erfurt, Deutschland
produktsicherheit@kolibri360.de